Contemporary Issues in Biomedical Ethics

Contemporary Issues in Biomedical Ethics

First Edition

Written And Edited By Meegan Zickus

Grand Valley State University

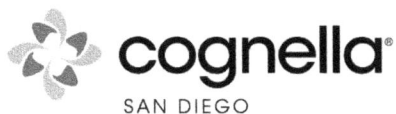

cognella®

SAN DIEGO

Bassim Hamadeh, CEO and Publisher
Craig Lincoln, Project Editor
Susana Christie, Senior Developmental Editor
Rachel Kahn, Production Editor
Emely Villavicencio, Senior Graphic Designer
Laura Duncan, Licensing Coordinator
Natalie Piccotti, Director of Marketing
Kassie Graves, Senior Vice President, Editorial
Alia Bales, Director, Project Editorial and Production

Contents

Acknowledgments

Writing a book is the coalescence of experience and inquiry, melded with support and inspiration. I would like to express my deepest gratitude to those who have contributed to the realization of this work.

To my mentor, Joseph Jacquot, your ability to help me dig in and out of holes is invaluable.

I owe a very special debt of appreciation to two exemplary former students, Karly Brouwer and Jonathan McCabe, who painstakingly helped with their intelligence and perspective at every level, every chapter, and every word.

To my mentors and colleagues in the field of ethics, especially those at the Michigan Department of Health and Human Services Crisis Standards of Care, Scarce Resource Allocation, and Palliative Care Committees, thank you for sharing your wisdom and expertise. Your insights have deepened my understanding and shaped the content of this book.

No finer group of educators, practitioners, and human beings exists than those I worked with at Butterworth ER and Emergency Care Specialists. Similarly, the legal acumen of "investing in the process" is owed to the attorneys I trained under and alongside.

I am deeply grateful to the Cognella team for their professionalism, dedication, meticulous attention to detail, and belief in this project.

To the twenty-five years of students who have faithfully followed the various discussions and tangents where the ideas in this book were refined and debated, your perspectives have enriched the discourse on ethical issues.

To all those whose names may not appear on these pages but whose support has been felt nonetheless, I extend my deepest gratitude.

To my husband and daughters, your unwavering support is a constant source of strength.

I extend a unique and resonating reflection to Dr. Margherita Milone, MD, PhD, at the Mayo Clinic. Thank you for saving my life and resurrecting my world. The irony of being a bioethicist zebra is not lost. You are bloody fantastic.

Finally, to the readers of this text, thank you for your curiosity and open-mindedness. These words were written to inspire you to think beyond a book and embrace the lessons of caregiving. May you remember to meet patients and people where they are at. They will not always be where you want them to be, expect them to be, or think they should be. They all, however, deserve care.

With profound gratitude,
Meegan Zickus

Introduction

Bioethics is a field of study that integrates philosophy, law, biology, and medicine. Bioethics helps to guide life science innovations and applications using moral principles. The survey of bioethics requires attention to three key areas: moral principles and theories, the governing law, and the application of ethical tests.

Moral principles guide a person's sense of right and wrong, behavior, and decision-making. They are the rules a person chooses to live by, so they believe they are doing the right thing. These are some common moral principles framed for the study of bioethics.

- **Autonomy:** respecting individuals' right to decide about their health care and treatment options. This principle emphasizes informed consent, ensuring individuals have the necessary information to make decisions that align with their values and preferences.
- **Beneficence:** acting in the patient's best interests and promoting their well-being. Health care professionals are ethically bound to provide care that maximizes benefit to the patient. This principle emphasizes the importance of considering medical interventions' potential benefits.
- **Nonmaleficence:** the principle of not harming patients. It requires health care providers to avoid causing harm to patients and to minimize the risks of adverse outcomes associated with medical interventions. This principle underscores the importance of harm prevention in health care practice.
- **Justice:** fair and equitable distribution of society's resources, benefits, and burdens. In bioethics, this principle requires that health care resources and services be allocated fairly. This distribution is based on medical needs rather than wealth, social status, or other arbitrary criteria.
- **Veracity:** Veracity, or truthfulness, provides a developed system of honesty and transparency in health care communication. Health care professionals are ethically obligated to provide accurate and truthful patient information, including their diagnosis, treatment options, and prognosis. Open and honest communication fosters trust and enables patients to make informed decisions.
- **Confidentiality:** respecting patients' privacy and excluding health information from third parties. Health care providers are ethically obligated to protect the confidentiality of patient information, whether diagnosis, treatment, or prognosis, and to only disclose information with the patient's consent or as required by law.

These moral principles provide a framework for addressing ethical dilemmas and making health care and biomedical research decisions. While these principles may sometimes conflict or require careful balancing, they collectively guide ethical practice and promote the well-being of individuals and society.

Moral Theories

Moral theories are frameworks that help people determine right from wrong. They are complex because they have criteria and tests that must be met to be satisfied to show rightness. The following theories are applied to analyze and address issues in health care, biomedical research, and the life sciences.

- **Utilitarianism:** the greatest good for the greatest number of people. Rule utilitarianism emphasizes the importance of following rules or principles that, when universally applied, lead to the greatest overall happiness or utility for society. Act utilitarianism evaluates the morality of actions based on their consequences.
- **Virtue Ethics:** focuses on the character traits or virtues that contribute to moral excellence and flourishing. Rather than focusing on rules or consequences, virtue ethics emphasizes compassion, honesty, and integrity. In bioethics, virtue ethics inform health care professionals' character development and guide their actions in promoting the well-being of patients and communities.
- **Feminist Ethics:** challenges traditional ethical theories by emphasizing the importance of relationships, care, and empathy in moral decision-making. Feminist bioethics critiques conventional approaches to health care and biomedical research for their emphasis on autonomy and individual rights, arguing for a more relational and contextually sensitive approach to ethics. Feminist ethics in bioethics highlights the importance of addressing power imbalances, social inequalities, and the experiences of marginalized groups in health care.
- **Kantian Ethics:** Immanuel Kant, a German philosopher, emphasizes the importance of moral principles, duties, and rationality in ethical decision-making. It prioritizes the inherent moral worth of actions, irrespective of their consequences. Fundamental principles of Kantian ethics include categorical imperatives, respect for persons, duty and obligation, goodwill, and rationality and universality.
- **Roman Catholic moral theology:** encompasses many thinkers and theorists who have contributed to developing ethical principles within the Catholic tradition. This includes the work of St. Thomas Aquinas, who emphasized the importance of natural law, human reason, and the pursuit of virtue in ethical decision-making.
- **Contract Theory:** John Rawls, an influential political philosopher, is best known for his theory of justice as fairness. Rawls's Contract Theory presents a hypothetical social contract that individuals would agree to under conditions of fairness where they are behind a "veil of ignorance," unaware of their social status, talents, wealth, or personal preferences. From this position of ignorance, individuals are rational and self-interested but are unaware of their specific attributes.

These moral theories provide diverse perspectives and frameworks for addressing ethical issues in bioethics, and they are often applied in combination to analyze complex ethical dilemmas and promote ethical decision-making in health care and biomedical research.

U.S. Legal System

The U.S. government is based on foundational beliefs that promote checks and balances, federalism, and the Bill of Rights. These components provide a developed system of elections and division of power between a central federal government and individual state governments. The foundation of the U.S. government is the Constitution, which was ratified in 1788 and has been amended 27 times since then. The first ten amendments are known as the Bill of Rights. It outlines the government's structure, delineates each branch's powers, and protects citizens' rights. The Constitution is the supreme law of the land.

The U.S. government is divided into three branches: legislative, executive, and judicial. The legislative branch enacts laws that the executive branch enforces. The judicial branch interprets the laws by ruling on court cases via a structure at both the federal and state levels.

The federal court system handles cases involving federal law, disputes between states, and cases the United States is part of. The U.S. Supreme Court is the highest court in the land that can interpret the Constitution and federal laws. The other three courts are courts of appeals, circuit courts, and district courts.

The state courts each have their own court system, separate from the federal system, which handles cases involving state law and criminal and civil matters that fall under state jurisdiction. State court systems vary in structure but generally include the state supreme court, which is the highest court in the state and responsible for interpreting the state constitution and laws. Appellate courts hear cases that are appealed from the trial courts. They are the two types of courts underneath the state supreme court. In addition to federal and state courts, specialized courts focus on specific cases or issues such as bankruptcy, taxes, military, and tribes.

The U.S. court system is meant to provide impartial resolution for legal disputes, ensuring that justice is administered efficiently and effectively at the federal and state levels. It does this under the principle of stare decisis. Stare decisis is a Latin term meaning "let the decision stand." Once a court has ruled on a particular legal issue, that decision becomes a binding precedent and must be followed by lower courts when deciding similar cases. This principle provides stability, consistency, and predictability in the legal system. It is not the absolute rule, however. Courts have the authority to depart from precedent under certain circumstances, such as when the precedent is incorrect, outdated, or inconsistent with societal values or legal developments.

Criminal and Civil Law

The two main branches of law in the United States are criminal and civil law. Criminal law deals with crimes against the state or society, where the state prosecutes individuals accused of violating criminal statutes. In contrast, civil law governs disputes between private parties and focuses on resolving conflicts and compensating individuals for harm suffered.

In criminal and civil law, the standards of proof refer to the level of evidence that must be presented in court to establish the truth of the facts in dispute. Both require the presentation of evidence, but their standards are very different. Criminal cases have more severe penalties, such as the loss of liberty through incarceration. Thus, they require proof beyond a reasonable doubt. Civil cases, however, involve financial compensation; therefore, the standard of proof is only a preponderance of the evidence.

Medical Malpractice

Medical malpractice is a civil wrong. It occurs when a provider breaches the duty of the standard of care and causes injury, illness, or death. It can happen in many ways, such as misdiagnosis, surgical errors, medication errors, birth injuries, failure to obtain informed consent, and other acts of negligence or recklessness.

For a medical malpractice case to be successful, the provider must have a duty of care to the patient, the provider must breach the duty of care when they violate the standard of care, the breach must directly harm the patient, and the patient must have damages. If this is all proven, the provider is held liable for medical malpractice and will be required to compensate the victim financially. Remember, medical malpractice is a civil wrong, not a criminal one. Thus, the provider is liable, not guilty, for medical malpractice and, therefore, pays damages. Crimes are punishable by incarceration when a defendant is found guilty beyond a reasonable doubt. Civil cases result in damages being paid when a defendant is found liable by a preponderance of the evidence.

Bioethics

While some scholars argue that there is no difference between morality and ethics, we will distinguish it for this book.

Morality is a personal determination between right and wrong. It is a set of beliefs based on culture, society, religion, family, and community. It is a concept of philosophy. A person's morality is their personal belief system. Morality can be expressed with moral principles of autonomy, beneficence, nonmaleficence, justice, veracity, and confidentiality.

Ethics are principles of conduct that guide a larger group. They are an analytical, scientific approach to a more formal system of individuals or groups. While morality is a concept of philosophy about the sense of what is right and wrong, ethics are specific rules or actions in a system. Ethics is a branch of philosophy. A larger group's ethics can be expressed with the moral theories of utilitarianism, virtue ethics, feminist ethics, Kantian ethics, Roman Catholic theorists, and Contract Theory.

Bioethics is a branch of applied ethics. It studies medical and biological technologies and policies with analysis, theories, principles, and law. The chapters in this book focus on contemporary issues in biomedical ethics, starting with the foundation of a person's autonomy. Confidentiality, informed consent, human research, genetic considerations, reproductive technology, abortion, death and dying, and allocation of resources are introduced with key terms, legal cases, applying major moral theories, and relevant articles for discussion. Unique to this textbook is the Special Classes of Persons and Considerations chapter, which focuses on the specific issues of vulnerable populations. The chapter on healthcare providers looks at the very particular set of concerns facing the profession and the people who work in it. Finally, Future Trends in Health Care pulls from history to consider the forecast of how morals, ethics, science, and law will shape our tomorrow.

Chapter 1

Patient Autonomy and Paternalism

Introduction to the Chapter

The most fundamental ideal of bioethics is patient autonomy. The belief that persons should be allowed free choice is also a hallmark of the United States' core values. However, like other foundational beliefs, autonomy is not without limits.

Paternalism is the concept of limiting free choice. For example, when a physician explains treatment options to a patient, it is presumed that the patient gets to make their own choice about the options. Paternalism is when the patient does not get to choose freely. It comes in two different forms: solid or weak paternalism. Strong paternalism limits free choice with no regard for the ability of a person to make a choice. Soft paternalism restricts free choice for the protection of patients because of age, disability, or other influences. These patients may need additional protection or assistance because of incapacity or incompetence. These concepts have become intertwined with medical futility when science/medicine has no viable treatment options or cures.

In the United States, patient autonomy, paternalism, and medical futility are interpreted by statutes and case law such as *Bouvia v. Superior Court* (1986) and *In re Wanglie (1991)*.

The *Bouvia* court held that a patient can refuse any medical treatment, even one that may save or prolong life. It is a basic, fundamental right of privacy protected by state and federal constitutions. Courts, doctors, and ethics committees cannot negate the patient's choice. The decision to stop life-sustaining treatment is not suicide but rather the exercise of a patient's right and a matter of personal dignity. Competent patients can refuse treatment based on their judgment and considerations about quality of life.

In the case In re Wanglie (1991), the court extended the right of competent adult patients to the patient's surrogate. The right to choose care was paramount and belonged to the patient or their legal representative.

Applying moral theories and principles to patient autonomy:

- Utilitarianism believes in doing the most good for the most people. This could allow some paternalistic actions, such as choosing a treatment for a patient.
- Kantian ethics would reject all paternalism because of respect for personal autonomy.

- Natural law theory would be even more paternalistic than Kantian ethics. The doctrine of double effect would deny the request to die, seeing it as a bad outcome, even if the intent were to end suffering.
- Roman Catholic theorists would find the right to refuse extraordinary life-sustaining treatment permissible if no other medical treatments are available. Attempts to diminish the suffering of the patient are paramount for Roman Catholics.

Learning Outcomes

After reading this chapter, students will:

1. Define and integrate key terms into discussion, writing, assignments, and prompts.
2. Analyze relevant case law and statutes to predict future trends.
3. Integrate moral theories and principles into corresponding points to consider, including patient autonomy; the Hippocratic Oath; physician autonomy; accepting, refusing, and withdrawing treatment; futile treatment; refusing treatment for children on religious grounds; Do Not-Resuscitate orders, health care Powers of Attorney, and living wills; provider conflicts; medical limitations; when hospitals/providers should intervene; patient control; substitute decision makers; courts and ethics committees; and physician-patient relationship.

Key Terms

The following key terms will be introduced and used in this chapter.

- **Autonomy:** independent and free choice
- **Medical Futility:** lack of viable scientific or medical treatments/options
- **Paternalism:** limiting independent and free choice
- **Strong Paternalism:** limiting independent and free choice without justification
- **Weak Paternalism:** limiting independent and accessible choice for the protection of others because of age, disability, or other considerations

Introduction to the Readings

The readings that follow focus on facets of patient autonomy.

"The Ethics of Respect for Persons: Lying, Cheating, and Breaking Promises and Why Physicians Have Considered Them Ethical," by Robert M. Veatch and Laura K. Guidry-Grimes, considers the fundamental respect for persons. Physician behavior impacts patient care. In fulfilling the various obligations to their patients, physicians and other providers can be put into a delicate balance of beneficence and nonmaleficence. Truth-telling and patient self-regulation can be at odds. As you read the material, consider the exceptions to both ends of

the spectrum. How does the ethical ideal of autonomy and respect for persons balance with truth-telling or veracity? Consider what is beneficial for the patient against the respect for that patient's very person.

The second reading, "*Physician Autonomy vs. Self-Regulation: You Can't Have One Without the Other*," by Amir A. Khaliq, Ari K. Mwachofi, and Robert W. Broyles, addresses the nature of the physician-patient relationship. The relationship is based on trust, but this is an ethical ideal with variants. The provider's quality of care, competence, and conduct are intrinsic to the patient's well-being. This is why licensing and discipline must protect society from those physicians who do not take the "privilege of self-regulation" seriously. When physicians break the trust, society must have legal recourse through civil, criminal, and licensing actions.

Selection from "The Ethics of Respect for Persons: Lying, Cheating, and Breaking Promises, and Why Physicians Have Considered Them Ethical"

Robert M. Veatch and Laura K. Guidry-Grimes

LEARNING OBJECTIVES FOR THIS [READING]

(1) Identify different obligations or principles that fall under *respect for persons*.

(2) Explain the relationship between rights claims and obligations, including negative and positive rights.

(3) Analyze ethical tensions that can arise in trying to respect persons while also satisfying other role-specific obligations in healthcare.

(4) Illustrate how the concept of autonomy can and should affect healthcare practices, such as when physicians are trying to obtain informed consent.

In the case [...] Dr. Browne felt justified (and indeed was exonerated by the British General Medical Council) in breaking a confidence because he followed the Hippocratic dictum that the clinician should always act in a way that he or she believes will benefit the patient and protect the patient from harm. Reflection on cases such as this one has increasingly led critics of the Hippocratic ethic to doubt that the physician's subjective judgment of patient benefit is the definitive standard for clinician action. The ethic focuses only on the welfare of the patient, that is, patient-centered beneficence and nonmaleficence, excluding any consideration of the welfare of other parties. [...] The Hippocratic principle also poses problems even if we focus only on the individual patient. Increasingly critics are insisting that medical ethics must take into account duties and rights in the patient–healthcare professional relation as well as benefits and harms. The general problem is one of whether sometimes an action can be morally wrong even if it produces good consequences.

An ethic based on duty is increasingly replacing or supplementing one focusing exclusively on consequences. When that ethic focuses on duties to individuals it is often called an ethic of respect for persons. The ethics of respect for persons is one that derives to a great degree from the philosopher Immanuel Kant (1724–1804). Kant stressed that it was important to treat persons as ends-in-themselves and not mere means. He affirmed the intrinsic and absolute value of persons, which means that persons cannot be traded off. Persons thus deserve respect independent of the consequences of actions. We show respect for them by observing certain duties toward them.

The ethic of respect for persons, being a type of ethic based on duty, differs from ethics that focus on production of good consequences and avoiding evil ones. While consequentialist ethics determines what is morally right by examining the consequences of actions, an ethic of respect for persons considers certain behaviors simply to be one's duty—regardless of the consequences. If an action includes a lie, a broken promise, or a violation of another's autonomy, then these features tend to make it morally wrong—even if the consequences are good. Such an ethic focuses on the intrinsic nature of the action, its moral structure or form, and hence is sometimes called formalism. According to this view, actions (or sets of actions) are right or wrong, not based on the consequences they produce, but on their inherent content or form. Certain actions are simply one's duty regardless of the consequences. Some people also call this kind of ethic **deontological**, derived from the Greek word for duty. Deontological or formalist approaches to ethics such as an ethic of respect for persons stand as a major alternative to ethics that decide what is morally right or wrong on the basis of consequences.

In modern Western society those who emphasize more deontological or formalist approaches sometimes use the language of *rights* rather than duties, but [...] there is a close connection between the two. If one person has a right—for example, a right to refuse medical treatment—then other people have a reciprocal duty—in this case, the duty to leave the individual alone when he or she refuses treatment.

For a discussion of the "basics of bioethics," we will present a shorter list of core principles (with the assumption that all of the UNESCO principles can be accounted for as specifications of this list). Figure 1.1.1 presents [...] the ethical principles at the level of interactions between individuals. It shows the principles of ethic of respect for persons as an alternative to the Hippocratic ethic. The figure indicates four principles that are sometimes included under the rubric of respect for persons. The first is the principle of fidelity; that is, fidelity to commitments made in relations with others, to promises made and contracts to be kept. Anyone who feels some moral duty to keep a promise, even if the consequences are not the best, is reflecting this principle. But this is only one aspect of respecting persons. The second is the principle of autonomy. The notion of informed consent can be derived from this principle. Third is the principle of veracity, or simply the duty to tell the truth. The fourth [...] is the principle of avoidance of killing. In some religious systems, this is referred to as the sacredness of life or the ideal that life is precious and to be respected. Kant derived from that the idea that not only should one not kill other people, but even that one should not take one's own life. So for Kant, suicide was prohibited because suicide was failing to show adequate respect for one's own person, for one's own life, or for failing to treat life as an end in itself.

	Consequentialist Principles	Duty-based Principles
Individual	**Subjective** 1. Beneficence 2. Nonmaleficence – –Hippocratic Utility– – **Objective** 1. Beneficence 2. Nonmaleficence	The Ethic of Respect for Persons 1. Fidelity 2. Autonomy 3. Veracity 4. Avoidance of Killing
Social		

Figure 1.1.1 Ethical Principles at the Individual Level

The ethic of respect for persons stands in contrast with the ethics of Hippocratic benefit. The problem was encountered in the case of Dr. Browne [...]. The general form of the problem is that one course of action is believed by the physician to be most beneficial for the patient while another course, often expressed in terms of either rights or duties, appears to be morally required by some principle related to respect for persons. The cases are ones in which the clinician feels required to do something other than what he or she believes is the most beneficial course.

Many people, when reflecting on Dr. Browne's choice to disclose the use of contraceptives to the young woman's father, believe he simply had a duty of confidentiality. Or to put it in other language that amounts to the same thing, the girl had a right to confidentiality. Whether duties or rights language is used, it conveys that Dr. Browne is obliged to do something other than merely do what he thinks will benefit his patient. This obligation appears to be related to the element of respect for persons that can be called the principle of fidelity. [...]

Selection from "Physician Autonomy vs. Self-Regulation: You Can't Have One Without the Other"

Amir A. Khaliq, Ari K. Mwachofi, and Robert W. Broyles

Abstract:

Physician autonomy is intricately linked with the quality of care and patient protection. Professional autonomy which gives physicians the freedom to exercise their judgment in the best interest of the patient without societal interference is based on the premise that physicians will act competently and will put the wellbeing of the patient ahead of their own personal interest. Since individual physicians cannot always be relied on to be competent and scrupulous, the social contract that gives the medical profession the privilege of autonomy goes hand in hand with the responsibility for effective self-regulation. Governments delegate their regulatory and policing power to the medical profession with the expectation that the profession will fulfill its self-regulatory obligation. For a variety of reasons, the medical profession has done a poor job in this regard and has been accused of complicity and complacency. Largely in response to negative media coverage and public pressure in various countries, the medical profession has undertaken initiatives in recent years to ensure continued physician competence, information sharing among different jurisdictions, increased transparency, greater public participation in the regulatory process, and more vigorous exercise of its policing power. Recertifica-

tion and revalidation requirements have helped address the issue of competence, but physician conduct still remains a source of concern. The progress toward effective self-regulation has been slow, and greater effort is necessary to allay public concerns in this regard.

Conceptual Background

The Declaration on Professional Autonomy and Self-Regulation adopted by the World Medical Association in October 1987 and revised in 2005 recognizes the "importance of professional autonomy and self-regulation" around the world.[1] The first principle in the declaration enunciates that "the central element of professional autonomy is the assurance that individual physicians have the freedom to exercise their professional judgment in the care and treatment of their patients." Whereas the central element of autonomy is the freedom to exercise professional judgment in the best interest of the patient, the central element of the medical profession's self-regulatory obligations is policing and punitive action.[2]

Physicians have long understood that professional autonomy can only be preserved by demonstrating effective self-regulation.[3,4,5] While physicians place a great deal of emphasis on professional autonomy, they also recognize society's interest in accountability and protection of patients against negligent, incompetent, and unethical practitioners. The authority of licensing boards, peer review organizations, and credentialing committees to license and regulate physicians stems from an implicit social contract between the medical profession and society regarding "reciprocal rights and obligations." The medical profession makes a commitment toward the wellbeing of patients, professional competence, and ethical conduct of physicians. In return, the society confers professional autonomy and "the privilege of self-regulation" upon the medical profession.[4,5]

Context and Purpose of Self-Regulation

The physician-patient relationship is based on trust[2] and an assumption of a high level of competence and ethical conduct on the part of the physician. Because of the complexity of medical information, the balance of power in the physician-patient relationship is tilted in favor of the physician. The fact that patients have to rely on the professional judgment and ethical conduct of the physician creates a situation in which patients are vulnerable to incompetent or unscrupulous physicians and at risk for great physical, mental, and economic harm.[4] To protect the wellbeing of patients, and to safeguard the autonomy of the physician,

1. The World Medical Association (WMA). 2005. Policy. Available at http://www.wma.net/e/policy/a21htm
2. Irvine D. The performance of doctors: professionalism and self-regulation in a changing world. British Medical Journal. 1997;314(7093):1540-2. Available at http://bmj.bmjjournals.com/cgi/content/full/314/7093/1540
3. Yeon H. B., Lovett DA, Zurakowski D, Herndon JH. Physician Discipline. Journal of Bone and Joint Surgery. 2006;88: 2091–6.
4. Cruess S. R., Cruess R. L. The medical profession and self-regulation: A current challenge. Virtual Mentor. 2005;7(4). Available at http://www.virtualmentor.ama-assn.org/2005/04/oped1-0504.html
5. Rothman D. J. Medical professionalism: focusing on the real issues. New England Journal of Medicine. 2000;342(17): 1284–6.

it is imperative for the medical profession to effectively deal with the small number of incompetent and unscrupulous physicians.[5] If the medical profession cannot guarantee the former, it stands to lose the latter as well.

Clearly, quality of care is a function of both the competence and the conduct of the provider. That is, the wellbeing of the patient is entirely dependent upon the competence and ethical behavior of the physician. Therefore, the obligations of the medical profession toward society boil down to these two elements. While competence deals with the attainment and exercise of requisite knowledge and skills, conduct deals with the observance and exercise of appropriate ethical and moral principles. Consequently, competence is gauged in terms of explicit standards of knowledge and skill, whereas conduct is assessed on the bases of prevailing societal norms, laws, and a code of professional conduct. Quite simply, the standards of competence, conduct, and quality require the physician to do the right thing for the right person at the right time in the right manner for the right reason.

Adoption of licensing and disciplinary procedures manifestly protects the interests of the medical profession by demonstrating to the society that the profession accords highest priority to the wellbeing of patients and does not tolerate misconduct or incompetence on the part of its members. By appropriately dealing with miscreants among its ranks, the medical profession avoids greater societal involvement in its affairs.[3,4] Thus, at the heart of regulatory procedures is the need to protect the patient ("first do no harm") and promote professional integrity. Driven by these needs, the licensing and disciplining mechanisms explicitly assess competence, quality of care, and adherence to a prescribed code of conduct. While quality assurance and patient protection are the primary objectives, these activities also help safeguard the autonomy of the medical profession. With varying degrees of success, licensing and credentialing procedures help ensure entry into the medical profession of only those who are appropriately trained.[6]

By requiring evidence of competence, licensing procedures protect the patients preemptively, whereas disciplinary procedures come into play only after an undesirable event has taken place. Disciplinary actions also serve as a deterrent against future acts of negligence or deviant behavior by setting precedence. At a societal level, licensing and disciplinary actions are implemented through a two-tiered system of judicial and prejudicial actions. Judicial actions can be taken only by law enforcement agencies, whereas prejudicial actions are the purview of the medical profession. Whereas judicial actions can result in both punitive and compensatory decisions, pre-judicial actions can only be punitive in nature. In other words, judicial actions can do both—punish the wrongdoer and compensate the victim, whereas prejudicial actions can only punish the wrongdoer by, for example, revoking a license.

[...]

6. Aarons D. E. Ethics, liabilities and licensing to practice. West Indian Medical Journal. 2007;56(30):208–12.

Review Questions

Directions: Refer to your readings to help respond to the questions and prompts below.

1. When can a wrong action, such as lying to a patient, produce good consequences?
2. Consider the strong paternalistic action of lying to a patient. Does this violate the duty-based principles of fidelity, autonomy, or veracity? Would it matter if there was no legal duty, only an ethical one? What is an example of a weak paternalistic lie?
3. The *Bouvia* case held that a patient's refusal of treatment is not the same as helping aid suicide, but that quality of life is a valid and essential consideration. Kantian ethics provides that one should not kill others or themselves. This was based on respect for persons, including one's own person. Considering that morality, ethics, and law are three different things, justify why each could result in a different outcome.
4. How does professional autonomy differ from personal autonomy or allowing patients to exercise it?
5. What are the consequences when a physician violates their professional autonomy? Are these consequences moral, ethical, and/or legal?

References

Bouvia v. Superior Court, 179 Cal. App. 3d 1127, 225 Cal. Rptr. 297. (1986)

Center for Practical Bioethics. (n.d.). The case of Helga Wanglie—futile treatment. https://www.practicalbioethics.org/wp-content/uploads/2021/10/Case-Study-The-Case-of-Helga-Wanglie-Futile-Treatment.pdf

In re Wanglie, No. PX-91-283, Minn. Dist. Ct., Probate Ct. Div. (July 1, 1991)

Chapter 2

Patient Confidentiality and Truth-Telling

Introduction to the Chapter

In 1996, Congress passed the Health Insurance Portability and Accountability Act (HIPAA). HIPAA is a federal law about personal health information (PHI). It organizes the management, restrictions, and oversight of a person's PHI use by providers. Contrary to public belief, HIPAA typically does not extend past those health care entities that process and use health insurance. For example, it is not a HIPAA violation to ask someone entering a public building if they have been vaccinated. HIPAA applies to health plans, not all entities and businesses.

HIPAA needed to be more apparent. Many patients required help understanding when or how it applied to their information. This confusion about patient confidentiality led many people to invoke HIPAA for unrelated health and privacy issues. This chapter will differentiate HIPAA, patient confidentiality, and other severe interrelated problems.

Patient confidentiality is the belief that information related to a patient, sometimes even their very identity, should only be known by providers who directly care for the patient. Patient confidentiality stems from the U.S. Constitution's right to privacy, a constitutionally protected fundamental right. They are tied to autonomy, liberty, and protection. Most U.S. citizens are familiar with the right to privacy when choosing to practice a religion, get married, and decide where to go to school. These privacy rights are based on the belief that privacy extends to certain confidentialities, especially for patients and health care. Like patient autonomy, patient confidentiality is an ideal. It has limits and can be somewhat unachievable in modern situations.

In 1976, the Supreme Court of California decided a landmark case, *Tarasoff v. Regents of the University of California*. This is a famous case about the duty to warn. The court determined that when a patient expresses a desire to hurt another person, the mental health professional is legally obligated to warn the other person. Failure to protect the other person breaches the duty of reasonable care. Furthermore, the court held that breaking patient confidentiality was necessary to protect another from harm.

When applying moral theories and principles to patient confidentiality:

- Kantian ethics would advocate for a duty to warn. They see any lie as a breach of trust and insensitivity and believe that treating people as a means to an end is unacceptable.

- Act and rule utilitarians would follow the act or the rule, maximizing the good for all. Providers should tell the truth to patients with thoughtfulness and sensitivity.
- Virtue ethics would also follow this belief. Honesty, understanding, faithfulness, and clarity would be fundamental in the physician-patient relationship.

Learning Outcomes

After reading this chapter, students will:

1. Define and integrate key terms into discussion, writing, assignments, and prompts.
2. Analyze relevant case law and statutes to predict future trends.
3. Integrate moral theories and principles into corresponding points to consider that extend from patient confidentiality, including truth-telling, duty to warn (transmissible disease and threats), disclosing the risk of inherited disease, lying to patients, cultural diversity, and cultural relativism.

Key Terms

The following key terms will be introduced and used in this chapter.

- **Covered Entities:** the HIPAA Rules apply to covered entities and business associates. Please refer to the chart in the link below.

https://www.hhs.gov/hipaa/for-professionals/covered-entities/index.html

- **Health Information Technology for Economic and Clinical Health Act of 2009:** promotes the adoption and meaningful use of health information technology and addresses the privacy and security concerns associated with the electronic transmission of health information, partly through several provisions that strengthen the civil and criminal enforcement of the HIPAA rules.

https://www.hhs.gov/hipaa/for-professionals/special-topics/hitech-act-enforcement-interim-final-rule/index.html

- **HIPAA 1996, Amended 2013:** first-time establishment of national standards for protecting certain health information.

https://www.hhs.gov/hipaa/for-professionals/privacy/laws-regulations/index.html

- **Office for Civil Rights:** branch of the U.S. Department of Health and Human Services (HHS) that enforces federal civil rights laws; conscience and religious freedom laws; the Health Insurance Portability and Accountability Act (HIPAA) Privacy, Security, and Breach Notification Rules; and the Patient Safety Act and Rule, which together protect your fundamental rights of nondiscrimination, conscience, religious freedom, and health information privacy.

https://www.hhs.gov/ocr/index.html

- **Patient Confidentiality:** limits access to Protected Health Information (PHI) while establishing privacy standards and standards of patient care.
- **Privacy Act of 1974:** principal law governing the handling of personal information in the federal government.

https://www.justice.gov/opcl/overview-privacy-act-1974-2020-edition/introduction

- **Protected Health Information (PHI):** individually identifiable health information transmitted or maintained in any form or medium (electronic, oral, or paper) by a covered entity or its business associates, excluding certain educational and employment records.

https://www.cdc.gov/phlp/publications/topic/healthinformationprivacy.html

- **Right to Privacy:** autonomous decision-making with freedom from interference or intrusion.

Introduction to the Readings

The readings that follow focus on a few facets of patient confidentiality.

"Patient Privacy in a Digital World," by Kristen J. Quinlan, considers people with behavioral health issues' sensitivity to sharing their health information and the rights attached to this issue.

"Privacy of Individual Health Information," by Susan D. Hosek and Susan G. Straus, discusses the impact of electronic medical records and health information. Concerns about the policies about information technology, the federal role, and security showcase factors for the privacy of medical data under HIPAA.

Patient Privacy in a Digital World

Kristen J. Quinlan

People with behavioral health problems may be particularly sensitive about having their health information shared

During the past decade, behavioral healthcare has seen the advent of new technologies for capturing patient data. In fact, the conversion of paper records to electronic medical records (EMRs) has been identified as a national healthcare priority by a presidential executive order. Such changes have generated many challenges and opportunities for behavioral healthcare organizations looking to capture information about their services' quality, ensure patient safety, and protect patient privacy in an electronic environment.

Legal Considerations

The federal government has set some ground rules for using patient data. Under the Health Insurance Portability and Accountability Act of 1996 (HIPAA) Privacy Rule, protected health information (PHI) may be disclosed for "primary" purposes, including treatment, payment, and program operations, without obtaining a patient's specific written authorization. However, the Privacy Rule does mandate that an organization's privacy policies and practices be explained in writing to patients prior to service.

The Privacy Rule also allows covered entities to disclose PHI for "secondary" purposes without patient authorization for a number of broad national priorities, including research. The

Privacy Rule grants law enforcement access to PHI without court approval or oversight. HIPAA defers to state privacy laws, including those that govern mental health or substance use treatment, if they provide more stringent patient privacy protections.

HIPAA isn't the only national regulation in town. The federal Confidentiality of Alcohol and Drug Abuse Patient Records law (42 CFR Part 2) was enacted decades earlier, providing significantly greater privacy protections for individuals receiving substance use treatment. The law prohibits the unauthorized disclosure of information about substance use treatment for purposes that would be permitted under HIPAA. There are few exceptions to the stringent privacy protections of 42 CFR Part 2.

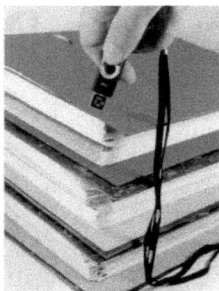

Image 2.1.1

Advantages of Using Patient Information

Dr. Eric Goplerud, director of Ensuring Solutions to Alcohol Problems in the Department of Health Policy at George Washington University Medical Center, notes that sharing personal health information for primary purposes has several recognizable benefits, particularly when substance use is involved. "A very important one is just straight patient safety," he explains. "There are any number of medications that interact very negatively with alcohol use." Dr. Goplerud points out that a patient can prohibit a provider from sharing information about his/her substance use treatment, but the law permits disclosure in medical emergencies without patient permission (Disclosure must be documented by the disclosing treatment provider).

Speaking specifically about the secondary use of health information, Harry Rhodes, director of practice leadership at the American Health Information Management Association, says, "It does help you to identify trends. It helps you to monitor treatment and the success of that treatment."

Privacy Concerns

Yet some advocates of patient privacy rights argue that regardless of whether information is being used for primary or secondary purposes, patients should have direct control over who sees their health record and how it's used. They have identified a host of problems around advertent and inadvertent data disclosure, and these problems may be compounded for individuals receiving treatment for mental health or substance use disorders.

Dr. Goplerud notes that "in a number of states, if a woman gives birth and tests positive for drugs, particularly cocaine, her baby may be taken away and put in foster care. ... Information about one's mental or substance use treatment can and is used in the courts around custody disputes. And so there's this retaliation that may take place." He adds that disclosure of substance use or mental illness can lead to difficulties in obtaining health or life insurance, could jeopardize employment, and could result in a loss of benefits. Thus, patients may feel the need to protect potentially pejorative types of their PHI from all but specifically designated caregivers or authorities.

Ensuring Privacy

Ensuring that advertent or inadvertent data disclosure will not occur is particularly challenging in an electronic environment, in which third-party vendors often develop and maintain provider databases. Dr. Deborah Peel, founder and chair of the nonprofit organization Patient Privacy Rights, suggests that to protect patient privacy, behavioral healthcare executives should closely examine their vendor contracts. "You should never use a vendor that ever wants to own or data mine protected health information," she says. "But a great many of them have that in their contracts as a way of helping to pay for the infrastructure."

You say EHR, I say EMR—what's the difference?

So just what *is* the difference between an electronic *health* record (EHR) and an electronic *medical* record (EMR)? The National Alliance for Health Information Technology has attempted to answer this question by drafting definitions on these and other ambiguous healthcare IT terms.

According to the Alliance, an EMR is "an electronic record of health-related information on an individual that can be created, gathered, managed, and consulted by authorized clinicians and staff within one health care organization." On the other hand, an EHR is "an electronic record of health-related information on an individual that conforms to nationally recognized interoperability standards and that can be created, managed, and consulted by authorized clinicians and staff across more than one health care organization."

These definitions and those for *personal health record, health information exchange, health information organization,* and *regional health information organization* are being presented to the American Health Information Community this month for final approval. For more information, visit www.nahit.org.

—Douglas J. Edwards

Rhodes agrees that contracts should contain clear agreements between parties on how the information will be used and shared. "Once a secondary database has the information, they could rationalize using it for different purposes, only to find out the original owner didn't agree with the use of the data for that purpose, because it was not clearly stated in advance," he says. If data are to be analyzed for secondary purposes,

Rhodes suggests making certain that third-party vendors agree to properly deidentify the data, "removing all of the data elements that HI PAA recommends."

Dr. Peel also suggests that behavioral healthcare organizations select a secure electronic system. She observes that protections against hacking in some systems are "almost worthless." However, she explains, "You can architect the databases so every record is essentially in a 'cubbyhole.' So even if someone breaks into the database system, the most they can get is one record."

To assist healthcare organizations in choosing a well-protected system, Patient Privacy Rights recently organized a consumer-led coalition for certifying health information systems and products. Dr. Peel estimates that the certification system will be in full operation in the next two to three months. Although the group has not yet developed a Website, www.patientprivacyrights.org will have information about the project in the meantime.

Dr. Peel also says that in an EMR "the consumer should be able to segment within that health record whatever they think is sensitive information."

Rhodes observes that because patient privacy often is compromised by "a lack of coherent policies and practices," employees should be given clear guidelines on proper data care. "You don't want the overworked employee to take work home on a laptop," Rhodes says. "Or, if you do, you need to be sure that the laptop has the proper encryption."

Dr. Goplerud suggests creating an organizational policy that ensures that a patient is truly informed about consenting to data sharing. "It is not sufficient to have the blanket HIPAA disclosure. ... Practitioners should offer information about both the costs and benefits of disclosing medical information, and should assist patients in making an informed decision," he explains. "A physician or the healthcare provider can, and probably should, say that it is good healthcare practice for [the patient] to provide consent so that [the provider] can share healthcare information. But it ought to be the patient's choice as to whether information can be disclosed and to whom."

Dr. Peel says that the only way the benefits of information sharing will ever truly be realized is if providers can assure patients that their information will not be released without their consent. She estimates that as many as 30 to 40% of people in need of mental health or substance abuse treatment refuse care because they fear that sensitive health information may be shared through an EMR system. By closely examining third-party vendor relationships and data systems, and by establishing clear organizational policies around using EMRs, behavioral healthcare organizations can help the field move toward secure, publicly trusted electronic systems, she suggests, adding, "If we're ever to get to really effective research about what works for mental illness and addiction, we're never going to get the data if 30 to 40% of the people are unwilling to participate in an electronic system."

Kristen J. Quinlan, PhD, is a freelance writer.

Suggested Reading

Beckerman JZ, Pritts J, Goplerud E, et al. A Delicate Balance: Behavioral Health, Patient Privacy, and the Need to Know. Oakland, Calif.: California Healthcare Foundation; 2008. www.chcf.org/documents/chronicdisease/ADelicateBalanceBehavioralHealthAnd-PrivacyIB.pdf

Calloway SD, Venegas LM. The new HIPAA law on privacy and confidentiality. Nurs Adm Q 2002;26(4):40–54.

Safran C, Bloomrosen M, Hammond WE, et al. Toward a National Framework for the Secondary Use of Health Data. Bethesda, Md.: American Medical Informatics Association; 2006. www.amia.org/inside/initiatives/healthdata/2006/finalpapertowardanationalframe-workforthesecondaryuseofhealthdata_09_08_06_.pdf

More Online

For more on this topic, visit www.healthcare-informatics.com/raths0508. To read about a privacy breach involving Britney Spears' mental health records, visit www.behavioral.net/edwards3152008.

Selection from "Privacy of Individual Health Information"

Susan D. Hosek and Susan G. Straus

Susan D. Hosek and Susan G. Straus, Selection from "Privacy of Individual Health Information," *Patient Privacy, Consent, and Identity Management in Health Information Exchange: Issues for the Military Health System*, pp. 19–23, 73–78. Copyright © 2013 by RAND Corporation. Reprinted with permission.

The shift from paper medical records to electronic records raises new concerns about privacy. Access to paper records for individual patients is limited to authorized personnel at the treating provider organization, including providers, clinical support staff, and administrative personnel. The same personnel may also access individual patients' electronic records. However, unlike paper records, electronic records can be disclosed in very large numbers, for example, through inadvertent loss or theft of computer storage devices. As more protected health information (PHI) is made available to networks of providers, the business associates of providers, and for secondary uses such as research and marketing, the risk of disclosure increases. With paper records, patients can be fairly certain that they know where their records are located and that only a limited number of people will see their information at this location. With increasing electronic storage, sharing, and use of PHI, patients cannot be certain of who has their information, how it is being used, or how well protected it is from inadvertent disclosure or security breaches.

Concerns about the privacy of PHI have been prominent in the policy debate regarding the federal role in health IT. A major report by the President's Council of Advisors on Science and Technology (2010) identified legitimate patient concerns about privacy and security as one of four major barriers to the development of effective health IT systems. It concluded:

Innate, strong, privacy protection on all data, both at rest and in transit, with persistent patient-controlled privacy preferences, is ... achievable, and must be designed in from the start. (p. 4)

The report identified four factors leading to concern about the privacy of medical data: (1) discrimination in health insurance coverage and employment based on health status, (2) exploitive use of the data for commercial interests, (3) the desire to keep government agencies from accessing private information, and (4) the unique nature of health information and the common desire to keep it private. Press reports of inadvertent disclosure of health records and other sensitive information draw public attention to the privacy risk associated with the growing adoption of health IT.

As we discuss below, the federal government mandated protection of PHI by health care organizations 16 years ago, before the widespread availability of health IT systems that enable providers to exchange electronic records. Growing awareness of the potential for health IT to improve the cost-effectiveness of health care has led to federal and state initiatives to promote adoption and to ensure appropriate access to and use of the information. Inadequately addressed privacy concerns could pose a barrier to adoption if providers and patients withhold information that would contribute to better care or lower costs. Therefore, the goal of policy is to design approaches that find a good balance between the beneficial use of electronic health records and privacy protection.

In this section, we review the requirements in the law for privacy protection in the United States, public opinion on issues related to the privacy of PHI, and frameworks laying out principles that should govern HIE. Privacy is a priority for all aspects of electronic health information collection, storage, and disclosure. [...]

Legal Requirements

HIPAA established standards for protecting health information (Office for Civil Rights, 2003). The standards were designed to safeguard individual health records while allowing for the exchange of information to ensure the quality of health care and public health. The requirements laid out in HIPAA were implemented by DHHS in the Privacy Rule.[1] The Privacy Rule applies to all health plans that provide or pay for health care; providers exchanging information for referrals to other providers, health care claims, business operations, or other specified purposes; health care clearinghouses; and certain business associates of covered entities. The HIPAA protections apply to health information in which the individual is identified directly or may be identifiable by inference, usually referred to as PHI. The rule permits disclosure for (1) treatment, payment, and health care operations and (2) a number of public-interest purposes, including specified government, law enforcement, and public health activities; military operations; and research. Disclosure for these purposes does not require patient consent, but disclosure for some other purposes does require consent. Patients may request access to and correction of their PHI and an audit trail of disclosures. They also may request restrictions on disclosure for the uses permitted under HIPAA, and, if an entity agrees to the restrictions, it is responsible for implementing the restrictions. Finally, HIPAA directed DHHS to develop standards for establishing

1. 45 CFR Part 160 and Subparts A and E of Part 164.

unique national identifiers for health providers, health plans, and patients. Concerns about privacy protection led Congress to withhold funding for developing the unique patient identifier system until the technology for ensuring the protection of health information is in place.

When HIPAA was enacted, health IT was in the earliest stage of development. More recently, recognizing the potential for health IT systems to improve the cost-effectiveness of care, Congress passed HITECH,[2] which strengthened the HIPAA privacy protections in several ways. First, it expanded the definition of business associates to include organizations that routinely access and transmit PHI, such as RHIOs and HIOs, and it subjected business associates to the same security requirements and penalties as health plans and health care providers. Second, it specified requirements for notifying those individuals whose PHI has been breached. Third, it directed DHHS to provide education to covered entities and individuals about their rights and responsibilities regarding the privacy and security of PHI. Fourth, it directed DHSS to issue guidance on the definition of minimum necessary information and gave patients more rights regarding their data in electronic format. Fifth, it prohibited the sale of EHRs or PHI, with some exceptions. Finally, HITECH mandated stronger enforcement of federal PHI privacy regulations and established stronger penalties for violations.

At the federal level, additional privacy requirements are levied for records of care provided in substance abuse treatment programs and for treatment of drug abuse, alcoholism or alcohol abuse, and, in the VA, infection with the human immunodeficiency virus (HIV) or sickle cell anemia.[3] However, these requirements do not apply to the exchange of PHI between DoD and the VA. DoD regulation allows for the disclosure of protected PHI for military personnel by any covered entity when it is "deemed necessary by appropriate military command authorities to assure the proper execution of the military mission" or upon separation from military service to support determination of benefits eligibility.[4]

States vary in their laws governing the privacy of PHI. Some states have no provisions or have adopted the HIPAA provisions, but other states have added restrictions on disclosure of PHI relating to especially sensitive areas such as mental health or HIV. The state provisions are not applicable to care provided in MHS or VA facilities, but civilian providers may feel bound by them except when they treat active-duty patients.

Researchers studying privacy and HIE have noted that federal privacy protections leave some gaps as information exchange capabilities grow, inhibiting trust in HIE (Greenberg, Ridgely, and Hillestad, 2009; McGraw et al., 2009). For example, network design characteristics and the oversight and accountability mechanisms have yet to be established and tested to ensure that PHI shared over a widely distributed network is appropriately protected once it leaves the control of the initial holder of the information. McGraw et al. (2009) also note the need for policy changes to strengthen privacy protections in HIPAA and instill trust in HIE; for example, by clearly defining health care operations, tightening restrictions on secondary uses of PHI for marketing purposes, and revisiting standards in the Privacy Rule to ensure that there is minimal risk of re-identifying de-identified data.[5]

[...]

2. Title XIII of Division A and Title IV of Division B of the American Recovery and Reinvestment Act (ARRA) of 2009 (Pub. L. 111–5).

3. 42 CFR Part 2 and 38 CFR Part 1.

4. DoD 6025.18-R, Section C7.11.1

5. HIPAA allows covered entities to provide de-identified data to third parties for uses such as research or business planning. If the recipient re-identifies the data, which is relatively easy to accomplish in some cases, the re-identified data are not subject to HIPAA.

Selections from "The Ethics of Respect for Persons: Lying, Cheating, and Breaking Promises and Why Physicians Have Considered Them Ethical"

Robert M. Veatch and Laura K. Guidry-Grimes

[...]

Non-Hippocratic Approaches to Confidentiality

A number of codes have more rigorous confidentiality requirements. They prohibit disclosure even if the healthcare professional believes the breaking of confidence is to benefit the patient. One might ask, "Why shouldn't a physician or other healthcare professional break confidence if he or she believes it would benefit the patient in the end?" Confidentiality, according to the respect for persons view derived from fidelity to commitments, involves more than patient benefit. The duty to keep medical information confidential is part of fidelity to the patient. A promise of confidentiality is, at least by implication, made when the relation is created. Views that find a duty of confidentiality that goes beyond patient benefit hold that there is a duty to keep confidences when confidentiality is promised.

The World Medical Association (WMA) Declaration of Geneva is generally Hippocratic; it is a rewriting and modernizing of the Hippocratic Oath. On this issue, however, it breaks with the Hippocratic Oath. It gives a flat pledge of confidentiality promising to "respect the secrets confided in me." No exception clauses are included.

In 1971, just after the Dr. Browne case, the BMA rewrote its code to deal with cases such as Dr. Browne's in which the physician believes it is in the patient's interest to disclose confidential information to a third party. In 1971 it said that in such cases "it is the doctor's duty to make every effort to persuade the patient to allow the information to be given to the third party, but where the patient refuses, that refusal must be respected."[1]

Some codes that are more recent go beyond the Hippocratic Oath in requiring or permitting disclosure of confidential information, not to benefit the patient, but to protect others from serious harm. The BMA, for example, says that, according to its opinion, confidences may be broken when the law requires it or when the physician has an overriding duty to society. Depending on the jurisdiction, this might include the legal duty to report gunshot wounds, venereal or other infectious diseases, or a diagnosis of epilepsy. It is the physician's obligation to make sure the patient understands that exception.

An issue of controversy today is whether the law should require reporting of HIV diagnoses. Some jurisdictions require reporting; others do not. When a physician is facing a patient in whom tests for HIV are contemplated in a jurisdiction that requires reporting, fidelity to the patient requires mentioning the reporting requirement. A physician who is committed to practicing within the constraints of the law and who is practicing in a jurisdiction with a reporting requirement will have to disclose a positive diagnosis. If the patient at that point cannot continue the relation on that basis, he or she has the right to end it.

The 2005 UNESCO Universal Declaration on Bioethics and Human Rights is unfortunately vague on the issue of confidentiality. Like the WMA, it offers no exceptions to the confidentiality requirement, but includes the statement that patient information should not be disclosed without patient consent "to the greatest extent possible." That offers no opening to disclose to protect third parties, but seems to imply that sometimes withholding information might not be possible.

If confidentiality is part of the ethics of promise-keeping, what is crucial is what the clinician promises the patient. The corollary is that healthcare professionals should not promise more than they can deliver. Consider the following case in which a physician may imply too much to his patients.

CASE 14: THE CASE OF THE HUSBAND WITH SECRET AFFAIRS

A family physician, Dr. Zane Abara, had seen Jim Park for years, even before Mr. Park married Janice Roberts. Ms. Roberts became a patient of Dr. Abara's soon after the marriage, almost a year ago. On a Tuesday morning, Mr. Park came into the office while his wife was at work. Mr. Park began the conversation asking if he could tell Dr. Abara something confidentially, to which Dr. Abara assured him without thinking too much about it that the doctor–patient relation was confidential. He told Dr. Abara that he believed he might have a sexually transmitted disease (STD) based on some recent symptoms. Mr. Park also revealed to his trusted physician that he had been having an affair for a number of months, and he was even taking her to Key West the following week. After a physical exam, Dr. Abara informed Mr. Park that he did likely have an STD, but he needed to run further tests to make sure. Mr. Park then asked, "All of this is just between us, right, doc? You can't tell my wife."

Dr. Abara began to realize he was facing a dilemma. If he followed the Hippocratic principle, it was his duty to do what he believed would be beneficial to the patient. In this case, the deceived wife was herself a patient who would benefit from knowing her spouse's sexual plans and decisions. On the other hand, if he had promised confidentiality, it was his duty to his other patient, Mr. Park, not to disclose without the man's permission.

At this moment the physician found himself in a bind. He believed that Ms. Roberts was at some risk. First, he knew that her husband had a sexually transmitted disease, which he could spread to her without her knowing. Second, the physician was rather confident that Ms. Roberts was in the middle of a marriage full of deceit and broken promises, and it was likely headed toward divorce.

Dr. Abara concluded it was his duty to Ms. Roberts to find out from Mr. Park whether his wife knew at all about his extramarital relations; if she didn't, Dr. Abara would urge Mr. Park to inform her. He might be lucky and discover that she already knew the situation or that Mr. Park was willing to have the physician help the couple discuss it. If, as seemed more likely, he was not willing to discuss it with his wife, then the physician's problem would remain because he also concluded that his duty to Mr. Park was to keep confidentiality.

The physician believed he had promised confidentiality to the male patient and Hippocratic beneficence to the female patient, but he could not deliver on both promises. He found himself in a spot in which he had two duties and had to determine which one should prevail. Once he has made two contradictory commitments, there is no ideal solution to the problem. If he had been more cautious in what he promised to either patient—for instance, if he had promised to Ms. Roberts that he would work for what was in her interests unless it involved breaching confidentiality with another patient, or, alternatively, if he had promised to Mr. Park to keep information confidential unless it was crucial to the welfare of another patient—then the problem would have been solved. But this physician had gotten himself into a bind by making commitments on which he could not deliver simultaneously.

The striking thing about this case is that the Hippocratic solution of doing what will benefit the patient does not satisfy most people. First, it poses a serious problem because the clinician has two patients who may have significantly different interests. In that case, it is impossible to be Hippocratic to both patients simultaneously. Second, even if that problem is avoided, as long as the clinician believes it is in Ms. Roberts's interest to know about her husband's ongoing affair and STD, he has a duty to tell her, and that does not square with his duty to keep the implied promise of confidentiality with Mr. Park.

Those who hold that the promise of confidentiality must be kept must yield on their commitment to the Hippocratic notion that the physician's primary duty is to benefit the patient. If there is reason to keep the confidence, it must stem from the obligation owed to Mr. Park, one best understood as deriving from a promise made. Respect for persons and the principle of fidelity under that notion appear to generate obligations, in this case the obligation of confidentiality, that cannot be overridden by mere considerations of the consequences to another patient.

There is another dimension to the confidentiality controversy. Even if confidences cannot be broken merely to do what the clinician believes will be beneficial to the patient, it is possible they may be broken in some cases to benefit others. The AMA Principles of Medical Ethics have been interpreted by its Judicial Council (American Medical Association, 1984, p. 19) to permit disclosure when "a patient threatens to inflict serious bodily harm to another person and there is a reasonable probability that the patient may carry out the threat." This is clearly not a Hippocratic paternalistic provision.[2] It could easily justify breaking confidence when it is not in the patient's interest to do so. Contrary to the Hippocratic perspective, it introduces a social dimension: consideration of other persons. [...] Now we need to see how, at the level of an individual patient, there may be other principles derived from the notion of respect for persons that place limits on the healthcare professional's duty to do what he or she thinks will benefit the patient.

[...]

Notes

1. Central Ethical Committee, *British Medical Journal Supplement* (May 1, 1971), p. 30. The BMA appears to have since backtracked on its overturning of the paternalistic exception, perhaps attempting to conform to the General Medical Council, which in Britain has the legal authority to discipline physicians. The BMA by the 1980s (British Medical Association, 1981, p. 12) was publishing a list of five exceptions to the duty of confidentiality. One was when the patient consented to disclosure. Three additional exceptions all involve disclosing to serve various interests of society (research, legal requirements to disclose, and "the doctor's overriding duty to society"). The fifth exception can only be seen as paternalistic: "When it is undesirable on medical grounds to seek a patient's consent, but is in the patient's own interest that confidentiality should be broken." This is compatible with the British General Medical Council's position, which reads, "only in exceptional cases should the doctor feel entitled to disregard his [the patient's] refusal." (See General Medical Council, 1990.)

2. In 1994, in a little-noticed modification, the AMA's Council on Ethical and Judicial Affairs (the new name for the Judicial Council) changed the wording to read "Where a patient threatens to inflict serious bodily harm to another person or *himself or herself* ...," thus reverting to the older notion of Hippocratic paternalism, while still including the non-Hippocratic authorization to break confidence to protect third parties (American Medical Association, 1994, p. 72).

Bibliography

American Medical Association. *Current Opinions of the Judicial Council of the American Medical Association—1984: Including the Principles of Medical Ethics and Rules of the Judicial Council.* Chicago, IL: American Medical Association, 1984.

British Medical Association. *Handbook of Medical Ethics.* London: British Medical Association, 1981.

General Medical Council. *Professional Conduct and Discipline: Fitness to Practise.* London: The Council, 1990.

Review Questions

Directions: Refer to your readings to help respond to the questions and prompts below.

1. When can a wrong action, such as breaking patient confidentiality, produce good consequences?
2. Consider the action of violating patient confidentiality. Refer to Chapter 1, Patient Autonomy and Paternalism. Is violating patient confidentiality an example of strong or weak paternalism?
3. The *Tarasoff* case held that a patient's confidentiality may be breached to protect an outside party. This is commonly known as the duty to warn. Third parties are owed this duty when their safety may be in danger. This is another example of respect for persons. Consider how respect for persons is honored morally, legally, and ethically if patient confidentiality is upheld (law before *Tarasoff* with no duty to warn) and broken (law after *Tarasoff* with a duty to warn).
4. How does professional autonomy differ from personal autonomy or allowing patients to exercise it?
5. What are the consequences when a physician violates their professional autonomy? Are these consequences moral, ethical, and legal?

Reference

Tarasoff v. Regents of the University of California, 17 Cal. 3d 425, 551 P.2d 334, 131 Cal. Rptr. 14 (1976)

Chapter 3

Informed Consent

Introduction to the Chapter

For people born after the mid-1970s, the principles of informed consent are routine. Doctors are expected to explain the diagnosis, prognosis, risks, and benefits. Providers counsel patients about their treatment options, and the patient typically understands their care well. After all, people who understand and agree to treatment are most likely to succeed. Before 1972, however, informed consent was not a law or routine practice in medicine.

Valid informed consent exists if and only if the patient is competent to decide, gets an adequate disclosure of information, understands the information, voluntarily chooses the treatment without pressure, and consents to the treatment. This is based on autonomy, beneficence, self-determination, and the belief that patients will benefit the most from the therapy they agree to. Strong paternalism is denied. Competent adults should make their own decisions with complete information and without interference.

This is an ideal that can be difficult in real situations. How is legal competence determined? What is adequate disclosure? What changes in an emergency? Is a waiver ever legal? One controversial idea is therapeutic privilege. While the laws vary, some believe that therapeutic privilege should be utilized when physicians fear upsetting or distressing the patient or in the case of an already debilitated patient. The doctor decides to withhold information from the patient to avoid harm or upset. It relies heavily on goodwill but is controversial because it denies patient autonomy, the most fundamental bioethics principle.

It is important to remember that informed consent is not standard in other countries and cultures. Autonomous decision-making is a belief upheld by U.S. courts and culture. Many other countries and cultures consider the family's needs paramount to that of an individual. Some continue to believe that women are not able to consent for themselves and require the male head of household to determine a woman's care. Scholars must be aware of these differences in their practice as the integration of people, cultures, and belief systems continues worldwide.

The prominent applicable cases address the development of informed consent, especially from the perspective of who is liable when a patient does not receive the legal ideal.

Canterbury v. Spence (1972) was the first time the courts acknowledged the patient's need to know and understand their treatment choice. The court held that doctors must share the information that a patient would have every reason to expect about risks, benefits, alternatives, expectations, and the understanding of the preceding treatment. The doctor should explain this in everyday terms. Adequate disclosure of informed consent depends on the patient's understanding of their needs and the physician's informing the patient of what a reasonable person would find necessary to decide whether the patient specifically asks for the information.

Schloendorff v. Society of New York Hospital (1914) held that when a physician operates on a patient without obtaining the patient's informed consent, they are liable for assault unless it is an emergency when the patient is unconscious.

When applying moral theories and principles to informed consent:

- Utilitarians would look at the overall good that would be produced for everyone. Thus, act utilitarians would consider each circumstance to determine if informed consent would benefit the patient and anyone else involved. rule utilitarians would consider what rule could be used that could help the most, paying attention to the outcome. Patients must be voluntarily treated and consented, and the choice must be fully autonomous.
- Kantian ethics demands that everyone be treated equally. It does not approve of therapeutic privilege but allows the idea of waiver. Contract Theory fully supports informed consent because liberty is primary. Lying, misconstruing, or controlling facts all disregard personal freedoms.

Learning Outcomes

After reading this chapter, students will:

1. Define and integrate key terms into discussion, writing, assignments, and prompts.
2. Analyze relevant case law and statutes to predict future trends.
3. Integrate moral theories and principles into corresponding points to consider that extend from informed consent, including conditions of informed consent, mandated disclosure of important information, decision-making capacity, adolescent informed consent, joint informed consent, and transparency.

Key Terms

The following key terms will be introduced and used in this chapter.

- **Competence:** legal capacity; the legal ability to act, reason, and decide. A judge, not a physician, determines it. Competency can factor in most legal decisions, such as the competency to stand trial, make a will, or determine health care decisions. A competent person must understand, consult, assist, deliberate, reason, and appreciate the circumstances.
- **Informed Consent:** a process detailing medical practitioners' legal and ethical obligations. It is based on autonomy and a person's right to determine their health care decisions and what happens to their body, such as treatment, procedures, research, and forgoing treatment. It must consist of

counseling between a physician and patient about specific interventions with an understanding of the risks, benefits, and alternatives. In some instances, a surrogate can give informed consent on behalf of a patient, or informed consent can be implied in the case of an emergency.

- **Therapeutic Privilege:** a robust and paternalistic belief that permits a provider to withhold information from a patient out of fear that the information would cause harm to the patient. It can be used to override informed consent and as a legal defense against battery or negligence, as it overrides patient autonomy because the patient's capacity is limited by disease or debilitation.
- **Waiver:** the legal act of forfeiting some or all of a person's rights by removing liability to a party. It must be made autonomously and be clear, mainly because of Health Insurance Portability and Accountability Act (HIPAA) regulations.

Introduction to the Readings

The readings that follow focus on a few facets of informed consent.

"Consent With Competence and Without," by Gary Seay and Susana Nuccetelli, focuses on surrogate decision-making. Valid consents can include advance directives or living wills. Substituted judgment, the best interest standard, decision-making for incompetent adults, and decision-making for children, including newborns, are analyzed.

"The Principle of Autonomy and the Doctrine of Informed Consent," by Robert M. Veatch and Laura K. Guidry-Grimes, discusses autonomy through the lens of fidelity, respect for persons, and integrity. Therapeutic privilege is highlighted in *Natanson v. Kline* (1960) and *Canterbury v. Spence (1972)*.

Selection from "Consent With Competence and Without"

Gary Seay and Susana Nuccetelli

[...]

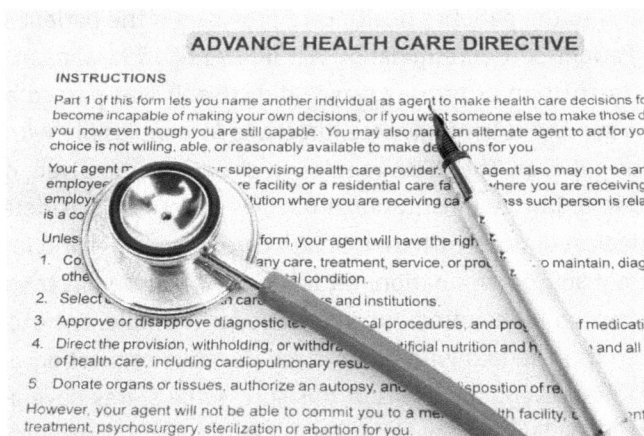

ADVANCE HEALTH CARE DIRECTIVE

INSTRUCTIONS

Part 1 of this form lets you name another individual as agent to make health care decisions fo... become incapable of making your own decisions, or if you want someone else to make those de... you now even though you are still capable. You may also name an alternate agent to act for you... choice is not willing, able, or reasonably available to make decisions for you

Your agent m... ...r supervising health care provider... agent also may not be an... employee... ...re facility or a residential care fa... where you are receiving... employe... ...tution where you are receiving ca... ...ss such person is relat... is a co...

Unless... ...form, your agent will have the righ...

1. Co... ...any care, treatment, service, or pro... ...o maintain, diag... othe... ...tal condition.
2. Select... ...n car... ...s and institutions.
3. Approve or disapprove diagnostic te... ...cal procedures, and pro... ...f medicatio...
4. Direct the provision, withholding, or withdra... ...tificial nutrition and h... ...and all c... of health care, including cardiopulmonary resu...
5. Donate organs or tissues, authorize an autopsy, an... ...sposition of re...

However, your agent will not be able to commit you to a me... ...th facility... ...nt treatment, psychosurgery, sterilization or abortion for you.

Image 3.1.1

Consent in the absence of Competence

Decisionmaking for Previously Competent Adults

Valid consents or refusals for medical interventions can also be obtained when patients lack maturity or suf-ficient mental competence. Here we consider standards for obtaining valid consent or refusal of treatment for previously competent adults who have lost medical decisionmaking capacity, owing to conditions such as dementia or permanent loss of consciousness. We refer to such patients as 'incompetent' or 'nondecisional' to signify that their decisionmaking capacity is below the threshold necessary for counting as autonomous.

Advance Directives

In surrogate decisionmaking for an incompetent adult, others make medical decisions on her behalf—usually next of kin in consultation with the attending physician. Respect for autonomy recommends that the surro-gate honor what the patient would have wanted, including any refusal of treatment. An instruction advance directive or living will, when available, is the best way of knowing this. Such a document, composed and signed while the patient was still competent, would state her treatment preferences (including nontreat-ment) in case she becomes incompetent. Such instructions may also be given orally to a surrogate who will, if needed, offer testimony. Living wills are considered the gold standard in surrogate decisionmaking (Capron, 1986).

But not all jurisdictions recognize decisionmaking by living wills. Some favor the proxy advance direc-tive, a medical durable power of attorney whereby a patient while competent officially designates someone else to make health care decisions on her behalf. The proxy, usually a relative, serves as her 'attorney' in the event she becomes incompetent or unable to convey her preferences. It is the responsibility of the patient to make sure the proxy is fully informed in advance about her wishes, and about the duty of the proxy faithfully to express those wishes to the patient's health care providers if the patient should become incompetent.

In the US, the Patient Self-determination Act (PSDA) of 1991 aims at promoting patient awareness of the right to have an instruction or proxy advance directive. It was passed after the Supreme Court decision in *Cruzan* [...] emphasized the role of advance directives in permissible withdrawals of life supports for per-manently unconscious patients. The PSDA requires that patients be given, on admission to a hospital, infor-mation outlining the state law and institutional policies governing self-determination, encouraging them to discuss end-of-life medical options with their health care providers—who in turn must be familiar with ques-tions concerning patient self-determination. Yet having an advance directive on file does not ensure that the patient's preferences would be honored. Emergencies, for example, are exceptions to informed consent. An emergency team, even if presented with an advance directive requesting no cardiopulmonary resuscitation might still initiate it[1]. To prevent situations of this sort, some states have adopted Physician Orders for Life Sustaining Treatment (POSLT) programs, whereby patients facing death within a year can decide, in consul-tation with their health care providers, about which treatments they consent to, and which they refuse. A POLST form is then completed by the patient and signed by a physician, becoming a standing medical order

---

1. See "Max Story," http://www.polst.org/advance-care-planning/polst-experiences/.

that must be recognized by any medical team when presented. The POSLT form supplements, rather than replaces, an advance directive. Among the differences between these two approaches are

- Advance directives express decisions for future care of any person aged 18 or older and does not have the force of a medical order.
- POLST forms have the force of medical orders and can be completed by patients of any age, provided they are seriously ill.

Substituted Judgment

Advance directives of either type can be the basis of a substituted judgment, or decision about medical treatment made by a previously competent patient's surrogate according to an interpretation of what the patient would have wanted. When there is no advance directive, the previously competent patient's point of view is reconstructed in approximation by the surrogate, preferably the person who knows her best (e.g., her spouse, next-of-kin, or significant other). In choosing among care-alternatives, the surrogate is expected to choose not the care-alternative *he* thinks best for the patient, but the one *the patient would choose*—that is, to adopt the alternative she would want for herself in the circumstances, given her values, beliefs, and plan of life. Occasionally, the courts may appoint a guardian *ad litem* to represent the interests of an incompetent patient. Here is one such occasion:

> *Claire Conroy*, an 84-year-old resident of the New Jersey Parkview Nursing Home, was declared incompetent in 1979, and her nephew appointed as guardian. She experienced periodic confusion caused by organic brain syndrome. By 1982 she had developed severe dementia, inability to speak, incontinence, arteriosclerosis, diabetes, hypertension, bedsores, and a gangrenous leg. She was hospitalized twice and fed by nasogastric tube. In 1983, her nephew requested that the tube be removed. The court granted his request, but the decision was stayed pending an appeal to the New Jersey Supreme Court. That court ruled that only a rigorous determination of a patient's incompetence, together with a joint decision by the guardian, an attending physician, and a state appointed ombudsman, could justify withdrawing life supports from an incompetent patient. While the case was on appeal, Ms. Conroy died.

According to financial records, there was no inheritance or other conflict of interest behind the nephew's decision. He visited his aunt regularly and everything suggested that he believed she would not have wanted to continue living in her condition.

But the courts act on behalf of the state, whose authority to protect life includes protecting incompetent patients vulnerable to surrogates' malicious or biased end-of-life decisions. They may also intervene when surrogates and health care providers disagree about forgoing life supports for a patient. I [... I]n connection with the landmark US Supreme Court decision in *Cruzan*, states have the right to set their own evidentiary standards for valid refusals by previously competent adults. Conflicts are easily resolved when the patient has an instruction advance directive. In its absence, substitute decisionmaking by next-of-kin may be morally dubious. Since end-of-life decisions rest in part on the patient's values concerning her quality of life, why think that the substitute decisionmaker would share those values? After all, kinship is an accident of birth. This might explain data suggesting that the probability that such decisionmakers are good predictors of what the patient might have wanted is mere chance (Seckler et al, 1991). Furthermore, as Kluge (2008) argues, substitute decisionmakers may not always have the patient's best interests at heart.

The Best-Interest Standard

Some of these problems for substituted judgment are avoided by the best-interest standard, sometimes viewed as its competitor. Instead of assuming that an incompetent patient should receive the medical care that she herself would have wanted, this standard assumes that she should receive the care that is in her true best interest, all things considered. The treatment decision is made by evaluating the patient's medical condition and relevant facts about her life. This has problems of its own, since treatment consent and refusals involve value judgments. Acting on the opinion of health care providers, justices might, for instance, decide that life-sustaining treatment is not in a patient's best interests. But this presupposes an evaluation of whether the patient's life is worth living. A patient with different values may consider their decision wrong or even harmful [...].

American and British courts have different views about the weight of the best-interest standard for incompetent adults when an advance directive is not available. In America, it is the last resort in the absence of substituted judgment. But sometimes the best-interest standard is the only option available because there is no advance directive and no one who knows the patient well enough to exercise substituted judgment on her behalf. And on occasion, courts asked to authorize removal of life-prolonging treatment have used the patient's best interests rather than substituted judgment by next-of-kin (as in *Conroy*). In Britain, however, the best-interest standard is the preferred approach to avoid possible conflicts of interest and selfish agendas of next-of-kin that might (sometimes unwittingly) taint a substituted judgment. In both countries, however, the courts prefer advance directives because they facilitate the previously competent patient's participation in end-of-life decisions.

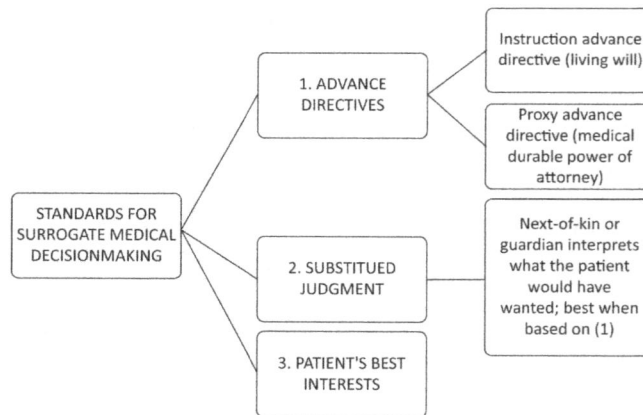

Figure 3.1.1   Medical Decisionmaking for Previously Competent Patients

Decisionmaking for Never Competent Adults

Unlike previously competent patients who might have expressed their medical preferences or completed an advance directive, some adult patients have, owing to profound cognitive impairment, never had decisional capacity. These patients pose a deeper challenge to informed consent, because substituted judgment is unachievable in their case: for reasons discussed below no one can interpret what they might have wanted. Yet in making treatment decisions for them, health care providers are constrained by the obligations to maximize wellbeing, minimize harm, respect patient autonomy and see that justice is done. Given the principles of autonomy and justice, reasonable criteria should be in place so that the never competent can, like other patients, consent to or refuse medical treatment. Furthermore, treatment decisions for them should be comparable to standard decisions for competent patients with similar clinical profiles. For example, if blood transfusions are a standard, life-prolonging procedure for competent patients with bladder cancer, then, other things being equal, justice requires them also for the never competent with bladder cancer. In addition, health care providers have a fiduciary obligation (i.e., an obligation based on trust) to intervene whenever they judge that a proxy decisionmaker's choice could harm the patient, especially if it involves forgoing life supports or administering aggressive treatments. Yet health care providers' decisions too rest not only on facts but also on values as is evident in two judgments delivered in 1981 by the same New York Court of Appeals:

> *Matter of Storar* and *Matter of Eichner*. John Storar, whose mental age was 18 months, was institutionalized and dying of bladder cancer at age 52. Health care providers started blood transfusions as a protection against other diseases, not as a cure, since his condition was terminal. His mother, 77, who visited him every day, was his only living relation. She sought to end the life-prolonging transfusions because of the physical pain and psychological suffering they inflicted on her son, who could not understand the treatment. But the court found for the health care providers because "a parent cannot deny a child all treatment for a life-threatening condition." In *Eichner*, a 53-year-old Catholic priest, Brother Fox, had suffered anoxic brain damage as result of a cardiac arrest during a hernia operation, and this left him in a permanent vegetative state, with breathing assisted by mechanical ventilation. The same court, invoking the hopelessness of the condition, compelling evidence that Brother Fox did not want his life prolonged in that way, and common law regarding self-determination and informed consent, authorized removal of the ventilator.

These rulings seem inconsistent, since both of the cases involve refusals of life supports on behalf of patients permanently incapacitated and thus unable to make their own decisions. Yet attention to the details may help explain why the Court authorized withdrawal only in *Eichner*. First, the court was deciding on behalf of the state. Brother Fox, owing to his injury, had no prospect of ever being conscious again, and thus, of ever having interests in need of the state's protection. Storar, however, though cognitively disabled, was conscious and therefore had interests eligible for state protection.

But, most important, Brother Fox was a previously competent patient with known preferences about his medical care. Decisions in such cases are commonly made by substituted judgment, or interpretation of what he might have wanted in that situation. But Storar never had competence to consent to, or refuse, medical treatment. Nobody could interpret what he wanted. As proxy decisionmaker, his mother refused further life-prolonging treatment for him that health care providers thought medically indicated. Evidently they judged that hastening Storar's death was a harm. Given nonmaleficence, they disregarded the mother's request—which, from their perspective, might also have appeared unjust. For justice required that Storar receive treatment analogous to what any nondisabled competent patient with the same clinical profile commonly receives. Yet their perspective is based on values. Furthermore, hastening a patient's death does not always conflict with obligations of nonmaleficence [...]. Note that, from the mother's perspective, the blood transfusions did conflict with nonmaleficence, for they brought uncompensated burdens (the pain) that Storar could not understand. From her perspective, what looked unjust was the court's decision. After all, Storar was denied the right that competent patients usually have to refuse a treatment. Since his mother had a history of deciding in his best interests and reasons to support her request, the court's ruling denied to an incompetent patient a right that competent patients may usually take for granted.

Storar illustrates the difficulties involving ethical decisionmaking for never competent patients. Substitute decisionmakers cannot capture what these patients might have wanted, because that requires approximating their decisions, and they are nondecisional. So, in such cases, decisionmaking relies on the patient's-best-interest standard. Since application of this standard in part involves values, hard conflicts may arise between next-of-kin and health care providers, with occasional interventions by the courts. There is no accepted protocol to resolve such conflicts objectively in a way consistent with all principles of biomedical ethics. But all agree that, when a proxy decision seems to violate one or more principles, health care providers have the fiduciary power and obligation to intervene on behalf of these patients.

Decisionmaking for Children

Children are among the never competent. Informed consent for them, therefore, is given by substitute decisionmakers—in the US, commonly their parents. We refer to such proxy decisionmaking as 'parental choice.' For neonates, however, their best interest is the decisionmaking standard. This section examines some problems facing parental choice and the best-interest standard. It also considers the case of *Ashley X*, a young child with profound cognitive deficits, for whom her parents requested a number of nonmedically indicated treatments that some considered morally unjustified, although they might have been in the interests of both parents and child.

Parental Choice versus Patient's Best Interests

In the 1970s and early 80s, the prevailing decisionmaking standard for neonates in the US switched from parental choice to the child's best interests. Not all agreed with that switch, which was in part prompted by some parental refusals of life-saving treatment for impaired newborns [...]. Opposition was evident during the 1995 trial of dermatologist Gregory Messenger of Lansing, Michigan.

> *Baby Messenger* was born by Caesarian section at 25 weeks of gestation when her mother went into premature labor as a result of pulmonary edema and hypertension. The neonatologist, Dr. Padmani Karna, predicted a 30% to 50% chance of survival for the infant, and if he survived, a 20% and 40% chance of severe impairments owing to intraventricular hemorrhage. The Messengers told Dr. Karna they did not want any heroic measures if the baby was born alive, including resuscitation. Yet she instructed the physician assistant (PA)

that if Baby Messenger looked "vigorous" and "active," critical care should be initiated. The baby was born hypotonic and hypoxic, purple-blue in color, and weighing only 780g. But he had an 80 to 90 beats/min umbilical cord pulse, so the PA resuscitated, intubated, and incubated him. Upon her return to the hospital, Dr. Karna saw the baby stable in the NICU and decided to run some tests. In the meantime, the baby's father, Dr. Messenger, who saw the baby in the delivery room, asked to be alone with his son and disconnected the respirator. The infant died later in his mother's arms. Pathologists determined that the baby would have survived had he not suffered respiratory failure as a result of his father's action. In 1995 Dr. Messenger was tried for manslaughter but acquitted.

The press followed the trial closely, with the *Chicago Tribune* running the headline "Jury to Weigh Father's Guilt in Premature Baby's Death."[2] Since it was a criminal case won by the accused, it set no precedent in the law. Yet it sent a clear message: juries and the public tend to question the morality of medical interventions that conflict with the parents' reasonable choices for their medically compromised newborns. This tendency is consistent with moral theory, especially utilitarianism, given the baby's bleak prospects. But the neonatologist was not unreasonable. She followed the 'initiate and reevaluate' protocol prevailing in the US and Britain for newborns with low survival chances, whereby critical care is started at birth and withdrawal contemplated later, depending on the infant's progress.

This case suggests that the pendulum marking where the law stands on informed consent for newborns had swung too far in the early 1980s: from absolute parental choice to absolute infant's best-interests. Fueling this change was the fact that reasonable parents sometimes fail to be objective judges of their infant's best interests, and their choices can flout bioethical principles of nonmaleficence and justice. The former recommends avoidance of harm to the newborn, the latter that it receive the care that other newborns with similar life prospects receive. Other things being equal, decisions resulting in the newborn's death or impairments flout nonmaleficence; those depriving it of due care flout justice. But the best-interest standard has the problems outlined above—namely, that the medical team decides, according to their own values and notion of a life worth living, what is best for the neonate, even though it is the parents who must care for the infant after it leaves the hospital.

Moral theory offers different perspectives on who should decide. For Kant, parents have a duty to avoid decisions that harm their newborns, provided these can develop a rational nature and thus acquire the absolute moral worth of persons. So he should give primacy to the infant's best interests, on the grounds that parents are poor judges of those interests. But utilitarians [...] think that, on the whole, the benefits of parental choice outweigh possible harms from making mistaken decisions, except when the neonate's life falls short of being worth living.

2. Roger Worthington, "Jury to Weigh Father's Guilt in Premature Baby's Death." *Chicago Tribune*, 1/30/1995.

BOX 3.1.2 DECISIONMAKING FOR NEWBORNS

Prevailing Standard: The infant's best interests, when clear.

Primary Decisionmaker: The parents, unless they are incapacitated or their decision conflicts with what reasonable people think is in the infant's best interest.

Health Care Providers' Role: (1) Developing protocols for decisions to forgo life supports, and for settling disagreements with parents. (2) Seeking judicial review for any nonemergency parental decision seriously at odds with the provider's view of the infant's best interest.

Conflict Resolution: End-of-life decisions are reviewed by an *institutional ethics committee*. When disagreement occurs, the committee (1) verifies that the parties have up-to-date, reliable information; (2) assesses the parents' decisional capacity and understanding of treatment options; and (3) if necessary, seeks a third party's intervention (usually the courts, charged with determining the infant's best interests).

Finding a Compromise

Even if parents are poor judges of what is best for their compromised infant, since the burdens of its care after it leaves the hospital fall on them, their choices shouldn't be ignored. In 1983, the President's Commission for the Study of Ethical Problems in Medicine provided an influential framework for a compromise between parental choice and the infant's best interests. It recognized the parents as primary judges of those interests and suggested that institutional ethics committees review each decision to forgo life supports from a newborn. When disagreement arises between parents and health care providers, the committee reviews the reasons on both sides, following the steps in Box 3.1.2 above. Although the burden of proof is on health care providers, when they have serious doubts about a parental decision, they should seek judicial determination of a child's best interests. As we see next, that was the upshot of heated deliberation about parental choice in a case involving invasive treatment for a severely disabled child.

[...]

Additional References

Capron, A.M., "Historical Overview: Law and Public Perception," in Lynn 1986, pp. 11–20.
Kluge, E.-H. W., "Severely Disabled Newborns," in Kuhse and Singer 2012, pp. 274–85.
Seckler, A.B., D. E. Meier, M. Mulvihill, and B. E. C. Paris, "Substitute Judgment: How Accurate Are Proxy Decisions?" *Annals of Internal Medicine* 115.2, 1991: 92–8.

Selection from "The Ethics of Respect for Persons: Lying, Cheating, and Breaking Promises and Why Physicians Have Considered Them Ethical"

Robert M. Veatch and Laura K. Guidry-Grimes

[...]

The Principle of Autonomy and the Doctrine of Informed Consent

Keeping faith in relations, called for by the principle of fidelity, is not the only principle entailed in respect for persons. But once one understands the relation between duties derived from fidelity and those derived from beneficence and nonmaleficence, the implications of the other principles under the rubric of respect for persons will be easy to grasp. The most visible principle of the bioethics of the past generation has been the principle of autonomy—another aspect of showing respect for persons. In fact, respecting autonomy is so central to respect for persons that some (see Beauchamp and Childress, 2013) are inclined to treat autonomy as the only principle of this sort. It seems clear, how-ever, that even persons who are not substantially autonomous can still command respect. For instance, the principle of fidelity requires that promises made to the nonautonomous still must be kept. Likewise, in the following sections, we shall see that many people hold that respect for persons implies two further principles: veracity and avoidance of killing. They entail duties to deal honestly and to avoid killing humans, even if those humans are not substantially autonomous or arguably may not be "persons" on some accounts [...].

The Concept of Autonomy

Etymologically, autonomy means "self-legislation," and it can refer to someone's mental capacity, the quality of a decision, or the moral principle that falls under respecting persons. Someone with the *capacity* for autonomy can make decisions that reflect his or her values, preferences, and sense of self; an autonomous *decision* is made freely on the basis of these considerations. The *principle* of autonomy comes, not from the Hippocratic tradition, but from the traditions of Kant and liberal political philosophy. Liberal political philosophy (the very term *liberalism* focuses us on liberty) has dominated the bioethics of the United States and much of the rest of the Western world since the radical rethinking of bioethics began about 1970. The liberty of the individual is very frequently a key part of the principle of autonomy. We see it dominating liberal political philosophy (although not medical ethics articulated by the medical profession) from the eighteenth century. We frequently see this kind of thinking represented by the use of "rights" language. [...R]ights have a reciprocal relation with duties. If one person has a right, then others normally have duties. Controversy remains over whether rights or duties are conceptually prior (Macklin, 1976), but they are clearly closely related. Normally, when an appeal is made to a *right*, this claim is seen as having a special priority or standing such that mere appeals to consequences cannot be used to override the right.

We often talk about the right of a patient to give informed consent before being touched, for example, prior to surgery. That's just an example of playing out this respect for the autonomy of the patient. We can either express this in duty language or rights language, but in either case, the language signals a priority for the claim being made. Sometimes philosophers will say that rights "trump" appeals to consequences, implying that they believe that the principles upon which the rights claim is based take priority over appeals to consequences. Thus, when philosophers say rights and duties are correlative, they mean that this priority might be expressed in two different ways. I can say that a physician has a duty to get informed consent before touching the patient, or I can say the patient has a right to give informed consent before being touched. They mean exactly the same.

Sometimes, in Western thought, people talk about a woman's *right* to procure an abortion. When a woman expresses this right, she is claiming that under the principle of autonomy she should be free to proceed. Of course, if one believes that the fetus has full moral standing so that duties such as the duty to avoid killing it apply, then the woman would be acting in a way that is depriving someone else of their rights. We would, once again, have a clash between two principles, in this case between the principles of autonomy and avoidance of killing.

[...]

Informed Consent, Autonomy, and Therapeutic Privilege

Informed consent is a critical element of any theory that gives weight to autonomy. Hippocratic beneficence might incorporate some minimal informed consent, but only when the clinician believes informed consent will benefit the patient. For example, if a physician is about to write a prescription for diphenylhydantoin, an anti-seizure medication, she might feel obliged to say to that patient that one of the side-effects of diphenyl-hydantoin is that it can make one drowsy. She might warn the patient not to drive a car or operate danger-ous equipment until he is sure he knows how he responds to this drug. This informing occurs, however, only because she is worried that the patient might injure himself or somebody else. The physician must provide certain information just to protect the patient.

In liberal political philosophy, the key idea is that meaningful information must be disclosed even if the clinician does not believe that it will be beneficial. By contrast, Hippocratic ethics includes what is known as therapeutic privilege. It is the privilege that a Hippocratic physician will claim when withholding information that the physician believes would be harmful or upsetting to the patient. That privilege makes sense in an ethic based on paternalistic patient benefit, but is contrary to an ethic giving important place to the principle of autonomy.

In the conflict between liberal political philosophy and Hippocratic ethics, a major clash emerges over informed consent. The case of *Natanson v. Kline* suggests the continuing evolution of the principle of auton-omy as a replacement for the Hippocratic ethic and the related doctrine of therapeutic privilege.

CASE 15

NATANSON v. KLINE: WHEN MAY INFORMATION BE WITHHELD?

In 1960 in the state of Kansas, a woman named Irma Natanson suffering from breast cancer needed radiation following a radical mastectomy. She suffered terrible radiation burns, after which she sued her doctor, Dr. John Kline, for the injury. One of the counts was that she had not consented to the risk of the radiation burn.

Dr. Kline defended himself claiming therapeutic privilege. He did not deny that he had failed to tell Mrs. Natanson about the risk of the burns. Often physicians in this posi-tion claim that such information might disturb the patient, perhaps even irrationally lead her to refuse consent to the needed treatment. Did Dr. Kline have the right to withhold this information if he believed it would upset her or make her do something irrational? Or, alternatively, did he have a duty to explain about those risks anyway?

Justice Schroeder, the judge in this case, gave the definitive response of Anglo-American liberal political philosophy. Although he used masculine pronouns fashionable in that day when the patient clearly was female, Justice Schroeder held:

Anglo-American law starts with a premise of a thorough-going self-determination. It follows that each man is considered the master of his own body, and he may, if he be of sound mind, expressly prohibit the performance of life-saving surgery or other medical treatment.

It followed that, if this information was relevant to her decision about whether she wanted the radiation, she had a right to be informed. When she charged Dr. Kline with failure to get informed consent, the dispute was not over whether she had signed a form. The issue was whether the consent was informed and voluntary. We don't really care, from the point of view of the ethics, whether a piece of paper has a signature. The piece of paper with a signature may help to demonstrate that the patient has at least seen the paper. It will not prove that the patient read the paper; much less that the signer understood it. The court will, in some cases, throw the consent form out if it is believed that the patient never understood what was on the paper.

Thus, back as far as 1960, Justice Schroeder appeared to be rejecting the therapeutic privilege. In 1960, we were just at the beginning of the era when liberal political philosophy was exerting its influence on medical ethics and challenging the therapeutic privilege. We were in a period of transition in which judges and others sometimes reverted to Hippocratic language and sometimes talked as if autonomy were all that counted. Additional text from Justice Schroeder's opinion reveals the confusion. In spite of the bold appeal to autonomy, Justice Schroeder also said:

> The physician's choice of plausible courses should not be called into question if it appears, all circumstances considered, that the physician was motivated only by the patient's best therapeutic interest and he proceeded as a competent medical man would have done under a similar situation.

That sounds very much like the therapeutic privilege doctrine of an earlier era and appears to reject a "thorough-going self-determination." It sounds like the judge is about to say that as long as the physician was worried about Mrs. Natanson's welfare, he had acted acceptably. Justice Schroeder said both that the patient has an absolute right to self-determination and that the physician should not be questioned if he had the patient's best therapeutic interest in mind and acted as competent medical men would have in the circumstances. The latter sounds like therapeutic privilege, the former, more like the principle of autonomy.

Just before the latter sentence, however, there is an opening clause that conveys that, even as far back as 1960, autonomy was really dominant in Justice Schroeder's mind. He introduced the therapeutic privilege language with the clause, "So long as the disclosure is sufficient to assure an informed consent." On balance he appears to be insisting on an adequately informed consent, not just a consent without potentially disturbing information. But in 1960 therapeutic privilege was so common that the judge was still inserting therapeutic privilege language. He was part of the way down the road toward a conversion to respecting autonomy, and he liked to talk self-determination language, but he still lapsed into the talk of therapeutic privilege. In the end, the judge insisted that the consent be informed. The case presents an ambiguous combination of two points of view and, on balance, it seems to be tipping in the direction of requiring information, even if it is upsetting to the patient and even if it is not the common practice among physicians of the day.

It was a series of cases from 1969 to 1972 that really set the pattern of the shift from the more paternalistic Hippocratic basis for consent to one grounded squarely in respect for patient autonomy (*Berkey v.*

Anderson, 1969; *Canterbury v. Spence*, 1972; *Cobbs v. Grant*, 1972). *Canterbury v. Spence* (1972) is a good example.

CASE 16

CANTERBURY V. SPENCE: INVOKING THERAPEUTIC PRIVILEGE

A 19-year-old youth named Jerry Canterbury suffered from back pain. He had an operation called a laminectomy to repair a ruptured disc. Afterwards he fell from bed and suffered an injury that resulted in lower-body paralysis. In the court case, the critical question was whether his physician, Dr. William Spence, should have explained to Mr. Canterbury the risk of falling out of bed. Dr. Spence made a therapeutic privilege claim, saying he did not think that disclosure was appropriate. Disclosure might have discouraged the patient from consenting to a procedure he needed and might have produced "adverse psychological reactions which could preclude the success of the operation."

The court affirmed the right of self-determination, holding that the patient needed to have the information necessary to make an informed decision. At this level the court did not say that Dr. Spence needed to inform about the risk of falling out of bed. That question was referred back to a lower court. What the higher court said was that Dr. Spence had to tell the patient everything that the patient would deem significant to his decision. Dr. Spence still had available the possibility that he could convince a lower court that falling out of bed was so rare or the risk so obvious that the patient would not need to be told about it to make a rational decision. What this court said was that the physician could not use therapeutic privilege to justify withholding of relevant information. [...]

Bibliography

Beauchamp, Tom L., and James F. Childress, eds. *Principles of Biomedical Ethics*, 7th ed. New York: Oxford University Press, 2013.
Berkey v. Anderson. 1 Cal. App. 3d 790. 82 Cal. Rptr. 67 (1969).
Canterbury v. Spence. United States Court of Appeals, District of Columbia, 464 F.2d 772, 150 U.S.App.D.C. 263 (1972).
Cobbs v. Grant. 502 P.2d 1, Cal. (1972).
Macklin, Ruth. "Moral Concerns and Appeals to Rights and Duties." *Hastings Center Report* 6, No. 5 (1976): 31–38.

Review Questions

Directions: Refer to your readings to help respond to the questions and prompts below.

1. Does the waiver of informed consent during emergencies best serve society? What is the difference between informed and implied consent?
2. Some countries have "opt-out" provisions for organ donation. This means a person is automatically considered an organ donor unless they sign to "opt out" of donating. Does this violate the principles of informed consent?
3. Consider if and when the solid paternalistic action of therapeutic privilege could be best. Does this violate the duty-based principles of fidelity, autonomy, or integrity? Would it matter if there was no legal duty, only an ethical one? What is an example of a weak paternalistic lie?
4. To understand case law, a person must consider the events and culture when the case was decided. Let your mind travel back to 1972 when the *Canterbury* case was settled. What was life like in the late 1960s and early 1970s? Describe how the history of that period directly affects the decision. How were things different then? How were things similar? Why does considering these realities make a difference in our understanding of the law? Consider the Vietnam War, civil rights, women's rights, technology, and news sources. What were the demographics of physicians? Of the United States?

References

Canterbury v. Spence, 464 F.2d 772, 150 U.S. App. D.C. 263 (D.C. Cir. May 19, 1972)
Schloendorff v. New York Hospital 211 N.Y. 125 (N.Y. 1914)

Chapter 4

Special Classes of Persons and Considerations

Introduction to the Chapter

Every human being is defined by more than one attribute. People identify by race, sex, choice, culture, age, and illness. The unfortunate part of how people remember is the related stigma. Negativity attaches to social dimensions, and structural and institutional discrimination results in misconceptions, resulting in horrible outcomes for people seeking medical care. Researchers from multiple disciplines offer suggestions to increase health care providers' structural and cultural competency but acknowledge that doing so does little to mitigate the infrastructure issues of access to food, health care, housing, and even defining health and sickness.

Veterans, Native Americans, immigrants, refugees, college students, and the uninsured or underinsured population make up special classes of persons with unique considerations. Others include the homeless, the impoverished, and the incarcerated. Chronically ill, invisible illness, and mental disability/illness populations are as complex as other vulnerable populations, like the elderly or incapacitated. People who have not reached the age of majority (18 years), commonly called minors, also require special medical and legal consideration. Thus, medical providers and bioethicists must continually respond to complex and varied needs arising from attributes and identifiers and disease, injury, illness, or condition. Beneficence and autonomy must guide the approaches that meet legal standards.

Accordingly, laws about discrimination and protections are vast and convoluted. The National Defense Authorization Act provides annual updates aimed at rectifying harms to veterans and service members, such as those exposed to "forever chemicals" and those suffering from mental health conditions, and even improving access for low-income or rural veterans.

The landmark decision *Estelle v. Gamble* (1976) guaranteed prisoners the constitutional right to medical care under the Eighth Amendment. Failure to respond to serious medical needs or unjustifiable pain by refusing or stalling medical care is a violation of civil rights.

In 1946, the Hill-Burton Act, which constructed public hospitals and long-term care facilities for all, allowed states to create separate and unequal care facilities for African Americans because of the Jim Crow Laws.

Mental health laws provide for "the involuntary detention and psychiatric treatment of persons with severe mental impairment." It thus interferes with the individual liberty and bodily integrity of those with mental illnesses and those who lack decision-making support. This law can be seen to infringe upon the right to equality, legal capacity, and ban on torture/cruel and unusual punishment.

When applying moral theories and principles to the topic of special classes of persons and considerations:

- Classic utilitarians would focus on overall happiness for all involved.
- Kantian ethics believe that any time a human being is treated as less than a person, it is unacceptable.
- Human beings should be saved, protected, and treated for their intrinsic worth.
- Natural law theorists contend that humans have intrinsic value and traits because they can make rational decisions, choosing right and wrong. It is based on being morally correct.
- Therefore, because of their unique attributes, most moral theories and principles would support actions that protect, serve, and honor special classes or persons and considerations.

Learning Outcomes

After reading this chapter, students will:

1. Define and integrate key terms into discussion, writing, assignments, and prompts.
2. Analyze relevant case law and statutes to predict future trends.
3. Integrate moral theories and principles into corresponding points to consider that extend from special classes of persons and considerations, including racial bias in health care, profiling versus reliance on known statistics about prevalence, biomedical research collection of race data, zebra patients, and continual awareness of emerging populations.

Key Terms

The following key terms will be introduced and used in this chapter.

- **Implicit Bias:** a form of bias, prejudice, or attitude that a person is unaware of, which occurs automatically and unintentionally. Implicit bias affects judgments, perceptions, decisions, and behaviors. It is thought to be influenced by experience and learned associations between particular qualities and social categories, including race, gender, age, or disability.
- Institutional Racis**m:** ways that policies and practices oppress and disadvantage racial groups. It can be interpersonal, cultural, or historical.
- **Invisible Illness:** a medical condition not easily seen by the casual observer that is often hard to diagnose; is difficult to treat; and features debilitating pain, fatigue, and obscure symptoms.
- **Race:** a group of people related by shared ancestry or heredity, often divided based upon physical traits regarded as typical for a particular racial group with related descent.
- **Racial Discrimination:** any distinction, exclusion, restriction, preference, or unequal treatment of an

individual or group based on race, skin color, or ethnic origin. It nullifies or impairs the recognition, enjoyment, or exercise on an equal basis of human rights and fundamental freedoms in the political, economic, social, cultural, or any other domain of public life.

- **Racial Prejudice:** an attitude held towards an individual or group that is not justifiable or based upon factual information but instead on unsupported generalizations. It creates a partiality that inhibits objective treatment of individuals, issues, or situations.
- **Racism:** a belief that individuals within a particular racial or ethnic group have distinct human characteristics, abilities, or qualities that determine cultural or individual achievement. It is an idea that one racial group is superior or inferior to other racial groups.
- **Structural Racism:** basis for all forms of racism and can be hard to see in institutions because it is so pervasive.

Introduction to the Readings

The following readings focus on a few special classes of persons and considerations.

"Children's Health Disparities," by Donald A. Barr, MD, PhD, offers statistics showing 20 percent of children living in poverty, 39 percent in substandard housing, high obesity rates, and a growing number of children with foreign parents increasing tenfold. The consequences of low-level education, lack of English language proficiency, and lack of health insurance speak to the needs of a growing demographic.

"Culture, Illness, and Mental Health: Conceptual Tools," by Peter J. Brown and Svea Closser, discusses conceptual tools neatly bullet-pointed to address culture, mental health conditions, labels, diagnosis, assumptions, structural violence, and psychosomatic illnesses. The focus is on how different cultures' views and anthropological interests affect mental health.

"Stigma and Coping with Chronic Illness: Conceptual Tools," also from Peter J. Brown and Svea Closser, addresses the often-overlooked population affected by long-term disability and illness using more conceptual tools about stigma, invisible illness, social dimensions, aging, and the interactions of the medical system. It points out how chronic illnesses become a part of people's core social identities and require adjustments for both the patient and providers.

"Structural Competency Meets Structural Racism" by Jonathan M. Metzl and Dorothy E. Roberts focuses on race, politics, and medical knowledge. Matters of diversity affect diagnosis and treatment but illustrate that many health-related facts also represent decisions from larger social contexts, such as food, infrastructure, and patient approaches. There is a "crisis of medical competence" in medical education and health care disparities.

Selection from "Children's Health Disparities"

Donald A. Barr

Donald A. Barr, Selection from "Children's Health Disparities," *Health Disparities in the United States: Social Class, Race, Ethnicity, and the Social Determinants of Health*, pp. 170–171, 309–346. Copyright © 2019 by Johns Hopkins University Press. Reprinted with permission.

[...]

The Changing Demographics of Children in the United States

Established in 1994, the Federal Interagency Forum on Child and Family Statistics publishes annual updates on the status of America's children. Their 2017 report provides an important perspective on the changing demographics of young Americans: "Racial and ethnic diversity have grown dramatically in the United States in the last three decades. This growth was first evident among children. This population is projected to become even more diverse in the decades to come. In 2020, less than half of all children are projected to be White, non-Hispanic. By 2050, 32 percent of U.S. children are projected to be Hispanic (up from 25 percent in 2016), and 39 percent are projected to be White, non-Hispanic (down from 51 percent in 2016)" (p. vii).

In 2015 20 percent of all children ages 0–17 lived in poverty; 59 percent of children lived in counties with air pollution above national standards; and 39 percent of children lived in substandard housing, based either on housing quality or affordability. In 2014 18 percent of children ages 6–11 and 21 percent of adolescents ages 12–17 were obese, with higher rates among

61

Mexican American (25 percent) and black (23 percent) children. In 2015 13 percent of children had been diagnosed with asthma at some time in their lives, while 8 percent of children were reported to currently have asthma. The rate of current asthma was higher among black (13 percent) and Puerto Rican (14 percent) children. It thus seems clear that health disparities among children differ among socioeconomic and racial/ethnic groups.

An important part of the changing demographics of children is the growing number of children with one or more parents who were born elsewhere and immigrated to the United States. The percentage of US children with at least one foreign-born parent grew from 15 percent in 1994 to 25 percent in 2016. Twenty-three percent of babies born in 2016 in the United States were born to a mother who was Hispanic. In California, 47 percent of all babies born in 2016 were Hispanic (Martin and colleagues 2018).

In 2009 the National Population Council of Mexico and the University of California, working in close collaboration, released a study of the heightened challenges faced by children of Mexican immigrants in the United States. At that time, immigrant children with parents from Mexico made up 37 percent of all immigrant children in the United States. As one of the fastest growing groups in the United States, these children nevertheless face a series of challenges. For 60 percent of these children, neither parent was a US citizen. For 49 percent, neither parent finished high school—by far the highest percentage among immigrant groups.

One of the principal consequences of having noncitizen, immigrant parents with low levels of education and associated low levels of English language proficiency is the likelihood that a Mexican immigrant child will not have health insurance, and as a consequence will have reduced access to health care. This often happens even if the child is fully eligible for publicly sponsored insurance such as Medicaid or the Children's Health Insurance Program (CHIP). At that time, 19 percent of Mexican immigrant children under age 6 were uninsured, while 27 percent of those aged 6–17 were uninsured. This compared to uninsured rates among US-born black children of 7 percent for those under 6 and 9 percent for those 6–17. The lack of health insurance means that many Mexican and other Hispanic immigrant children have no regular source of medical care. As a consequence many parents delay care for their child, and then rely on the hospital emergency room for care. In addition, many of these children do not get needed prescription medicines, glasses, or dental care.

The percentage of children without health insurance has decreased since that time, with 4.3 percent of white children, 4.9 percent of black children, 4.6 percent of Asian children, and 7.7 percent of Hispanic children lacking health insurance in 2017 (Berchick et al. 2018). However, of the 3.3 million children who were uninsured in 2016, 57 percent were eligible for either Medicaid or CHIP but had not been enrolled by their parents or caregivers. Among children eligible for Medicaid or CHIP, 7.3 percent of white children, 3.9 percent of black children, 5.2 percent of Asian children, and 6.5 percent of Hispanic children remained un-enrolled despite their eligibility for these programs (Haley et al. 2018).

[...]

References

Berchick, E. R., Hood, E., Barnett, J. C. 2018. Health Insurance Coverage in the United States: 2017. Available at https://www.census.gov/library/publications/2018/demo/p60-264.html, accessed September 30, 2018.

Federal Interagency Forum on Child and Family Statistics. 2017. America's Children: Key National Indicators of Well-Being, 2017. Available at https://www.childstats.gov/americaschildren/index.asp, accessed August 13, 2018.

Haley, J. M., Kenney, G. M., Wang, R., et al. 2018. Uninsurance and Medicaid/CHIP Participation Among Children and Parents: Variation in

2016 and Recent Trends. Available at https://www.urban.org/research/publication/uninsurance-and-medicaidchip-participation-among-children-and-parents-variation-2016-and-recent-trends, accessed October 4, 2018.

Martin, J. A., Hamilton, B. E., Osterman, M. J. K., et al. 2018. Births: Final Data for 2016. *National Vital Statistics Reports* 67(1). Available at https://www.cdc.gov/nchs/data/nvsr/nvsr67/nvsr67_01.pdf, accessed August 13, 2018.

National Population Council of Mexico and the University of California. 2009. Migration and Health: The Children of Mexican Immigrants in the U.S. Available at http://healthpolicy.ucla.edu/publications/search/pages/detail.aspx?PubID=98.

Culture, Illness, and Mental Health: Conceptual Tools

Peter J. Brown and Svea Closser

Peter J. Brown and Svea Closser, "Culture, Illness, and Mental Health: Conceptual Tools," *Understanding and Applying Medical Anthropology: Biosocial and Cultural Approaches*, pp. 298–299, 449. Copyright © 2016 by Taylor & Francis Group. Reprinted with permission.

- Culture defines normality, and cultural rules determine who is crazy. How do you know if you're normal? How do you know if your emotional feelings are appropriate or if your thought processes are disturbed? These are difficult questions because we have to compare ourselves with others, and yet there are no cross-culturally universal standards for normal behavior or thinking. Historical and cultural contexts vary. Saintly behavior in one context may be considered deranged in another. Before the Civil War in the United States, there was a mental illness affecting African American slaves called drapetomania. The symptoms of this illness included repeated attempts to run away from the owner's plantation, and slaves with this "illness" had less value. In more recent history, homosexuality was officially diagnosed as a mental illness, and then, in a revision of the *Diagnostic and Statistical Manual* (*DSM*) of the American Psychiatric Association, it was decided that homosexuality was no longer an illness. The powerful novels of Aleksandr Solzhenitsyn, such as *The Gulag Archipelago* (1973), show how psychiatry can become a powerful tool of social control by the state—when any political dissidence becomes de facto evidence of insanity. The problem of the definition of normality is exactly the same as the problem of cultural relativity: Although we need to be tolerant of a range of variation of the definitions of normal thought and behavior, absolute relativism—an "anything goes" approach—is not acceptable. Boundaries of health and illness are difficult to set. Recognition of this cultural relativity and the function of mental illness categories as agents of social control have played a role in labeling theory and the antipsychiatry movement (Szasz 1974).

- Some mental conditions may be more pronounced or elaborated in particular cultural settings; these conditions have been labeled "culture-bound" or "culture-specific" syndromes (Simons and Hughes 1985). This concept in medical anthropology and cross-cultural psychiatry has caused significant debate. Culture-bound syndromes (CBSs) seem exotic and usually have vernacular ethnomedical labels depending on the locality where they were first described. For example, *latah* is an elaborated startle response that is founded in Malaysia (Simons 1985, 1996). People (usually older women) who have *latah* are often startled several times a day, because their response is so extreme and entertaining. Sometimes their attention can be captured and they mimic their tormentors; sometimes they say colorful obscenities. Another CBS is *koro*, an extreme anxiety reaction affecting males. A victim fears that his penis is shrinking up into his abdomen and that when it ascends all the way he will die. Epidemics of *koro* have been reported in China and Malaysia. Other CBSs include *pibloktoq* (arctic hysteria), *amok* (sudden mass assault), and the folk illness *susto* (soul loss or magical fright). Some anthropologists have argued that the criteria for culture bound syndromes fit particular conditions in the United States, including premenstrual syndrome (PMS) (Johnson 1987) and obesity (Ritenbaugh 1978). Most medical anthropologists do not believe that mental disorders can actually be limited to a particular society with a particular culture; rather, society *constructs* illness labels, and social customs may function to put people at elevated risk for certain kinds of stressors that may result in mental illness (Hahn 1995). And these labels sometimes have complicated social histories: for example, Dutch colonial administrators in Java talked about *amok* in a way that promoted perceptions of Malays as impulsive and violent—and thus perhaps not able to govern themselves.

- Some cross-cultural psychiatrists believe that there are a very small number of universal mental illnesses, two of which correspond to biomedical labels of "schizophrenia" and "depression." In contrast to labeling theorists who emphasize cultural relativity, some cross-cultural epidemiological studies of mental health have focused on commonalities of serious mental disorders. Schizophrenia-type illnesses—including cognitive impairment, auditory hallucinations, and inappropriate behaviors—appear to have some cross-cultural validity. There is also persuasive evidence that there is a genetic component to these illnesses. Depression-type illnesses are common throughout the world, although the local expression of the affective (emotional) disorder varies (Kleinman and Good 1985). Risk of depression-type illnesses also appears to have a genetic component. Evolutionary theorists have speculated as to why genes involved in the etiology of severe mental illnesses seem to persist in human populations (Allen and Sarich 1988). It is possible that mild expressions of these illnesses—for example, in creativity or social sensitivity—may be advantageous.

- Different cultures have their own ethnopsychiatric systems for diagnosing and curing mental illness. All ethnopsychiatric systems are based on cultural assumptions and social role expectations. In ethnomedical studies, it is difficult to separate psychiatric practice from other kinds of medical interventions, because other cultures may not rely on the same philosophical assumptions—for example, the separation of mind and body in Euro-American medicine. The cross-cultural study of ethnopsychiatric systems is very interesting (Gaines 1992), and more epidemiological studies of the effectiveness of traditional therapies is warranted. For example, H. Kristian Heggenhougen (1984) has shown the effectiveness of religious healers in treating heroin addiction in Southeast Asia. Medical anthropologists have also examined the cultural assumptions embedded in a psychiatric category system like the *DSM's* definitions of personality disorders. Charles Nuckolls has shown that U.S. psychiatrists often arrive at diagnoses of personality disorders in the first few seconds of an interaction and that personality disorder categories hinge on definitions of appropriate gender attributes (Nuckolls 1996).

- Because mental illnesses are so difficult to define, it is sometimes difficult to know if they are increasing or decreasing. It is difficult to do epidemiological studies on stigmatized conditions using standardized methods like surveys. Recently it has become clear that rates of "common mental disorders" (primarily anxiety and depression) are more common than previously thought. There are similar questions about ADD and autism-spectrum disorders. Do increased numbers just mean earlier and more sensitive diagnoses?

- Social stress is a serious cause of illness. Generations of psychosomatic researchers have demonstrated that feelings of distress and hopelessness affect physical well-being. Although stress is difficult to define, its importance is obvious. Studies of stress show the interconnectedness of the physical, psychological, and social aspects of an individual. Recent studies by medical anthropologists have shown that the stresses of modernization and a growing discrepancy between rich and poor are serious world health problems (Desjarlais et al. 1995).

- Mental health problems are not limited to the developed world. Problems such as unipolar depression are widespread throughout humanity, in rich and poor nations alike, and they result in a great deal of suffering and disability. In the field of global health, a new measure of the burden of disease focuses on disability-adjusted life years (DALYs) that are lost because of a specific health problem. On this measure, mental health problems rank very high. World mental health problems have been studied by some medical anthropologists (Desjarlais et al. 1995) and pose a major global challenge.

- Structural violence is related to trauma and Post Traumatic Stress Disorder (PTSD). There is increasing anthropological interest in mental health issues related to violence. Medical anthropologists have long been interested in the diagnosis of PTSD (Young, 1997) and especially in recent years with the wars in Afghanistan (Finley 2011) and the tragedies of HIV/AIDS (Nguyen 2010).

References

Allen, J. S., and Sarich, V. M. 1988. Schizophrenia in an Evolutionary Perspective. *Perspective in Biology and Medicine* 32: 132–53.

Desjarlais, R., Kleinman, A., et al. (Eds.). 1995. *World Mental Health: Problems, Priorities and Responses in Low Income Countries*. Oxford: Oxford University Press.

Finley, E. P. 2011. *Fields of Combat: Understanding PTSD among Veterans of Iraq and Afghanistan*. Ithaca, NY: Cornell University Press.

Gaines, A. 1992. *Ethnopsychiatry: The Cultural Construction of Professional and Folk Psychiatries*. Albany: State University of New York Press.

Hahn, R. A. 1995. *Sickness and Healing: An Anthropological Perspective*. New Haven, CT: Yale University Press.

Heggenhougen, H. K. 1984. Traditional Medicine and the Treatment of Drug Addicts: Three Examples from Southeast Asia. *Medical Anthropology Quarterly* l6(os) (1): 3–7.

Johnson, T. 1978. Premenstrual Syndrome as a Culture-Specific Disorder. *Culture, Medicine, and Psychiatry* 11: 337–56.

Kleinman, A., and Good, B. (Eds.). 1985. *Culture and Depression: Studies in the Anthropology and Cross-Cultural Psychiatry of Affect and Disorder.* Berkeley and Los Angeles: University of California Press.

Nuckolls, C. 1996. *The Cultural Dialectics of Knowledge and Desire.* Madison: University of Wisconsin Press.

Ritenbaugh, C. 1978. Obesity as a Culture Bound Syndrome. *Culture, Medicine, and Psychiatry* 6: 347–61.

Simons, R. C., and Hughes, C. C. (Eds.). 1985. *The Culture-Bound Syndrome.* Dordrecht: D. Reidel.

Solzhenitsyn, A. 1973. *The Gulag Archipelago, 1918–1956.* New York: Harper & Row.

Szasz, T. 1974. *The Myth of Mental Illness: Foundations of a Theory of Personal Conduct.* New York: Harper & Row.

Stigma and Coping with Chronic Illness: Conceptual Tools

Peter J. Brown and Svea Closser

- Stigma is the negative social attribution placed on people because of their disability or illness. The famous work of Erving Goffman (1963) defines *stigma* as a sociological phenomenon in which an individual is devalued and shunned because some illness or disability makes her or him different or "not normal." The stigmatized condition becomes the "master status" that overpowers all other social attributes. This is especially the case when a chronic condition is obvious and public. Stigma creates long-lasting suffering.

- When stigmatized conditions are "invisible," they involve the dilemma of disclosure. Some illnesses, such as genital herpes and deafness, as seen in the articles in this section, require a person with the affliction to decide when or if to disclose his or her status to another person. Disclosure risks not only social rejection for an individual but also the possibility that the negative information will become widely known.

- Chronic illnesses have different and more complex social dimensions than acute illnesses do. The rights and responsibilities of the "sick role" usually refer to time-limited illness experiences, when an individual is sick and then is cured. Chronic illnesses or disabilities do not follow the conventions of the sick role. Instead, chronic illnesses become part of people's core social identities. The illness experience is a continuing one, to which an individual must adjust. These adjustments can be difficult, especially because of sociocultural expectations about being "normal."

- The anthropological study of aging has much in common with medical anthropology. Aging is a normal part of the human life cycle. In American society, however, the process of aging has been medicalized. A significant number of anthropological studies of communities of the elderly, including the particular contexts of nursing homes (Savishinsky 1991; Sokolovsky 1983), have shown how the lives of the elderly are shaped by their interactions with the medical system. In addition, the elderly often live in circumstances of age segregation, separated from their families, almost as if old age itself was a stigmatized condition.

- Stigma is often the result of fear. Stigma is a type of xenophobia that possibly, in the historical past, functioned to encourage people to avoid contagion. Widespread fear in social groups, however, can result not simply in scapegoating and discrimination against individuals but also in violence and forced displacement of large groups of people. Social tensions between groups can lead to a lack of trust and cooperation in times of emergency. Fear of new diseases or fear of government entities can hamper the reporting of disease outbreaks. Combatting new emerging diseases, which can spread rapidly throughout the world because of airline travel, requires mutual trust and international cooperation.

Selection from "Structural Competency Meets Structural Racism: Race, Politics, and the Structure of Medical Knowledge"

Jonathan M. Metzl and Dorothy E. Roberts

Jonathan M. Metzl and Dorothy E. Roberts, Selections from "Structural Competency Meets Structural Racism: Race, Politics, and the Structure of Medical Knowledge," *Virtual Mentor*, vol. 16, no. 9, pp. 674–675, 683–689. Copyright © 2014 by American Medical Association. Reprinted with permission.

Physicians in the United States have long been trained to assess race and ethnicity in the context of clinical interactions. Medical students learn to identify how their patients' "demographic and cultural factors" influence their health behaviors.[1] Interns and residents receive "cultural competency" training to help them communicate with persons of differing "ethnic" backgrounds.[2] And clinicians are taught to observe the races of their patients and to dictate

---

1. Association of American Medical Colleges. Tool for Assessing Cultural Competence Training (tacct). https://www.aamc.org/initiatives/tacct. Accessed July 17, 2014.
2. Pérez MA, Luquis RR. *Cultural Competence in Health Education and Health Promotion.* 2nd ed. New York: Jossey Bass-Wiley; 2008.

these observations into medical records—"Mr. Smith is a 45-year-old African American man"—as a matter of course.[3]

To be sure, attention to matters of diversity in clinical settings has been shown to affect a number of factors central to effective diagnosis and treatment.[4] Yet an emerging educational movement challenges the basic premise that having a culturally competent or sensitive clinician reduces patients' overall experience of stigma or improves health outcomes. This movement, called "structural competency,"[5] contends that many health-related factors previously attributed to culture or ethnicity also represent the downstream consequences of decisions about larger structural contexts, including health care and food delivery systems, zoning laws, local politics, urban and rural infrastructures, structural racisms, or even the very definitions of illness and health. Locating medical approaches to racial diversity solely in the bodies, backgrounds, or attitudes of patients and doctors, therefore, leaves practitioners unprepared to address the biological, socioeconomic, and racial impacts of upstream decisions on structural factors such as expanding health and wealth disparities.[6]

In 1968, the U.S. civil rights activist Stokely Carmichael famously assailed racial bias embedded, not in actions or beliefs of individuals, but in the functions of social structures and institutions. "I don't deal with the individual," he said. "I think it's a copout when people talk about the individual."[7] Instead, speaking to a group of mental health practitioners, Carmichael protested the silent racism of "established and respected forces in the society" that functioned above the level of individual perceptions or intentions and that worked to maintain the status quo through such structures as zoning laws, economic policies, welfare bureaucracies, school systems, criminal law enforcement, and courts. Institutionalized racism, he argued, "is less overt, far more subtle, less identifiable in terms of specific individuals committing the acts, but is no less destructive of human life."[7]

Attention to structure as an organizing principle in U.S. medical education is particularly important at the current moment because the forces Carmichael described have become more pressing and recognizable. Indeed, U.S. physicians have never known more about the ways in which the inequities of social and economic systems help to shape the material realities of their patients' lives. Epidemiologists tie the daily experience of racial discrimination to damaging levels of chronic stress, illuminating how racism is "embod-

3. Peek ME, Odoms-Young A, Quinn MT, Gorawara-Bhat R, Wilson SC, Chin MH. Race and shared decision-making: perspectives of African-Americans with diabetes. *Soc Sci Med.* 2010;71(1):1–9.

4. Stepanikova I, Zhang Q, Wieland D, Eleazer GP, Stewart T. Non-verbal communication between primary care physicians and older patients: how does race matter? *J Gen Intern Med.* 2012;27(5):576–581.

5. Metzl JM, Hansen H. Structural competency: theorizing a new medical engagement with stigma and in equality. *Soc Sci Med.* 2014;103:126–133.

6. Deaton A. Health, income, and inequality. *NBER Reporter.* Spring 2003. http://www.nber.org/reporter/spring03/health.html. Accessed July 17, 2014.

7. Carmichael S. Black Power, a critique of the system of international white supremacy and international capitalism. In: Cooper DG, ed. *The Dialectics of Liberation.* New York: Penguin; 1968:151.

ied."[8,9] Neuroscientists show neuronal linkages of social exclusion and poverty with hampered brain functioning.[10,11] Epigenetic researchers explain, at the level of gene methylation, how high-stress, resource-poor environments can produce risk factors for disease that may last for generations if not interrupted by social interventions.[12] And economists prove that people with low incomes can reduce their rates of diabetes and major depression by moving to safer, more affluent neighborhoods.[13] These are but a few examples of the types of research that doctors can now access to understand how disadvantages stemming from social and economic infrastructures can impair health.

On the other hand, evidence also suggests that inattention to these forces has caused a crisis of competence for which American medical education is ill-prepared. Eighty-five percent of primary care providers and pediatricians polled in a 2011 Robert Wood Johnson survey agreed with the statement that "unmet social needs are leading directly to worse health for all Americans" while at the same time voicing concern that they did not "feel confident in their capacity to meet their patients' social needs," and that their failure to do so "impedes their ability to provide care."[14]

Building on scholarly work from fields including law,[15] public health,[16,17,18] history,[19,20] and sociology,[21] structural competency addresses these "social needs"—and their links to race and racism[22]—by increasing clinician recognition of the health-related influences of institutions, markets, and health care delivery systems. This, in turn, shapes doctors' diagnostic knowledge, influencing what happens in the clinic in profound ways.

8. Krieger N. Embodying inequality: a review of concepts, measures, and methods for studying health consequences of discrimination. *Int J Health Serv.* 1999;29(2):295–352.

9. Roberts D. *Fatal Invention: How Science, Politics, and Big Business Re-Create Race in the Twenty-First Century.* New York: New Press; 2011:123–146.

10. Evans GW, Schamberg MA. Childhood poverty, chronic stress and adult working memory. *Proc Natl Acad Sci USA.* 2009;106(16):6545–6549.

11. Buwalda B, Kole MH, Veenema AH, et al. Long-term effects of social stress on brain and behavior: a focus on hippocampal functioning. *Neurosci Biobehav Rev.* 2005;29(1):83–97.

12. Johnstone SE, Baylin SB. Stress and the epigenetic landscape: a link to the pathobiology of human diseases? *Nature Rev Genetics.* 2010;11(11):806–812.

13. Ludwig J, Sanbonmatsu L, Gennetian L, et al. Neighborhoods, obesity, and diabetes—a randomized social experiment. *New Engl J Med.* 2011;365(16):1509–1519.

14. Goldstein D, Holmes J. 2011 Physicians' daily life report. http://www.rwjf.org/content/dam/web-assets/2011/11/2011-physicians-daily-life-report. Accessed July 17, 2014.

15. Roberts DE. *Killing the Black Body: Race, Reproduction, and the Meaning of Liberty.* New York: Vintage Books; 1999.

16. Hatzenbuehler ML, Link BG. Introduction to the special issue on structural stigma and health. *Soc Sci Med.* 2014;103:1–6.

17. Farmer P, Castro A. Understanding and addressing aids-related stigma: from anthropological theory to clinical practice in Haiti. *Am J Public Health.* 2005;95(1):53–59.

18. Farmer PE, Nizeye B, Stulac S, Keshavjee S. Structural violence and clinical medicine. *PLoS Med.* 2006;3(10)e449:1686–1691.

19. Raz M. *What's Wrong with the Poor?: Psychiatry, Race, and the War on Poverty.* Chapel Hill: University of North Carolina Press; 2013.

20. Metzl JM. *The Protest Psychosis: How Schizophrenia Became a Black Disease.* Boston: Beacon Press; 2009.

21. Bonilla-Silva E. Rethinking racism: toward a structural interpretation. *Am Sociol Rev.* 1997;62(3):465–480.

22. Bradby H. What do we mean by "racism"? Conceptualising the range of what we call racism in health care settings: a commentary on Peek et al. *Soc Sci Med.* 2010;71(1):10–12. 23

This [reading] uses three historical case studies to illustrate how extraclinical stigma, socioeconomic factors, and politics can shape diagnostic and treatment disparities. We then explore how attention to structure helps explain the role of race in clinical encounters. Finally, we draw some lessons for medical education that take account of structure.

[...]

Concrete Ways for Health Care Professionals to Become More Structurally Competent

Specific steps include:

1. *Be skeptical of race-based differences in diagnosis.* Findings such as the overdiagnosis of schizophrenia in African American men or of neurologic syndromes in Latin American populations were initially held to result from biological differences among "ethnic" groups, only to later be discovered to have social or structural etiologies. [23,24]

2. *Create alliances between doctors and other professionals who serve the same vulnerable patients* to better address the multiple and entangled structural forces that affect patients' health. Programs that partner doctors and lawyers, such as the Medical-Legal Partnership in Boston, integrate legal assistance as a core component of patient health care to address the complex needs of low-income patients and ensure that they can meet their basic needs of food, housing, employment, family stability, and safety.[25] Medical-legal partnerships also "go beyond curing an individual" by working to improve conditions, such as dangerous housing, for entire communities.[26] Similarly, clinician Mindy Fullilove partners doctors with community-based organizations, urban planners, and architects to "treat" cities that have been "fractured and wounded" by racial segregation, urban renewal, and redlining policies that discriminate against inner-city neighborhoods, with the ultimate aim of creating healthy spaces for use by all city residents.[27]

3. *Be creative in addressing extraclinical structural problems.* For instance, when medical students in Tennessee observed that minority and low-income patients failed to comply with instructions to take their medications after meals because they had to travel more than two hours to reach the nearest grocery stores, they created a social enterprise program called Nashville Mobile Market that partnered with community organizations to deliver food and other items to impoverished areas in refrigerated food trucks.[28] So too, Health Leads, an organization founded by Rebecca Onie while she was an undergraduate at Harvard University, provides

23. Metzl JM, Franklin J. Race, civil rights, and psychiatry. *Atrium.* 2011;9:12–16.
24. American Association of Physical Anthropologists. aapa statement on biological aspects of race. *Am J Phys Anthropol.* 1996;101:569–570.
25. Medical-Legal Partnership, Boston website. www.mlpboston.org. Accessed March 25, 2014.
26. Rosenberg T. When poverty makes you sick, a lawyer can be the cure. *Opinionator.* http://opinionator.blogs.nytimes.com/2014/07/17/when-poverty-makes-you-sick-a-lawyer-can-be-the-cure/. Accessed July 30, 2014.
27. Fullilove M. *Urban Alchemy: Restoring Joy in America's Sorted-Out Cities.* Oakland, CA: New Village Press; 2013.
28. Nashville Mobile Market website. http://www.nashvillemobilemarket.org. Accessed March 25, 2014.

resource desks in the waiting rooms of urban health centers. At these sites, doctors "prescribe" a wide range of basic resources, like food assistance or heating fuel subsidies, which Health Leads' volunteers "fill."[29]

4. *Learn from social science and humanities disciplines such as sociology, anthropology, history, and critical race theory to be more aware of the ways racism is embedded in institutions and operates apart from the blatant acts of individual bias.* As sociologist Eduardo Bonilla-Silva notes in his classic *Racism without Racists*, seemingly colorblind policies that focus on individuals can leave in place the structural roots of racial inequality. [30]

5. *Draw lessons from other professions that have taken active steps toward addressing structural racism.* For instance, the National Association of Social Workers convened a presidential task force subcommittee on institutional racism. The report produced by the subcommittee, "Institutional Racism and the Social Work Profession: A Call to Action," urged social workers to develop a "knowledge base, theories, and values to understand relevant social issues," understand historical notions of race and racism, and "look in the mirror" as a means of self-reflection.[31] The report ultimately called for a series of short- and long-term steps aimed at investigating and challenging structural racism, including "dialogue and inclusion/become partners and allies," "interpersonal capacity and collaboration," "social work organizations becoming antiracist entities," and "focus on client, community, and social policy." Meanwhile, the Grassroots Policy Project produced a workbook for "Dismantling Structural Racism" that includes a guide to "Racial Justice Policy Development."[32] And the city government of Seattle, Washington, approved funding for "technical assistance" to Seattle's network of human services agencies to build their capacity to address structural racism.[33]

6. *Speak up more vocally about structural issues that impact patients—politically.* In the current U.S. political landscape, the loudest political voices that emerge from medicine are often unfortunately those that argue for dismantling many of the social-support networks and infrastructures that ameliorate the effects of structural stigma and racism.[34] Meanwhile, organizations such as Physicians for a National Health Program (pnhp) that speak out against the inadequacies of health insurance and advocate for single-payer national health insurance are frequently marginalized. Given this climate, the U.S. vitally needs coherent voices from within medicine to argue for the medical and moral necessity of assuring equitable health and health care for everyone.

[...]

29. Health Leads website. http://www.healthleadsusa.org. Accessed March 25, 2014.

30. Bonilla-Silva E. *Racism without Racists: Color-Blind Racism and the Persistence of Racial In equality in America*. Lanham, MD: Rowman & Littlefield; 2006.

31. National Association of Social Workers. Institutional racism and the social work profession: a call to action. http://www.socialworkers.org/diversity/institutionalracism.pdf. Accessed March 25, 2014.

32. Grassroots Policy Project. Race, power and policy: dismantling structural racism. http://www.strategicpractice.org/system/files/race_power_policy_workbook.pdf. Accessed March 25, 2014.

33. City of Seattle Office for Civil Rights. Structural racism technical assistance for human service agencies request for proposals (rfp). http://www.seattle.gov/docs/2014-Structural-Racism-TA-RFP-2-7-14.pdf. Accessed March 3, 2014.

34. Peters JW. Is there a doctor in the House? Yes, 17. And 3 in the Senate. *New York Times*. March 8, 2014:A1. http://www.nytimes.com/2014/03/08/us/politics/doctors-confident-in-their-healing-powers-rush-for-congress.html. Accessed July 18, 2014.

Review Questions

Directions: Refer to your readings to help respond to the questions and prompts below.

1. Visit your school's online library. You should have access to a few legal search engines. If you need help, ask the reference librarian for guidance researching any new case law about discrimination in access to health care. Have any new cases been decided?
2. Consider the idea of patient autonomy covered in the preceding chapter. How does this theory apply to special classes of persons? Is autonomy always able to reach the ideal of personal choice? Does assisting or caring for these populations abridge mercy, beneficence, or autonomy?
3. Capacity and competence address whether a person can make his or her own decisions. How is capacity different from competence? Should there be a distinction between the two terms? How does this affect how these special classes of persons are treated legally and medically?
4. Compare and contrast two of the laws discussed in the introduction. Which of them is more aligned with autonomy? Mercy? Beneficence? Would you add anything to the laws that would impact the populations? Why or why not?

References

Estelle v. Gamble, 429 U.S. 97 (1976)

Chapter 5

Human Research

Introduction to the Chapter

Human research often evokes apprehension and caution: images of manipulative, forced experiments to visions of sickly, bedridden patients hoping for a cure. Notable experiments such as Dr. Josef Mengele's genetic testing on concentration camp prisoners and radiation experiments performed in the United States prove the horrible truth of unguarded science. Human research has also provided state-of-the-art medicine and treatments to ease suffering.

Human research is a relatively new branch of study, and researchers must learn from their discoveries, both scientifically and, even more importantly, ethically. Autonomy, beneficence, and nonmaleficence should be more valued than any scientific discovery. How society treats other members, especially the most vulnerable, is a litmus test for the future.

One of the most outrageous experiments is the Tuskegee Study. Conducted in Macon County, Alabama, from 1932 to 1972, the U.S. Department of Public Health studied approximately 400 African American males who were infected with syphilis. Even when penicillin became available as a treatment, these men were not treated so that researchers could follow the development of latent syphilis. Notably, this experiment continued for many decades after the atrocities discovered following World War II and long after the establishment of the Nuremberg Code. The Nuremberg Code is the most essential document in the history of medical research, as it sets ethical research principles for human experimentation.

Despite the Nuremberg Code's existence and its explicit provisions, human research has continued to run afoul. The UCLA Schizophrenia Stud (1983) human radiation experiments (1944–1974), and the Willowbrook State School cases (1956) continued horrible, unguarded, and unethical instances of human research abuses.

Applicable case law addresses fiduciary duty to patients and research subjects, unjust enrichment, and treatment of donated research specimens.

Moore v. Regents of University of California (1990) concerns informed consent and profit. The court held that a patient surrenders ownership of removed cells, forfeiting ownership. It was not a breach of fiduciary duty or conversion when the cells were used in research. The patient's informed consent was not violated.

*Gre*enberg v. Miami Children's Hospital Research Institute (2002) held that there was no duty to obtain informed consent from people who donated blood and other samples to research, even when the research resulted in a patent. It is neither fraud nor unjust enrichment.

When applying major moral theories and principles to human research:

- Utilitarianism considers beneficence and what would maximize the good for all, believing that human research is acceptable if there is proper informed consent. Otherwise, any benefit of the actual research is questionable if personal liberties are ignored.
- Kantian ethics would discourage human research if people are not treated equally or similarly. Persons must be allowed to make autonomous decisions without deception or force, especially protecting human beings from being used as a means to an end.
- Contract Theory advances the belief that those who are better off should not benefit more than those who are not. Research should help all, especially those in undeveloped countries.

Learning Outcomes

After reading this chapter, students will:

1. Define and integrate key terms into discussion, writing, assignments, and prompts.
2. Analyze relevant case law and statutes to predict future trends.
3. Integrate moral theories and principles into corresponding points to consider that extend from access to care, including beneficence, placebos, informed consent for research projects, research on the vulnerable, research on women, the reasons for entering a clinical trial, stopping clinical trials, randomized clinical trials, the Belmont Report of 1974, the National Commission for the Protection of Human Subjects of Biomedical and Behavioral Research, and equipoise.

Key Terms

The following key terms will be introduced and used in this chapter.

- **Blinding:** a technique that shields both the researcher and subject from the intervention being administered or received. Much like randomization, this method reduces bias in a research study.
- **Clinical Trial:** a standardized way of investigating the effectiveness of a medical intervention or medication.
- **Placebos:** inactive treatments used to simulate getting a medical intervention or medication. It has been shown that when patients think they are receiving a medication, even if that medication does not have any physiological impact, symptoms can sometimes improve.
- **Randomization:** a research tool that controls bias by randomly placing subjects in control and experimental groups. This reduces the chance that unconscious researcher bias impacts the research outcome.

Introduction to the Readings

"Experiment or Treatment? Histories of Medical Care Research and Regulation," by John A. Lynch, discusses the Nuremberg Code, the history of its impact on American research studies, and the push for research regulation. Notorious cases of medical research are provided, as well as a discussion of Dr. Henry K. Beecher's 1966 exposé in the *New England Journal of Medicine*.

"Research on Human Tissue Samples: Balancing Autonomy vs. Justice," by David Korn and Rachel E. Sachs, continues the analysis of human research consent through documents such as the 1964 Declaration of Helsinki and the 1978 Belmont Report. Autonomy, the Common Rule, societal benefits, and multiple legal cases are examined with a focus on informed consent.

"Social Ethics of Medicine: Allocating Resources, Health Insurance, Transplantation, and Human Subjects Research," by Robert M. Veatch and Laura K. Guidry-Grimes, examines many terms of art, including innovative therapy, social utility, respect for persons, justice, and treatment of vulnerable patients. It asks: What is acceptable to ask patients to do, especially the very sick ones? What is a considerable burden for a sick or dying person?

Selection from "Experiment or Treatment? Histories of Medical Care Research and Regulation"

John A. Lynch

[...]

Medical Research during and after World War II

World War II intensified the trends of earlier medical research. Benevolent paternalism, the drive to usability, and the confusion of therapy and research continued. These concerns became more prominent as medical research burgeoned during the war and after the Nazi medical atrocities were revealed. During the war, medical research was overseen by the Committee on Medical Research (CMR), established in the summer of 1941. The CMR organized contracts with universities to conduct medical research, and by the end of the war, it had funded 593 contracts worth $24 million that involved the work of more than five thousand investigators. The accomplishments of the CMR were impressive. Peni-cillin was refined and distributed to the European and Pacific Theaters, as well as hospitals in the United States. Other accomplishments included developing gamma globulin (a treatment for hepatitis), blood transfusion and blood substitutes, other treatments for dysentery and malaria, and the production of insecticides to control mosquitoes and other pests. Much of the disease research in World War II repeated the most problematic aspects of pre-World War II research. For example, studies on dysentery and influenza used patients in institutions for the developmentally disabled, and research on malaria used prisoners as research subjects. Wartime necessity reinforced the need to render all bodies useful. The war made experimentation "a patriotic necessity for all Americans. Men, women, and children were pressed into service as research subjects as researchers joined the war efforts ... moral qualms about using these populations [i.e., developmentally disabled, orphans, and prisoners] in nontherapeutic studies faded in the harsh light of wartime necessity." Researchers, the government, and the public all saw the success of medical research and considered the costs acceptable, to the degree that they knew the costs.

The federal government continued funding and providing intellectual direction to medical research after the war. This was part of the broader vision for American investment in basic science articulated by Vannevar Bush in a report titled *Science, the Endless Frontier.* Medical research was primarily supported by the National Institutes of Health (NIH), but additional research (primarily focused on understanding the effects of radiation) was supported by the Atomic Energy Commission, the Department of Defense, and the Department of Energy.

The Nuremberg Code

While the American research enterprise expanded, some politicians, lawyers, and physicians grappled anew with the ethics of medical research in light of the Nuremberg trial of Nazi physicians who experimented on people in concentration camps. While they were not the first example of willfully harmful research in medical history, "the Nazi experiments were in many respects unprecedented in the extensiveness and extremity of the harm and suffering to which they knowingly exposed their victims." Experiments included exploring "the effects of ingesting poisons, intravenous injections of gasoline, immersion in ice water ... infection with epidemic jaundice and spotted fever virus," among others. An American military tribunal tried the Nazi physicians. The trial ran from December 9, 1946, to August 19, 1947, and in their verdict against the physicians, the military tribunal articulated a set of ten standards for medical experimentation. They included requirements for informed and voluntary consent, prior experimentation on animals, and a balancing of risks to participants and potential benefits for the participants and society.

Yet, the impact of the Nuremberg Code on American research practices was uneven at best. The trials and the code did lead to the creation of several policy documents in the United States. In December 1946, as a result of reports from consultants to the Nuremberg prosecutors, the American Medical Association revised its code of ethics to require voluntary consent of research participants. While the rules were published and were disseminated to most American physicians, "these rules were not published prominently; they were set in small type along with a variety of other miscellaneous business items.... Only an exceptionally diligent member [of the AMA], or one with a special interest in medical ethics, is likely to have located this item." In 1947, the Atomic Energy Commission's general manager created a series of statements outlining requirements that university contractors solicit verbal consent from participants, but the "statements were not routinely communicated in response to requests for guidance from non-AEC researchers." Finally, in 1953, Department of Defense secretary Charles Wilson established that the Nuremberg Code would be the operating ethical policy for DOD research; but the memorandum outlining this policy was classified top secret and not circulated widely, limiting its impact.

At roughly the same time, the NIH's Clinical Center, a 500-bed research hospital on the NIH's Bethesda campus, adopted a policy for research on human participants. The policy required at least verbal consent from all research participants and "written consent from healthy subjects and from only certain patient-subjects," as well as prior review of research protocols by other physicians and researchers at the Clinical Center. While the NIH had participated in the DOD's deliberations over human subjects, the extent to which the Nuremberg Code influenced NIH policy is not clear. Charles McCarthy argues that the policy was rooted in changes "in the appreciation of ethical issues in medical research" without specifying the basis for those changes. Regardless of the impetus, the NIH Clinical Center developed a policy that mirrored many of the principles of the Nuremberg Code. Yet, that policy was limited to the Clinical Center, not all NIH-funded research, and it never included clear standards for what researchers needed to disclose to participants about risks and benefits, details of procedures, etc.

Policies based on the principles of the Nuremberg Code were developed by many of the agencies involved in human subjects research, but those policies were not disseminated widely to the researchers who needed to implement them. Even if the policies had been disseminated, it is not clear what influence they would have had with researchers and funding agencies. First, issues of usability influenced the degree to which the federal government enforced its existing policies, especially in the context of DOD research. For example, since the time of Walter Reed, research by the armed services had a tradition of informed consent, but as the Advisory Committee on Human Radiation Experiments (ACHRE) noted, the imposition of ethical limits on researchers "depended on the nature of its [DOD's] interest in the research being done." In other words, the needs of the state determined whether ethical considerations trumped usability.

Second, American medical researchers did not see the Nuremberg Code and its principles as relevant to their activities. David Rothman states that American researchers viewed the Nazi physicians as "Nazis first and last; by definition, nothing they did, and no code drawn up in response to them, was relevant to the United States." Similarly, Allan M. Brandt and Lara Freidenfels argued that in the immediate aftermath of World War II, "researchers cited Nazi science as an example of the potential abuses of government oversight and control." In other words, outside forces—the government and Nazis—produced the experiments in the Nazi concentration camps, not medical researchers directly.

Third, concerns about maintaining the sanctity of the doctor-patient relationship and ongoing confusion of clinical treatment with research impacted how researchers and funding agencies understood research regulation policies. During the period from 1946 through the following decade, medical researchers and the government agencies funding research viewed research through the lens of the doctor-patient relationship, where "patient trust and medical beneficence were viewed as the unshakeable moral foundations on which meaningful interactions between professional healers and the sick should be built." The paternalistic legacy of Hippocrates guaranteed that judgments of beneficence were the purview of the individual physician: If a physician believed a course of treatment was beneficial and risks trivial, there was no pressing need to acquire consent from patients or research participants. Because a great deal of medical research involved people who were already ill, physicians and many other groups believed "that the researcher-subject relationship was identical to the doctor-patient relationship." Since the doctor-patient relationship was a *private* one, government funding agencies were leery of interfering with it, and physician-researchers would regularly argue that requiring consent, especially written consent, violated their relationship with patient-subjects. Overall, the confusion of research and treatment within the context of the paternalistic doctor-patient relationship, along with the state's willingness to use some people to further research of military and medical interest, was the context of normal medical research for most of the twentieth century. This created the space for medicine to go obviously and publicly wrong in the 1960s.

The Push for Research Regulation

Starting in the 1960s, politicians, philosophers, and the lay public generally became concerned about medical practice, especially medical research practices. Scholars offer two overlapping reasons for this change. First, the protest movements of the 1960s and 1970s—civil rights, women's rights, LGBT rights, the consumer movement, etc.—focused attention on individual rights, choice, and autonomy, among other broader issues, and these movements often included concerns about health care and medicine. Second, these movements also encouraged a distrust of authority and paternalism, which were the cornerstones of medical practice. The demand to respect individual patients and their choices, along with the distrust of authority were crystallized by a series of scandals.

In 1961, American trust in medicine and the "miracles" medical research provided were shaken by the thalidomide scandal. Doctors had prescribed the sedative thalidomide to countless pregnant women in Canada, across Europe, and to a lesser degree in the United States. Thalidomide produced countless birth defects, primarily children born with missing or deformed limbs. According to ACHRE, the thalidomide disaster was widely covered by the media, especially television, and "the visual impact of these babies stunned viewers and caused Americans to question the protections afforded those receiving investigational agents [i.e., experimental drugs and medical treatments]." The scandal led Congress to empower the Food and Drug Administration to test new medications for safety and efficacy, and also to require informed consent for individuals involved in testing the new drugs.

In 1963, one of the first notorious cases of medical research in the post–World War II era came to light, the Jewish Chronic Disease Hospital (JCDH) cancer study. Dr. Chester M. Southam led this study where twenty-two patients at the JCDH in Brooklyn, New York, were injected with live cancer cells. According to Faden and Beauchamp, "Southam had convinced [JCDH medical director Emmanuel E.] Mandel that although the research was entirely nontherapeutic, it was routine to do such research without consent." Most of the patients were poor, and some of them were senile or had dementia. Even those patients who could have given informed consent were not told they would be injected with cancer cells "because to do so might agitate them unnecessarily." Three junior physicians at the hospital refused to participate in the study and resigned a few weeks after the study was initiated without them. As news of the research and the resignation of the three residents percolated through the hospital and New York medical community, medical authorities tried to contain and downplay the event until William E. Hyman, a lawyer and JCDH cofounder and board member, sued the hospital to get details from internal committees about the research. Amidst the hostile public reaction to revelations of the study, the New York State Board of Regents "suspended the licenses of Drs. Mandel and Southam, but subsequently stayed the suspension and placed the physicians on probation for one year." Medical researchers rallied around Southam; in fact, a few years later, they elected him president of the American Association for Cancer Research. Overall, this incident highlights medical paternalism in Southam and Mandel's reliance on Southam's judgment of risk alone, ignoring oversight committees and the concerns of junior colleagues, as well as the willingness to render indigent elderly patients with dementia usable for the nation-state through research.

While medical researchers generally rallied around Southam and defended their professional prerogatives to determine the course of research, leaders of medical research, especially NIH director James Shannon, were disturbed by the details of Southam's research and the negative public reaction to it. As a result, Shannon pushed for the development of guidelines for clinical research that recognized for the first time that the researcher-participant relationship differed substantially from the doctor-patient relationship. Shannon's efforts led to the creation of a Public Health Service (PHS) policy published in 1966 that recognized that "patient-subjects, like healthy subjects, should be included in the consent provisions for federally sponsored human experimentation." The PHS tried to balance federal regulation and local control of research. As a result, "the new rules were neither as intrusive as some investigators feared nor as protective as some advocates preferred."

While the NIH and PHS were developing new standards for research, Henry Beecher, an anesthesiologist from Harvard, published what is considered the most important medical publication on medical ethics in the mid-twentieth century. Beecher published an account of twenty-two anonymized cases of medical research that he felt "endangered the health and well-being of subjects without their knowledge or approval." The research was conducted at prominent medical institutions: "Four came from Harvard Medical School, three from the NIH Clinical Center, and the rest from other prominent institutions." To help disseminate his findings and his concerns, Beecher distributed an earlier version of the article to journalists in 1965, but refused to give interviews: "This was the beginning of Beecher's strategy of speaking directly in the medical literature only, but making sure that the public heard about his criticisms second-hand. That way, he gave the appearance that he was prompting a discussion within the medical profession, which the public happened to be observing, rather than inviting the public to join the discussion." For all his concern about unethical research, Beecher's suggested course of action still reinforced the professional prerogatives of medical researchers. He was opposed to outside regulation and ethical codes, including the Nuremberg Code. He doubted "the ability of a formal code of ethics to shape researchers' behavior" and called for researchers to be more responsible in their conduct of research.

One of the twenty-two studies identified by Beecher was Saul Krugman's study of hepatitis at the Willowbrook State School. Yet, while the study was easily identified from Beecher's description despite his attempt to anonymize it, the study did not receive much attention in 1966. The study finally became notorious after Beecher offered an expanded discussion of it in his 1970 book and after the publication in *The Lancet* of criticism by Stephen Goldby. This debate and the research continued until the public outrage about conditions at the school started the process of the school's closure in 1972.

Then, in 1972, alongside the controversies over the Willowbrook hepatitis study, there was the public revelation of the Tuskegee Syphilis Study. Despite the PHS creating guidelines for research in 1966, the study had continued. Individuals, like Henry Beecher and Jay Katz, who had been concerned about informed consent in medical research missed the study in their canvass of medical publications for questionable research. Public revelation of the study brought outrage, and in the face of that outrage, the Department of Health, Education, and Welfare (DHEW) created the Tuskegee Syphilis Study Ad Hoc Advisory Panel, consisting of nine men and women from a range of professions, of whom five were black and four were white. Their purpose was "to review the study as well as the Department's policies and procedures for the protection of human subjects in general." The panel declared that the study should be terminated at once, the men remaining in the study should receive all health care necessary to treat disabilities that resulted from their participation, and better protections for human subjects were needed in all DHEW research, which included the work of the NIH and the PHS.

Other stories of dubious medical research percolated through medical and public discourse, like the Cincinnati Whole Body Radiation (WBS) study, but most of those received substantially less attention at the time. These three scandals—JCDH, Willowbrook, and Tuskegee—received the most attention, and it was Tuskegee that in many ways guaranteed congressional action. The earliest attempts at congressional oversight of research occurred in 1968. Walter Mondale introduced a bill for a Commission on Health, Science, and Society. The bill faced "unbending opposition" from medical researchers who "fought doggedly to maintain their authority over all medical matters." The opposition was so virulent that it left Mondale "disgusted" with medical practitioners, and he continued fighting for research regulation with little success through 1973. His quest was successful after he was joined by Senator Edward Kennedy. Kennedy chaired the hearings on the syphilis study at Tuskegee. The hearing featured testimony from men in the study, their attorney Fred Gray, and members of the DHEW Ad Hoc Panel. David Rothman argues, "Kennedy, more artfully than Mondale earlier, structured the hearings to demonstrate the need for outside intervention." During these hearings and later, Kennedy would repeatedly invoke "the great scandals in human experimentation—Willowbrook, Tuskegee, Brooklyn Jewish Chronic Disease Hospital." Kennedy's efforts, along with Mondale's, led to the successful passage of the National Research Act in 1974: It established a National Commission that "did pioneering work as it addressed issues of autonomy, informed consent, and third-party permission, particularly in relation to research involving vulnerable subjects such as prisoners, children, and people with cognitive disabilities." While the commission produced multiple reports, perhaps the most important is the Belmont Report, which defined the fundamental values that should guide the ethical conduct of research. The values and processes of risk-benefit calculation and informed consent have shaped research regulation in the United States since 1981.

[...]

Selection from "Research on Human Tissue Samples: Balancing Autonomy vs. Justice"

David Korn and Rachel E. Sachs

David Korn and Rachel E. Sachs, Selection from "Research on Human Tissue Samples: Balancing Autonomy vs. Justice," *Specimen Science: Ethics and Policy Implications*, ed. Holly Fernandez Lynch, et al., pp. 95–101,104–105. Copyright © 2017 by MIT Press. Reprinted with permission.

[...]

Balancing Autonomy with Justice

Bioethics' focus on the centrality of Autonomy dates back to the founding documents of the field, all of which enshrine the importance of consent. Indeed, the very first sentence of the Nuremberg Code, a set of research ethics principles composed in 1947 in response to atrocities committed in the name of "experimentation" by Nazi physicians during World War II, avers that "the voluntary consent of the human subject is absolutely essential" (Nuremberg Code 1947). Autonomy similarly took precedence in the 1964 Declaration of Helsinki, adopted by the World Medical Association, that particularly emphasized and added content to the requirement that the patient not merely give consent, but give fully free, informed consent (World Medical Association 1964).

But the US biomedical research establishment would not adopt its own set of ethics principles until the Belmont Report, issued in 1978 by the National Commission for the Protection of Human Subjects of Biomedical and Behavioral Research. In the wake of Henry Beecher's famous 1966 expose in the *New England Journal of Medicine* (Beecher 1966) drawing attention to American research abuses of human subjects, and the 1972 revelations of the Tuskegee Syphilis Study (Jones 1993), the Belmont Report similarly focused on the importance of the ethical principle of Autonomy, phrased here as "respect for persons" (Belmont Report 1979).

When first promulgated, none of these three documents referred specifically to research involving human biospecimens, referring only more generally to research involving human subjects. That has changed only very recently, with the latest revision of the Declaration of Helsinki in 2013. The Declaration now devotes a single paragraph to research on human tissues, noting that "[f]or medical research using identifiable human material or data, such as research on material or data contained in biobanks or similar repositories, physicians must seek informed consent for its collection, storage and/or reuse. There may be exceptional situations where consent would be impossible or impracticable to obtain for such research. In such situations the research may be done only after consideration and approval of a research ethics committee" (World Medical Association 2013).

This passage encapsulates the general view of many bioethicists on the topic of research involving human biospecimens. The problem, of course, is that key terms in the paragraph are open to debate and dispute. In particular, scholars and policy makers have hotly debated what it means to give "informed consent" for future research on a given biospecimen. Views about the proper definition of this term span a continuum from highly specified, iterative requirements to little or no requirements at all.

Some scholars stand close to one end of the spectrum, advocating highly specified consent forms that would inform potential research subjects not only that their tissues might someday be used for research, but that would list specific ways in which those tissues might be used and require the subjects to select, in checklist fashion, only those uses to which they consent (Tomlinson 2013; Arnason 2004). Also specified may be the researchers or institutions that will have access to the specimens, and with whom they could or could not be shared. Many of these authors would also require researchers to gain consent anew each time they wished to use an identified specimen, a requirement that becomes more difficult (and then impossible or meaningless) the older the specimen.

This position is fundamentally rooted in the value of Autonomy. In the views of these scholars, taking the principle of Autonomy seriously requires that specimen sources complete this set of finely specified consent procedures. For them, the value of Autonomy is not simply a formality to be observed. Giving it meaning requires potential research subjects to be informed not merely that their tissues may be used, but when and how they will be used, by whom, and to what end. In practice, this would require repeated notices and consent forms to be signed, and it isn't clear whether the specimen would be accessible at all for research after the death of the source. As we discussed in the previous section, such detailed consent poses the threat of insurmountable barriers to the permissible scope and time span of potential research on human specimens.

Rejecting the implications of this extreme position, many ethicists and policy makers have adopted a less restrictive interpretation of what informed consent requires. These views range from the argument that a general, broad consent at the time of donation is sufficient to the view that even no consent may often be appropriate, possibly in opposition to the Declaration of Helsinki's recent pronouncement (Grady et al. 2015; Edwards et al. 2014; Wendler 2013).

We agree with those rejecting the position requiring specific consent for different research uses of banked tissue. But we write to provide another justification for our position: specifically, we argue that advocates for the most extreme informed consent requirements have placed far too much emphasis on the principle of Autonomy embodied in the founding documents of bioethics, to the exclusion of the principle of Justice. Like Autonomy, Justice is one of the four principles of American bioethics famously articulated by Beauchamp and Childress (Beauchamp and Childress 2012), along with Beneficence and Non-maleficence. Although in our view these advocates also ignore the Principle of Beneficence, the *obligation* to act in the best interests of others, this topic is taken up elsewhere in this volume.

With their focus on Autonomy above all else, these advocates have seriously distorted the integrity of the Belmont Principles and shattered the carefully reasoned balance intended by the Belmont Report's framers. They ignore that the principle of Justice also has pride of place in the Belmont Report, which frames the concept as requiring the equitable distribution of the burdens and benefits of scientific experimentation. One of the Report's paradigmatic examples of injustice is the Tuskegee syphilis study, which not only "used disadvantaged, rural black men to study the untreated course of a disease that is by no means confined to that population" (Belmont Report 1979) but continued even after the discovery of penicillin made effective treatment of syphilis possible. More generally, where the benefits of a particular scientific study accrue broadly, it is unjust to permit the burdens of research to fall on disadvantaged societal groups, which in the United States have often been prisoners, the mentally disabled, racial minorities, or institutionalized children.

The principle of Justice has a straightforward application in research based on human tissue specimens. Typically, this research is performed to increase the store of medical knowledge that will redound to the benefit of society as a whole. Sometimes a particular population must be targeted because they are directly or uniquely relevant to the problem being addressed, or because they would reap particular benefits from the research. But when that is not true, researchers have an ethical obligation not to target particular disadvantaged populations to bear the burdens of research.

In our view, this duty of researchers imposes a reciprocal ethical duty on potential subjects to participate in research when opportunities arise that do not thereby put them at undue risk. Put simply, because every individual will inevitably benefit from the accumulation of medical knowledge from research on human tissues, we are all obligated to avoid letting the burdens of that research fall solely on others. This duty is surely limited to cases in which opportunities arise—we do not contend that individuals are obligated to make regular donations to tissue banks (excluding blood banks) or undergo more invasive procedures such as bone marrow donation *sua sponte*. But where individuals are having or have had tissue removed from their bodies and banked, as many of us have, we argue that refusal to consent to that tissue's use in research is typically unjust.

Although our argument largely rejects the prioritization of Autonomy above all, it is useful to consider a real-world example in which our views would reach the same ethical conclusions, although for different reasons: the Havasupai case. [...T]he rate of diabetes among the Havasupai is extremely high, and researchers have been interested in studying the tribe to learn more about the various potential causes of this disease, with the ultimate aim of contributing to the development of preventive behavioral practices and possibly effective therapies. In the early 1990s, the Havasupai tribe consented to the collection and use of their blood samples for a set of research projects on diabetes. But in 2003, they were dismayed to find that researchers had used their samples in addition to study migration patterns, reaching conclusions that contradicted the Havasupai's traditional spiritual beliefs about the site of the tribe's origin.

In 2004, the tribe sued the researchers involved. Although the case was settled and did not result in a precedential opinion addressing the legal rights of each party, we agree with other scholars that the researchers who used the tribe's samples for migration research without consent acted unethically. In our view, though, the reason is not simply that members of the tribe were not asked for permission to conduct the study, but also that the principle of Justice imposes heightened consent requirements in cases involving populations who are marginalized or hold particular cultural and religious beliefs. Especially in the case of research specifically involving Native American tribes, respect requires researchers to obtain consent from the tribal leadership before approaching individual members of the tribe. In the case of the diabetes research, the tribe itself stood to gain from the knowledge gained about the genetic causes of the disease, even though that benefit would obviously be distributed more broadly. But in the case of the migration research, the tribe gained nothing—indeed, it was harmed—solely in pursuit of knowledge.

In this case, the researchers exploited the fact that the samples were accessible to them and displayed a lack of sensitivity to and respect for the Havasupai and their beliefs, as well as respect for their tribal governance. We do not argue there is never a need for any type of consent in research with stored samples. But in our view, "informed consent" must be given content not merely by the principle of Autonomy but also by the principle of Justice. And the term can be interpreted permissively, rather than narrowly, to permit a scope of research on these specimens that is much broader than commonly believed. As we explain in the next section, any concerns about the legitimacy of research or the privacy policies implemented can be mitigated through a robust IRB review process that not only assures privacy, but can also serve as a surrogate for incomplete or missing consent.

The Legal Landscape

The legal cases regarding ownership and control of human tissue specimens are more closely aligned with our recommendation than they are with the views of scholars urging a more extreme version of informed consent. The published decisions in the well-known cases involving John Moore, the Greenberg family, and Dr. William Catalona all agree with our view of the absence of residual rights possessed by individuals in tissues removed from their bodies. [...]

The facts of the John Moore case are well-known to lawyers and ethicists alike. Moore's physician, in the course of treating him for hairy-cell leukemia, used tissue removed from Moore in repeated visits to produce what became a multi-billion-dollar cell line—all without Moore's knowledge or permission (*Moore v. Regents of University of California*, 125). Moore sued on a range of legal theories, most notably arguing that his physician should have disclosed his financial interest in Moore's tissues, on theories of breach of fiduciary duty and informed consent, and that his physician should be liable for "conversion," as he had deprived Moore of a property interest in his tissues.

The California Supreme Court's 1990 opinion ruled in Moore's favor on the first count, and against him on the second. First, the court held that treating physicians have a fiduciary obligation to their patients to disclose any research or financial interests they may have in those patients (*Moore v. Regents of University of California*, 131). Importantly, though, this duty did not extend to other researchers working with Moore's physician who were not themselves involved in patient care. Second, the court went on to hold that Moore lacked a sufficient ownership interest in his excised cells to support a claim for conversion. Not only did the court conclude that existing law did not grant Moore such an interest; it went on to hold that creating such an interest would have deleterious policy consequences, impeding "activities that are important to society, such as research" (ibid., 146).

The next canonical case, *Greenberg v. Miami Children's Hospital*, involved more agency on the part of the research subjects. A group of families affected by Canavan disease had donated their tissues (as well as financial resources through related nonprofits) to researchers interested in studying the disease and specifically, in creating a prenatal test for the condition. When the test was developed, and was patented by the researchers' institution and made available only on a limited basis, the families and nonprofits sued (*Greenberg v. Miami Children's Hospital*, 1067).

In the *Greenberg* case, much as in the *Moore* case, the federal district court concluded that the researchers involved, who were not the plaintiffs' treating physicians, did not have a duty to disclose their economic interests to the plaintiffs. In the court's view, doing so would be "unworkable and would chill medical research as it would mandate that researchers constantly evaluate whether a discloseable event has occurred" (*Greenberg*, 1070). Similarly, the court ruled that the plaintiffs had "no cognizable property interest in body tissue and genetic matter donated for research" (*Greenberg*, 1074). The decision was not entirely in the researchers' favor—the court declined to dismiss the plaintiffs' allegations of unjust enrichment, which the plaintiffs then used to extract a favorable settlement (Colaianni et al. 2010).

More recently, the Court of Appeals for the Eighth Circuit decided *Washington University v. Catalona*. During his decades as a urologist and researcher at Washington University, Dr. William Catalona had initiated and overseen a prostate cancer tissue repository that had amassed many thousands of surgically excised specimens that he and other members of the faculty used in their many independent research projects on prostate cancer. When Dr. Catalona accepted a position at Northwestern University, he—without any IRB approval—sent forms to his former patients requesting their consent to transfer their stored biological materials to Northwestern. Washington University sued Catalona to enjoin him from taking the biorepository to Northwestern, because the collection had become a widely used institutional research asset at Washington University.

The Eighth Circuit put the legal question presented by the case as follows: "whether individuals who make an informed decision to contribute their biological materials voluntarily to a particular research institution for the purpose of medical research retain an ownership interest allowing the individuals to direct or authorize the transfer of such materials to a third party" (*Catalona*, 673). The answer, quite simply, was that they do not. The research subjects surely had the right to decline to donate more materials in the future or to decline to answer other research queries, but in the court's view, they retained no right to control their tissues after donation.

These several courts were tasked with resolving questions of law and policy, not of ethics. It may be that the legality of the situation does not always accord with the ethics involved. Accordingly, we do not argue that our ethical argument is necessarily correct because it leads to the same conclusions reached by these courts. However, to the extent that laws and legal decisions often track the ethical views of society, the consistency of courts on this question over the past several decades is noteworthy.

A recent legal development—the September 2015 release by the Office of Human Research Protection (OHRP) of a Notice of Proposed Rulemaking (NPRM) to amend the Common Rule—is more overtly linked to the ethical questions we address here. The term Common Rule refers not only to the legal rules protecting human subjects involved in research, but also is generally thought to instantiate the ethical principles promulgated in the Belmont Report. The NPRM aimed comprehensively to overhaul the rules governing human research with biospecimens, as well as human subjects research more generally.

In some ways, the NPRM's proposed rules regarding biospecimen research were more restrictive even than the Declaration of Helsinki, as they proposed to require informed consent for research "even if the investigator is not being given information that would enable him or her to identify whose biospecimen it is" (NPRM 2015). Because of the rapid pace of technological progress, especially in genomics, and the fact that even de-identified data can be used to identify individuals in ways which were "simply not possible, or even imaginable" when the Common Rule was first adopted, this provision sought to protect individuals out of an abundance of caution. Importantly, the final rule did not include this provision about non-identified biospecimens.

But, critically, even the NPRM did not adopt the extreme view encouraged by many scholars of what "informed consent" requires. Specifically, for de-identified biospecimen research, informed consent "could be obtained using a 'broad' consent form in which a person would give consent to future unspecified research uses." The NPRM explicitly stated that consent does not need to be obtained for each specific study seeking to use a given biospecimen, as long as general consent has been provided up front. In reaching this conclusion, the NPRM specifically considered the ways in which the principle of Autonomy relates to the principle of Justice.

[...]

References

Arnason, Vilhjalmur. 2004. Coding and consent: Moral challenges of the database project in Iceland. *Bioethics* 18 (1): 27–49.

Beauchamp, Tom L., and James F. Childress. 2012. *Principles of Biomedical Ethics*, seventh edition. Oxford University Press.

Beecher, Henry K. 1966. Ethics and clinical research. *New England Journal of Medicine* 274 (24): 1354–1360.

Colaianni, Alessandra, Subhashini Chandrasekharan, and Robert Cook-Deegan. 2010. Impact of gene patents and licensing practices on access to genetic testing and carrier screening for Tay-Sachs and Canavan Disease. *Genetics in Medicine* 12 (4): S5–S14.

Edwards, Teresa P., R. Jean Cadigan, James P. Evans, and Gail E. Henderson. 2014. Biobanks containing clinical specimens: Defining characteristics, policies, and practices. *Clinical Biochemistry* 47 (0): 245–251.

Grady, Christine, Lisa Eckstein, Dan Brock Ben Berkman, Robert Cook-Deegan, Stephanie M. Fullerton, Hank Greely, Mats G. Hansson, et al. 2015. Broad consent for research with biological samples: Workshop conclusions. *American Journal of Bioethics* 15 (9): 34–42.

Greenberg v. Miami Children's Hospital Research Institute, Inc., 264 F. Supp.2d 1064 (S.D. Fla. 2003).

Jones, James H. 1993. *Bad Blood: The Tuskegee Syphilis Experiment*. Free Press.

Malkin, H. M. 1993. *The Foundation of Medicine and Modern Pathology During the Nineteenth Century*. Vesalius Books.

Moore v. Regents of University of California, 51 Cal.3d 120, 793 P.2d 479 (1990).

National Commission for the Protection of Human Subjects of Biomedical and Behavioral Research. 1979. *The Belmont Report: Ethical Principles and Guidelines for the Protection of Human Subjects of Research*.

Notice of Proposed Rulemaking: Federal Policy for the Protection of Human Subjects. 2015. *Federal Register* 80: 53936.

Nuremberg Code. 1949. *Trials of War Criminals before the Nuremberg Military Tribunals under Control Council Law No. 10*, volume 2. Government Printing Office.

Tomlinson, Tom. Respecting Donors to Biobank Research. 2013. *Hastings Center Report* 43 (1): 41–47.

Washington University v. Catalona, 490 F.3d 667 (8th Cir. 2007)

Wendler, David. 2013. Broad versus blanket consent for research with human biological samples. *Hastings Center Report* 43 (5): 3–4.

World Medical Association. 1964. Declaration of Helsinki. Helsinki, Finland.

World Medical Association. 2013. Declaration of Helsinki. Fortaleza, Brazil.

Selection from "Social Ethics of Medicine: Allocating Resources, Health Insurance, Transplantation, and Human Subjects Research"

Robert M. Veatch and Laura K. Guidry-Grimes

[...]

Research Involving Human Subjects

A fourth area in which bioethics inevitably becomes social is research involving human subjects (Brody, 1998; Katz, 1972; Lederer, 2009; Levine, 1988; Veatch, 1987). It is striking that a physician committed whole-heartedly to the Hippocratic ethic of doing whatever will benefit the patient is logically committed to the view that all research involving human subjects—that is, all interventions for the purpose of producing generalizable knowledge rather than for the benefit of the patient—is unethical.

Distinguishing Research and Innovative Therapy

Here it is important to distinguish between true research and what is sometimes called innovative therapy. Throughout history when a patient has had a condition that did not respond to standard treatments, physicians have felt compelled to try something that can be called innovative therapy. Through most of history, new treatments were attempted without any systematic scientific plan or intention. The goal was to try to help the patient. Risks were considered acceptable given the bleak alternatives. Medical research is a much more recent phenomenon, dating from only the nineteenth century. Its goal is not to benefit the patient, but to advance scientific knowledge. Research that involves randomization between two different treatments is ideal for isolating the critical variable being studied. It is morally justified only when researchers honestly do not know which of two treatments is preferable—when they are at or near what is called the indifference point or equipoise. In those situations, placing a patient in the randomized design cannot be to the patient's advantage compared to simply receiving the standard treatment since there is no basis at the inception of the study for believing anything other than the standard treatment is superior.

Medical research involving human subjects must meet all the ethical criteria [...]. A potential subject must give an adequately informed consent meeting the standards [...]. The subject's autonomy must be respected. If private information is collected about the subject, the rules of confidentiality grounded in the principle of fidelity must be followed. The principle of veracity must be followed as well. Hence, psychological studies built on the intentional deception of the subject have long been controversial. Based on traditional individually focused principles of beneficence and nonmaleficence, risks to the subject must be minimized. But here medical research departs from traditional clinical medicine. The obvious way to protect subjects from harm from procedures that cannot be known in advance to be beneficial to them is to avoid doing the research. If researchers have no reason in advance to believe the experimental treatment is better than the standard treatment, the subject would always be protected by simply not doing the study. This is true even more obviously in the case of research on normal, healthy subjects. If medical research is justified at all, it must be by appeal to some ethical principle other than maximizing benefit to the individual patient or subject.

Social Ethics for Research Involving Human Subjects

Social Utility

An examination of the standard guidelines for research involving human subjects will always reveal that the first, minimal condition for justifying studies on humans is that they are believed to offer hope of producing knowledge valuable to the society that cannot be obtained in any other manner. Thus, the study must be supported by the principle of social utility. Although it may justify innovative therapy, Hippocratic utility—patient-centered concern about benefits and harms—will not do to justify research. It is generalizable, scientific knowledge that is being pursued, not patient welfare. At the same time, terrible abuses of human subjects have occurred in the name of promoting social utility. We have now learned that these occurred not only in the Nazi concentration camps, but also in other societies including the United States (Moreno, 2000).

Respect for Persons

The Nuremberg Code makes clear that social utility is not the only criterion for justifying medical research involving human subjects. [...I]t gives a strong commitment to self-determination or what is now in ethical theory normally called *autonomy*. Since the time of the writing of the Nuremberg Code, the most important document summarizing the ethics of human subjects research is the Belmont Report of the U.S. National Commission for the Protection of Human Subjects of Biomedical and Behavior Research (1978). It is built on three ethical principles: beneficence (which it treats as if it were social utility—including duties to avoid harm as well as benefit), respect for persons, and justice. From *respect for persons* it builds a consent doctrine and could as well have developed commitment to confidentiality and honesty. Respect for persons in research also requires that there be a right of exit (that is, participants can leave the study freely and without fear of retribution or retaliation). The Belmont Report states that this principle is not merely a matter of respecting autonomy; it also involves protecting persons with diminished autonomy. Prisoners, for example, can be particularly vulnerable to undue influence and coercion, even with intact cognitive faculties. Extra protective measures could thus be called for whenever prisoners are included in research. For similar reasons, compensation strategies to recruit research participants have to be carefully scrutinized; the amount should not be so extravagant that would-be participants feel like they cannot freely say "no" to taking part in the study.

Justice

From the principle of justice, the Belmont Report recognizes a duty to ensure fairness in recruiting subjects. No study can recruit subjects solely from wards serving low-income patients or from prisons, psychiatric hospitals, or other institutions that would produce inequity in subject selection (unless the nature of the study requires that only these subjects participate). More recently, the principle of justice has been understood to require adequate recruitment of subjects to apply the findings across racial and gender differences. Other advocates of the principle of justice have claimed that the requirements of justice must go further.

Federal guidelines for human subject research have classified some groups as *vulnerable*, which prompts researchers and reviewers to ensure additional protections are in place as needed, and there has been a general presumption against including vulnerable persons in research. These protections encompass a number of ethical concerns, including respect for persons and nonmaleficence, but they also reflect a commitment to just treatment of research participants who might be particularly susceptible to harm or unable to advocate for themselves. This protective stance has also been challenged as being *unjust* in those cases where entire groups of people, such as pregnant women, are systematically excluded from research from which they could potentially benefit (Lyerly et al., 2008).[1] It is also controversial when researchers from a wealthy country plan on conducting research in an impoverished area of the world without access to scientific or medical advancements that could result from the research. A central question is: Why are the researchers going to *this* population to carry out their research? Other countries might not have as many regulatory protections or oversight, and informed consent barriers can vary substantially. The confidentiality protections might be different for a relatively small tribe, for example, where normal deidentification methods could prove inadequate for protecting participants' identity. Intentionally or not, researchers could end up exploiting participants—that is, taking unfair advantage of participants' vulnerability (Carse & Little, 2008).

Consider the following case, where questions of *just* research design comes to the fore:

CASE 28: JUSTICE IN DESIGN OF RESEARCH

Some years ago, researchers at a major medical center wanted to test several chemotherapeutic agents for toxicity and make an initial estimate of the effectiveness of the combination of drugs. One of the agents, methotrexate, can have serious side-effects, but the protocol called for giving it in the high dose followed the next day with a dose of leucovorin, which would neutralize the methotrexate. The methotrexate would be administered every 21 days at the hospital, followed by the leucovorin for three days. The controversy was over whether the leucovorin could be prescribed for the subjects to take at home, which would pose the risk of patients accidentally or intentionally omitting a dose—a mistake that could prove fatal.

Those who favored administering the leucovorin in the hospital argued that it would be safer for the patients if they were hospitalized for three days out of every 21, while they take their medication. They pointed out it would also provide for more carefully controlled science. Researchers would maintain better control over the amount of medication and timing of its administration. They also were concerned that researchers not inadvertently be a party to a suicide by means of refusing to take the leucovorin.

On the other hand, defenders of permitting the leucovorin to be taken at home emphasized the burden of making sick patients come to the hospital for three days out of every 21 of their remaining time. Some suggested that because they were particularly sick, they had a special claim to have the research design as convenient and pleasant for them as possible. As long as they knew the risks of taking the medication at home, they should be permitted to do so or given a choice whether to come to the hospital. It seemed that the safest course was also the best science, but that advantage would come at what some subjects would take as an additional burden of an already very difficult life.[2]

If the only ethical principle guiding this study were social utility, it seems obvious which research design should be chosen. Hospitalizing the patients for three days out of every 21 ensures better control and closer monitoring of the subjects. Moreover, it seems to provide better protection for patients against the risk that they will not take the rescue agent. If the alternative is to send a professional staff person from the study to the patient's home to administer the leucovorin, hospital administration might even be cheaper. From a utilitarian perspective, hospitalization seems the clear choice.

But these are very sick patients. Asking them to spend three out of 21 of the few days they have remaining seems a considerable burden for them. Many patients might legitimately prefer to stay at home and take their leucovorin without having to be in the hospital or under the watch of the researchers. If these subjects are among the worst off—as they well might be—then those who subscribe to a needs-based theory of justice could conclude that they have a special claim to have their interests served even if doing so does not maximize social utility. Especially, if these advocates of the principle of justice also minimized concern about the risk of the patients committing suicide and held a strong commitment to self-determination, they may well conclude that the morally correct protocol was at-home administration. Although at-home administration would sacrifice social utility, it would promote the well-being of these particularly needy persons. The choice of the proper research design will depend on how we resolve the conflict between social utility and justice.

[…]

Notes

1. The revised Common Rule, the set of federal regulations that govern human subjects research in the United States, went into effect in 2018. In this revision, pregnant women are no longer listed as a vulnerable population. Vulnerability is instead described as susceptibility to coercion or undue influence.
2. The case is based on Veatch (1979).

References

Brody, Baruch. *The Ethics of Biomedical Research: An International Perspective.* New York: Oxford University Press, 1998.

Carse, Alisa L., and Margaret Olivia Little. "Exploitation and the Enterprise of Medical Research." In *Exploitation and Developing Countries: The Ethics of Clinical Research*, ed. Jennifer Hawkins and Ezekiel J. Emanuel. Princeton, NJ: Princeton University Press, 2008, pp. 206–245.

Katz, Jay. *Experimentation with Human Beings.* New York: Russell Sage Foundation, 1972.

Lederer, Susan E. "The Ethics of Experimenting on Human Subjects." In *The Cambridge World History of Medical Ethics*, ed. Robert B. Baker and Laurence B. McCullough. New York: Cambridge University Press, 2009, pp. 558–565.

Levine, Robert J. *Ethics and Regulation of Clinical Research*, 2nd ed. New Haven, CT: Yale University Press, 1988.

Lyerly, Anne Drapkin, Margaret Olivia Little, and Ruth Faden. "The Second Wave: Toward Responsible Inclusion of Pregnant Women in Research." *International Journal of Feminist Approaches to Bioethics* 1, No. 2 (2008): 5–22.

Moreno, Jonathan D. *Undue Risk: Secret State Experiments on Humans.* New York: W. H. Freeman and Company, 2000.

National Commission for the Protection of Human Subjects of Biomedical and Behavioral Research. *The Belmont Report: Ethical Principles and Guidelines for the Protection of Human Subjects of Research.* Washington, DC: U.S. Government Printing Office, 1978.

Price, David, ed. *Organ and Tissue Transplantation.* Aldershot, Hampshire and Burlington, VT: Ashgate, 2006.

Veatch, Robert M. *The Patient as Partner: A Theory of Human-Experimentation Ethics.* Bloomington, IN: Indiana University Press, 1987.

Zenios, Stefanos A., E. Steve Woodle, and Lainie Friedman Ross. "Primum Non Nocere: Avoiding Harm to Vulnerable Wait List Candidates in an Indirect Kidney Exchange." *Transplantation* 72, No. 4 (2001): 648–654.

Review Questions

Directions: Refer to your readings to help respond to the questions and prompts below.

1. *The Immortal Life of Henrietta Lacks* (2010) by Rebecca Skloot tells the complicated story of HeLa cells, the immortal cell line taken from the body of Henrietta Lacks. Physicians and researchers profited immeasurably from this cell line, which is still used in labs worldwide. Do a bit of research about this story. How does it compare to other human research cases? Does it matter if the instances involve one person or thousands? Considering the millions of dollars made from her cells, does justice play a more significant role?

2. Consider the vulnerable persons in the world, such as those in third world countries, children, the incapacitated, or the imprisoned. Why were so many of these marginalized groups targeted for human research? Should reparations be made to them or their lineage? If so, who should pay?

3. With the onset of many new diseases, very ill patients are often asked to participate in research studies. Should special considerations be given to them, considering the severity of their illness and the presumably shorter life or quality of life? Would you consider participating in a research study if you were unfortunately ill? Why or why not? What moral principles would affect your decision?

References

Greenberg v. Miami Children's Hospital Research Institute, 208 F. Supp. 2d 918 (N.D. Ill. 2002)
Moore v. Regents of University of California, 51 Cal.3d 120, 271 Cal. Rptr. 146, 793 P.2d 479 (Cal. 1990)
Skloot, R. (2010). The immortal life of Henrietta Lacks. Crown.

Chapter 6

Genetic Considerations

Introduction to the Chapter

Direct-to-consumer DNA databases such as 23andMe and AncestryDNA search for genetic genealogy matches. People purchase packages, delving into the curiosity of their origins. However, these services have taken lineage to a fascinating forensic level.

Forensic genetic genealogy compares millions of DNA markers with a suspect's DNA sample. Family trees can be built by analyzing these DNA markers, comparing results against genetic genealogy databases, and finding people who share matching or similar DNA patterns. Investigators can build a family tree of a suspect's second, third, or potentially even fourth cousins, thus eventually determining the suspect's identity. However, privacy, consent, and notice to consumers that law enforcement may use these service sites complicate the landscape.

The laws about the application of this technology are evolving. The Food and Drug Administration (FDA), the Centers for Medicare and Medicaid Services (CMS), and the Federal Trade Commission (FTC) are three federal agencies that regulate genetic testing. Tests are critiqued via analytical validity, clinical validity, and clinical utility via the National Library of Medicine's Genetics Home Reference. The Genetic Information Nondiscrimination Act of 2008 (GINA) is a federal antidiscrimination statute prohibiting employment discrimination based on genetic information. The regulation of the direct-to-consumer DNA databases is uncertain, leaving it mostly up to the private sector.

This has solved many cold cases, most notably the Golden State Killer. In 2018, Joseph James DeAngelo Jr., a former police officer, was captured after committing 13 murders, 51 rapes, and 120 burglaries across California between 1974 and 1986. Three separate crime sprees in three separate parts of the state remained unsolved for over 20 years until genetic genealogists were able to use a DNA sample and construct a family tree that led them, literally, to DeAngelo's doorstep.

The Netflix documentary *Our Father* tells the story of Dr. Donald Cline, an Indiana fertility specialist who inseminated patients without their knowledge or consent with his sperm. To date, 94 children have been discovered, yet Dr. Cline did not have to answer in court because there was no law against his actions at the time. Alternatively, the documentary *Filling in the Blanks* tells the story of Jon Baime, whose DNA test kit showed he was the product of a sperm donation his parents had kept hidden but also resulted in joyous discoveries of siblings and family.

When applying moral theories and principles to genetic considerations:

- Utilitarians would likely support testing/therapy if it benefits society because people should have information about their risks. Still, the information should not be used against them. Prenatal testing, gene therapy, and positive eugenics would also be acceptable if suffering were eased.
- Kantian ethics would accept the use of embryonic stem cells from any source if it benefits society. Positive eugenics would also be viewed in this manner, and thus, genetic testing would be fair if no one was discriminated against or harmed.
- Roman Catholic theorists would disapprove of prenatal testing because selective abortion violates an embryo's right to life.
- Natural law theorists would agree with this but support somatic gene line therapy because it could have therapeutic outcomes that help human life.

Learning Outcomes

After reading this chapter, students will:

1. Define and integrate key terms into discussion, writing, assignments, and prompts.
2. Analyze relevant case law and statutes to predict future trends.
3. Integrate moral theories and principles into corresponding points to consider that extend from including genetic genealogy DNA databases such as 23andMe, forensic genetic genealogy, the Human Genome Project, designer babies, wrongful handicaps, embryonic versus stem cell use, screening for disability, limiting access to certain testing, genetic enhancement, germ line gene therapy, eugenics, a child's right to an open future, morality of having children with known risks/disabilities (having deaf children), and respect for embryos.

Key Terms

The following key terms will be introduced and used in this chapter.

- **Chromosome:** a collection of DNA wound together within a cell. Organisms can have varying numbers of chromosomes, but humans generally have 23 pairs of chromosomes, equating to 46.
- **Eugenics:** a pseudoscience movement that looks to improve the human genome by excluding "unfit" characteristics or disabilities from reproducing.
- **Gene:** a section of an individual's DNA that codes for a specific protein that manifests in ways that may result in disease.
- **Gene Therapy:** explores ways to treat disease by using an individual's genome by removing or replacing genes.
- **Genetic Discrimination:** denial of employment, insurance, or other means because of a person's

genome.

- **Genetic Testing:** analyzes a person's genetic information, usually to look for disease, irregularities, or mutations.
- **Genome:** the entirety of a living organism's genetic information, from single genes to each pair of chromosomes.

Introduction to the Readings

The readings that follow focus on a few facets of genetic considerations.

"Human Control of Life: Genetics and Modifying Human Nature," by Robert M. Veatch and Laura K. Guidry-Grimes, focuses on genetic counseling, aspiring to the ideal of being "nondirective" and not trying to show their feelings and ideas to clients. This permits clients to be independent. Direct-to-consumer genetic testing, broad consent, and genetic databases are described.

"Taking the Race Out of Human Genetics: Engaging a Century-Long Debate about the Role of Race in Science," by Michael Yudell, Dorothy Roberts, Rob DeSalle, and Sarah Tishkoff, addresses the convoluted aspects of racial research and inequality. Taxonomy or ancestry, phylogenetic methods or classifications, populations or cultures: how do we use race as a tool instead of a classification?

"Managing Patient Information," by Gary Seay and Susana Nuccetelli, explores the Human Genome Project, genetic pseudo-knowledge, and nondirective genetic counseling. The right to genetic ignorance is analyzed as a liberty in a democratic society to remain unaware of their offspring or genetics.

Selection from "Human Control of Life: Genetics and Modifying Human Nature"

Robert Veatch and Laura K. Guidry-Grimes

Robert M. Veatch and Laura K. Guidry-Grimes, Selection from "Human Control of Life: Genetics and Modifying Human Nature," *The Basics of Bioethics*, pp. 202–205, 212–215. Copyright © 2020 by Taylor & Francis Group. Reprinted with permission.

[...]

Dilemmas for Counselors

Genetic counselors and others who discuss options with prospective parents professionally, such as clergy and physicians, also face moral choices in the context of genetic counseling. A basic question for them is how they should interact with their clients. Many now take the position that they should be "nondirective"; that is, they should not attempt to transmit their own moral views to their clients. Instead, they maintain, they should provide them with scientific, social, and psychological information and leave the evaluative choices up to the client. These genetic counselors are aware of [...] how difficult and subjective it is to determine what counts as a good outcome. They give priority to client autonomy, interpreted as maximizing patient control and free choice, encouraging clients to make their own value judgments.

However, this value-neutral position is increasingly being called into question. Contemporary philosophy of science now suggests that value neutrality is impossible, that counselor values will inevitably seep into the information they transmit, and that deciding which information is important enough to provide will necessarily require some value judgments on the counselor's part. Moreover, some evaluations seem to pose such clear-cut choices that many

107

would consider it unethical to fail to voice an opinion about them. For example, parents can now decide to abort a fetus simply because it is not the preferred sex. They can also choose to carry a pregnancy to term in spite of the expectation that the child would experience nothing more than severe pain and imminent death. Many genetic counselors consider either of these sorts of choices so obviously wrong that it would call for more directive counseling. Deciding whether to be directive in these situations will depend not only on one's views about abortion and autonomy, but also about how one feels about intervening into life's most mysterious and important processes.

This suggests a serious problem for the future of genetic counseling. If counselors believe that some choices are so obviously immoral that they cannot in good conscience refrain from conveying their disapproval, how can prospective parents and others being counseled protect themselves from undue and distorting influences from their counselors? The moral beliefs of genetic counselors should not determine decisions made by counselees who are regarded as autonomous and self-determining moral agents, and yet these people cannot make their decisions without the assistance of such counseling. Genetic counselors grapple with this tension in their training and practice (see Berliner, 2015; Davis, 2001; Stern, 2012).

One approach would be to strive to have counselors try to be as fair and unbiased as possible while still realizing that their communications will inevitably contain value perspectives. Genetic counselors could make a concerted effort to keep their value judgments to themselves, but any aspect of giving information, interpreting results, and answering questions could reveal their personal values. If those being counseled understood that all counseling conveys value judgments, and if counselors openly expressed their points of view, clients could ideally pick their counselors and the institutions in which the counselors work on the basis of compatibility of values as well as availability of factual information. For important decisions they might seek out other counselors for second opinions, intentionally pursuing counselors whose values are quite different. For example, a traditional Catholic might first get counseling from someone from within that religion's tradition and then seek out a counselor whose values and beliefs are different. Even if these counselors try to present "just the facts" and present them as fairly as possible, in at least some cases, the messages are bound to be quite different.

Direct-to-Consumer Genetic Testing

The twenty-first century has witnessed the advent of relatively affordable genetic testing kits, delivered directly to consumers' doors. Whole genome sequencing can be requested from private companies, although a cheaper alternative is to pay for genotyping services that reveal genetic markers for certain diseases and other traits such as bald-headedness. 23andMe, one of the most successful companies in this business, offers testing for ancestry (including a relative finder tool), limited information regarding genetic health risks (e.g., three targeted mutations in BRCA1/2 common to those of Ashkenazi Jewish ancestry and the APOE e-4 gene variant for Alzheimer's), wellness (e.g., lactose intolerance and the ability to fall into a deep sleep), carrier status for select conditions that could be passed to children (e.g., cystic fibrosis and sickle cell anemia), and other traits (e.g., sensitivity to bitter taste and fear of heights). Consumers swab their cheek or send saliva to the company that analyzes the data and sends a report. Consumers are encouraged to get their family members to sign up for testing as well, and many of these companies regularly request consent for additional research.

There are many attractions to direct-to-consumer genetic testing. The service is available to anyone with the money and an address, including minors with consenting parents/guardians. There is no "gate-keeper" to genetic information—an interested person does not need a referral from a physician, for example (Hercher, 2015). The genetic information might seem more private, since it is not part of their medical record, which can also reduce the chances of unwanted disclosures and discrimination. These tests offer a way for people to learn more about themselves, plan for the future to some extent, and be proactive in their health-care. It also provides a way for people to connect with others, such as through the ancestry service and relative locator. 23andMe facilitates the creation of Genetics Clubs for college students, so their customers can discuss their tests and learn more about genetic discoveries together. Genetic tests can also be a form of self-expression, as seen in the advertised art prints based on a person's unique genetic traits.

Direct-to-consumer genetic tests have also raised significant concerns. Sensitive genetic information is being communicated through a company's report instead of through a trained healthcare professional, which means that customers will not have the benefit of expert conversations, educational support, or psychosocial assistance at the time they learn their results. 23andMe has a number of accessible educational videos and information available online for free, but these cannot replace the one-on-one attention that a genetic counselor can provide. Genetics is a complex science, and detailed reports are generally ineffective in facilitating informed decision-making. Consumers can easily overestimate and underestimate their genetic risks, which can lead to misguided health behavior changes. The results can also be misleading for people who are not experts in genetics; for example, the BRCA 1/2 testing is limited to mutations common in the Ashkenazi Jewish population but not helpful to others, which could lead to a false sense of security (and possibly skipped mammograms or other preventive care). While some companies are careful about offering any advice based on the results, other companies are more directive in their recommendations. For example, several emerging companies promise to give customers detailed advice on meal planning, vitamins, dental care, athletic training, and stress management—all based on genetic tests. These recommendations vary in their reliability and scientific validity, especially as they become more specific and detailed. The recommendations also necessarily require value judgments. For example, a recommendation about meal planning requires value judgments about how enjoyable certain foods are and how important it is to avoid undesirable consequences of eating the wrong foods. Nonetheless, these companies are offering a seductive service by increasing customers' sense of control over their health. Moreover, the pervasiveness of genetic essentialism compounds these concerns, since consumers might be mistakenly expecting more complete answers about their identity, their behavior, and their future than these tests could possibly reveal.

These companies can also sell people's genetic information, which raises concerns about consumers' privacy and control over their information. In 2018, 23andMe announced that the pharmaceutical company GlaxoSmithKline invested hundreds of millions of dollars in 23andMe, which allows GlaxoSmithKline to access customers' genetic data as part of their pharmaceutical research. Any breaches of identifiable data expose not only the customer but potentially their family members as well. Although 23andMe asks for consent before adding a customer's genetic results to their research database, this broad consent does not detail what the research could involve. Bioethicist Art Caplan has also made the point that the pharmaceutical research will be skewed toward the demographic that can take advantage of genetic testing services, which is likely not representative of the general population, which means that any pharmaceutical advancements might not be relevant to significant portions of the population.

We have seen other ways in which direct-to-consumer genetic testing has unforeseen consequences. People can discover shocking secrets related to their family tree, which can change their sense of family and ethnic heritage. For example, people could learn that they are genetically unrelated to their parents or that they do not have the genetic ties to a particular culture that they thought they did.

Genetic databases can be used for a variety of purposes that are not explicitly covered by a consent form, terms of agreement, or legal regulation. In 2018, law enforcement officials used an open-source genetic database to find matches to a genetic sample from the Golden State Killer. The serial rapist and murderer had eluded law enforcement for decades because his DNA was not in any criminal database, but the open-source genetic database found a match that led to a positive identification of a family member and subsequent arrest. This case led to public discussions about the expected and unexpected uses of genetic data and whether expanded access (e.g., to law enforcement) could be beneficial to the public good.

[...]

Bibliography

Berliner, Janice L., ed. *Ethical Dilemmas in Genetics and Genetic Counseling: Principles through Case Scenarios*. New York: Oxford University Press, 2015.

Davis, Dena S. *Genetic Dilemmas: Reproductive Technologies, Parental Choices and Children's Futures*. New York: Routledge, 2001.

Hercher, Laura. "Is That a Threat or a Promise? Direct-to-Consumer Marketing of Genetic Testing." In *Ethical Dilemmas in Genetics and Genetic Counseling: Principles through Case Scenarios*, ed. Janice L. Berliner. New York: Oxford University Press, 2015, pp. 135–158.

Stern, Alexandra Minna. *Telling Genes: The Story of Genetic Counseling in America*. Baltimore, MD: Johns Hopkins University Press, 2012.

Taking Race Out of Human Genetics: Engaging a Century-Long Debate about the Role of Race in Science

Michael Yudell, Dorothy Roberts, Rob DeSalle, and Sarah Tishkoff

In the wake of the sequencing of the human genome in the early 2000s, genome pioneers and social scientists alike called for an end to the use of race as a variable in genetic research.[1,2]

Unfortunately, by some measures, the use of race as a biological category has increased in the postgenomic age.[3] Although inconsistent definition and use has been a chief problem with the race concept, it has historically been used as a taxonomic categorization based on common hereditary traits (such as skin color) to elucidate the relationship between our ancestry and our genes. We believe the use of biological concepts of race in human genetic research—so disputed and so mired in confusion—is problematic at best and harmful at worst. It is time for biologists to find a better way.

Racial research has a long and controversial history. At the turn of the twentieth century, sociologist and civil rights leader W. E. B. Du Bois was the first to synthesize natural and social

1. F. Collins. *Nat. Genet.* 2004;36(suppl.):S13.
2. M. W. Foster, R. R. Sharp. *Nat. Rev. Genet.* 2004;5:790.
3. P. A. Chow-White, S. E. Green Jr. *Int. J. Commun.* 2013;7:556.

scientific research to conclude that the concept of race was not a scientific category. Contrary to the then-dominant view, Du Bois maintained that health disparities between blacks and whites stemmed from social, not biological, inequality.[4] Evolutionary geneticist Theodosius Dobzhansky, whose work helped reimagine the race concept in the 1930s at the outset of the evolutionary synthesis, wrestled with many of the same problems modern biologists face when studying human populations—for example, how to define and sample populations and genes.[5] For much of his career, Dobzhansky brushed aside criticism of the race concept, arguing that the problem with race was not its scientific use but its nonscientific misuse. Over time, he grew disillusioned, concerned that scientific study of human diversity had "floundered in confusion and misunderstanding."[6] His transformation from defender to detractor of the race concept in biology still resonates.

Today, scientists continue to draw wildly different conclusions on the utility of the race concept in biological research. Some have argued that relevant genetic information can be seen at the racial level[7] and that race is the best proxy we have for examining human genetic diversity.[8,9] Others have concluded that race is neither a relevant nor accurate way to understand or map human genetic diversity.[10,11] Still others have argued that race-based predictions in clinical settings, because of the heterogeneous nature of racial groups, are of questionable use,[12] particularly as the prevalence of admixture increases across populations.

Several meetings and journal articles have called attention to a host of issues, which include (i) a proposed shift to "focus on racism (i.e., social relations) rather than race (i.e., supposed innate biologic predisposition) in the interpretation of racial/ethnic 'effects'"[13]; (ii) a failure of scientists to distinguish between self-identified racial categories and assigned or assumed racial categories[14]; and (iii) concern over "the haphazard use and reporting of racial/ethnic variables in genetic research"[15] and a need to justify use of racial categories relative to the research questions asked and methods used.[6] Several academic journals have taken up this last concern and, with mixed success, have issued guidelines for use of race in research they publish.[16] Despite these concerns, there have been no systematic attempts to address these issues and the situation has worsened with the rise of large-scale genetic surveys that use race as a tool to stratify these data.[17]

It is important to distinguish ancestry from a taxonomic notion such as race. Ancestry is a process-based

4. W. E. B. Du Bois. *The Health and Physique of the Negro American*. Publ. no. 11. Atlanta, GA: Atlanta Univ. Publications; 1906.

5. T. Dobzhansky. *Genetics and the Origin of Species*. New York: Columbia University Press; 1937.

6. M. Yudell. *Race Unmasked: Biology and Race in the 20th Century*. New York: Columbia University Press; 2014.

7. E. G. Burchard et al. *N. Engl. J. Med.* 2003;348:1170.

8. Y. Banda et al. *Genetics*. 2015;200:1285.

9. C. E. Powe et al. *N. Engl. J. Med.* 2013;369:1991.

10. D. Roberts. *Fatal Invention: How Science, Politics, and Big Business Re-Create Race in the Twenty-First Century*. New York: The New Press; 2012.

11. D. Serre, S. Pääbo. *Genome Res.* 2004;14:1679.

12. P. C. Ng, Q. Zhao, S. Levy, R. L. Strausberg, J. C. Venter. *Clin. Pharmacol. Ther.* 2008;84:306.

13. J. S. Kaufman, R. S. Cooper. *Am. J. Epidemiol.* 2001;154:291.

14. T. R. Rebbeck, P. Sankar. *Cancer Epidemiol. Prev.* 2005;14:2467.

15. L. M. Hunt, M. S. Megyesi. *J. Med. Ethics*. 2008;34:495.

16. A. Smart, R. Tutton, P. Martin, G. T. H. Ellison, R. Ashcroft. *Soc. Stud. Sci.* 2008;38:407.

17. G. Lettre et al. *PLoS Genet.* 2011;7:e1001300.

concept, a statement about an individual's relationship to other individuals in their genealogical history; thus, it is a very personal understanding of one's genomic heritage. Race, on the other hand, is a pattern-based concept that has led scientists and laypersons alike to draw conclusions about hierarchical organization of humans, which connect an individual to a larger, preconceived geographically circumscribed or socially constructed group.

Unlike earlier disagreements concerning race and biology, today's discussions generally lack clear ideological and political antipodes of "racist" and "nonracist." Most contemporary discussions about race among scientists concern examination of population-level differences between groups, with the goal of understanding human evolutionary history, characterizing the frequency of traits within and between populations, and using an individual's self-identified ancestry to identify genetic risk factors of disease and to help determine the best course of medical treatments.[6]

If this is what race in contemporary scientific and medical practice is about, then why should we be concerned? One reason is that phylogenetic and population genetic methods do not support a priori classifications of race, as expected for an interbreeding species like *Homo sapiens*.[11,][18] As a result, racial assumptions are not the biological guideposts some believe them to be, as commonly defined racial groups are genetically heterogeneous and lack clear-cut genetic boundaries.[10,11] For example, hemoglobinopathies can be misdiagnosed because of the identification of sickle-cell as a "Black" disease and thalassemia as a "Mediterranean" disease.[10] Cystic fibrosis is underdiagnosed in populations of African ancestry, because it is thought of as a "White" disease.[19] Popular misinterpretations of the use of race in genetics also continue to fuel racist beliefs, so much so that, in 2014, a group of leading human population geneticists publicly refuted claims about the genetic basis of social differences between races.[20] Finally, the use of the race concept in genetics, an issue that has vexed natural and social scientists for more than a century, will not be obviated by new technologies. Although the low cost of next-generation sequencing has facilitated efforts to sequence hundreds of thousands of individuals, adding whole-genome sequences does not negate the fact that racial classifications do not make sense in terms of genetics.

More than five decades after Dobzhansky called on biologists to develop better methods for investigating human genetic diversity,[21] biology remains stuck in a paradox that reflects Dobzhanky's own struggle with the race concept: both believing race to be a tool to elucidate human genetic diversity and believing that race is a poorly defined marker of that diversity and an imprecise proxy for the relation between ancestry and genetics. In an attempt to resolve this paradox and to improve study of human genetic diversity, we propose the following.

Scientific journals and professional societies should encourage use of terms like "ancestry" or "population" to describe human groupings in genetic studies and should require authors to clearly define how they are using such variables. It is preferable to refer to geographic ancestry, culture, socioeconomic status, and language, among other variables, depending on the questions being addressed, to untangle the complicated

18. K. Bremer, H. E. Wanntorp. *Syst. Biol.* 1979;28:624.
19. C. Stewart, M. S. Pepper. *Genet. Med.* 2015.
20. G. Coop et al. *New York Times*. August 8, 2014:BR6.
21. T. Dobzhansky. *Mankind Evolving: The Evolution of the Human Species.* New Haven, CT: Yale University Press; 1962.

relationship between humans, their evolutionary history, and their health. Some have shown that substituting such terms for race changes nothing if the underlying racial thinking stays the same.[22,23] But language matters, and the scientific language of race has a considerable influence on how the public (which includes scientists) understands human diversity.[24] We are not the first to call for change on this subject. But, to date, calls to rationalize the use of concepts in the study of human genetic diversity, particularly race, have been implemented only in a piecemeal and inconsistent fashion, which perpetuates ambiguity of the concept and makes sustained change unfeasible.[16] Having journals rationalize the use of classificatory terminology in studying human genetic diversity would force scientists to clarify their use and would allow researchers to understand and interpret data across studies. It would help avoid confusing, inconsistent, and contradictory usage of such terms.

Phasing out racial terminology in biological sciences would send an important message to scientists and the public alike: Historical racial categories that are treated as natural and infused with notions of superiority and inferiority have no place in biology. We acknowledge that using race as a political or social category to study racism and its biological effects, although fraught with challenges, remains necessary. Such research is important to understand how structural inequities and discrimination produce health disparities in socioculturally defined groups.

The U.S. National Academies of Sciences, Engineering, and Medicine should convene a panel of experts from biological sciences, social sciences, and humanities to recommend ways for research into human biological diversity to move past the use of race as a tool for classification in both laboratory and clinical research. Such an effort would bring stakeholders together for a simple goal: to improve the scientific study of human difference and commonality. The committee would be charged with examining current and historical usage of the race concept and ways current and future technology may improve the study of human genetic diversity; thus, they could take up Dobzhansky's challenge that "the problem that now faces the science of man [sic] is how to devise better methods for further observations that will give more meaningful results."[21] Regardless of where one stands on this issue, this is an opportunity to strengthen research by thinking more carefully about human genetic diversity.

22. S. M. Fullerton, J. H. Yu, J. Crouch, K. Fryer-Edwards, W. Burke. *Hum. Genet.* 2010;127:563.
23. L. Braun, E. Hammonds. *Soc. Sci. Med.* 2008;67:1580.
24. W. C. Byrd, M. W. Hughey. *Ann. Am. Acad. Pol. Soc. Sci.* 2015;661:1.

Selection from "Managing Patient Information"

Gary Seay and Susana Nuccetelli

[...]

Genetic Information

The rapidly changing field of genetics has made innumerable contributions to medical science, including improvements in our understanding of the pathogenesis of health conditions affecting individuals, families, and sometimes groups. Genetic testing now allows patients to acquire information about the risks for them and their future children of developing certain diseases. But that information is not always welcome. After folk-singer Woody Guthrie died of Huntington's disease in 1967, his son Arlo reportedly decided to remain ignorant about whether he carried the gene himself. (He later learned that he didn't.) Genomic testing can also reveal one's risk of developing Alzheimer's disease by showing which variant of a gene one has inherited. Variant E4 triples that risk. Some eminent researchers have chosen not to learn which variant they carry, among them James Watson, who shared the Nobel Prize with Francis Crick for discovering the structure of DNA, and Harvard psychologist Stephen Pinker (see his 2009). In some circumstances, health professionals may need to know about the genetic makeup of some patients, and this can conflict with the patient's right to remain ignorant.

Before discussing which circumstances these might be, we need some clarity about genetic knowledge, as well as about two misunderstandings of human genetics. One of these reduces all factors for health, disability, and disease to genetics; the other to environment.

Genetic Knowledge

Developments in genetics have helped to advance scientific knowledge of health, disability, and disease, while also debunking some misconceptions about their genetic components. Early in this century, genomics, the specialization within genetics and molecular biotechnology devoted to the study of the structure and function of genes, mapped the partial or entire DNA sequences of many species. A species' genome is the sum total of the DNA sequence of an organism of that species, and thus contains all the information necessary to construct and maintain the organism. A turning point in genomics occurred with the Human Genome Project's (HGP) mapping of the entire sequence of human DNA. The HGP, completed in 2003 by two groups of researchers working independently (one with private funds, the other with funds from the US government), revealed that the human genome contains approximately 20,000 genes, depending on how 'gene' is defined. By making all their findings available to researchers and clinicians in public databases, the HGP opened the way, at least in principle, to the identification of each gene and its function in health, disability, and disease. Before the HGP, genomics had yielded limited results, usually restricted to knowledge of congenital disorders with a clearly inherited basis, such as sickle cell anemia, Tay-Sachs disease, and cystic fibrosis. With the HGP's basic genome map, researchers saw an opportunity to advance knowledge of the genes and genetic variations and mutations that may contribute to the onset of other conditions, such as certain cancers, cardiovascular disease, and some neurodegenerative disorders. For example, in 2005 the US National Institutes of Health launched The Cancer Genome Atlas (TCGA), a multi-center research study of the genomic alterations in the tumors of ovarian, brain, and lung cancers. By 2015, TCGA was well underway and had expanded its scope to explore the genetic bases of other cancers.

Parallel to these developments were advances in genetic testing. Clinicians now hope this area of genetics will soon contribute to better treatment outcomes by revealing the most efficient therapies for a disease on the basis of gene changes. Current methods of genetic testing, however, do not always mean better therapy outcomes. In addition, the tests are commonly provided as part of a genetic consultation and involve some expense. Less costly are home-based, genetic test kits marketed online. But this option leaves users without proper direction for understanding the possible benefits and limitations of the tests, and so for making autonomous decisions about using them. Furthermore, without intervention by a genetic counselor, users are in the dark about how to interpret results. Worse, it leaves them vulnerable to the misconception we'll consider next.

Genetic Pseudo-Knowledge

Consider cancer again. Genetics in part accounts for having an increased risk of developing certain cancers, the resilience of some of them, and typical mutations in some cancer cells. As a result, screening and diagnostic tests can now be used for early detection of high risks of, for example, breast cancer in women who have inherited the gene mutations BRCA1 and BRCA2. When these mutations are present, health care professionals present the woman with possible measures aimed at prevention. Among the most radical options are elective mastectomy and hysterectomy, which involve bodily mutilation, possible psychological harms, and the risks of surgery. Each may have profound consequences for the woman's future quality of life. An informed decision then requires weighing all of these with the information provided by genetic counselors about the actual risk of having inherited the mutation.

In any case, it is important to keep in mind that, with conditions such as hereditary breast cancer, a woman's mutation for this disease, passed on to her by female ancestors, is only *one* of the factors that may contribute to the development of the disease. Other factors include age, having given birth, the full history of recent breast cancers in the family, changes in breast tissue, and even ethnic background. More generally, a weighing of all contributing factors should be done for any hereditary health condition that depends not only on genetics but also on diet, life-style, environment, etc. This requires rejecting the following pseudo-scientific assumption:

Genetic Determinism
All risk factors for hereditary diseases or disorders reduce to genetic makeup.

There is no science supporting this widespread misconception, which may have harmful consequences, such as the stigmatization of individuals at risk of genetically related illness, a common attitude justifiably feared by people at risk of genetic disease. The medical and research communities, together with the rest of society, should strive to educate the public by exposing genetic determinism as little more than superstition.

Likewise, there is no science supporting a contrary misconception holding that,

Environmental Determinism
All risk factors for allegedly hereditary diseases or disorders reduce to environment.

This generalization is false, as is shown by what is now known about exclusively hereditary conditions such as Huntington's—a rare, progressive, neurodegenerative disease that is invariably fatal if the sufferer lives long enough. Huntington's genetic basis, long suspected in medicine, was established beyond doubt in 1983 with the mapping of the disease's gene to human chromosome 4p. Later genomic discoveries paved the way for new studies ultimately designed to develop some therapies for Huntington's. At present, it can be neither cured nor prevented. When a patient has inherited this disease, some brain nerve cells will eventually stop working, usually in adulthood. This will severely impair intellectual abilities, movements, and emotions. With the onset of symptoms, a person has a life expectancy of 10 to 20 more years. The gene for the disease is present at birth, inherited from a parent. Anyone carrying it will eventually develop symptoms. Since an affected parent has a 50/50 chance of passing Huntington's on to offspring regardless of sex, patients with a family history of it can learn by genetic testing whether they carry the gene. If they do and wish to have children, a genetic counselor is equipped to explain their options.

Thus neither genetic determinism nor environmental determinism can capture the facts about the complex relations between hereditary disease, genetics, and the environment. Only genetics can, by developing branches concerned with studying those relations scientifically. Consider behavioral genetics, the branch devoted to studying behavioral variations in animals, including humans, resulting from complex interactions between genes and environment. It tells us that it is neither true that our mind is a 'blank slate' at birth (so that conditioning is the only cause of mental illness), nor that mental disorders are encoded in our genes in a straightforward way (so that it can be known by genetics whether a person will develop, for example, bipolar disorder). The truth lies in complex interactions between genes and the environment that are not yet fully understood.

Nondirective Genetic Counseling

According to the current standard, genetic counseling for patients at risk of genetic conditions should be nondirective or value-neutral. It should outline all the options available to the person, who is called the 'client,' without letting the counselor's values influence the final decision. Consider the case of a patient with a family history of Huntington's disease, who is pre-symptomatic but plans to have a child. Health care providers will likely recommend elective testing to see whether the patient has the gene that causes the disease. The patient will then be better informed to make a reproductive decision. Yet the predominant view in the genetic community is that the counselor should avoid offering any reproductive advice but instead simply present all options for having a healthy, genetically related baby. These include undergoing prenatal testing and therapeutic abortion to prevent the birth of a carrier child, or in-vitro fertilization in combination with preimplantation genetic testing to select embryos for implantation that do not carry the gene.

Note that, given nondirective genetic counseling, the client-genetic counselor relationship stands out as very different from that of the patient-medical team relationship. For one thing, only in the latter relationship is professional advice part of what patients generally expect. There is consensus among genetic counsellors that nondirective counseling is necessary to promote autonomous decisionmaking by clients. But some bioethicists question whether being nondirective is the right standard for genetic counseling. They also question an assumption that underlies that standard: that clients have a right to remain ignorant about important facts of their own genetic makeups.

Is There a Right to Genetic Ignorance?

Some persons at risk of genetic health conditions may wish to remain ignorant of their actual risk. This is particularly troublesome when genetic information about them can be of benefit to their relatives or to a larger group. For example, a woman from a family with a history of breast cancer may understandably say, "I don't want to be tested," or "I don't want to know the results of my test." That is, she refuses to participate in a so-called linkage study, or she might participate but prefer not to learn its results. Similarly, a person from an ethnic group with a high gene-disease association may refuse participation in a population genetics study. Or an individual with a family history for a genetic disease who is planning to become a parent may refuse genetic diagnosis, invoking a right to genetic ignorance (recall the *Arlo Guthrie* case). Clinicians and genetic counselors generally think that

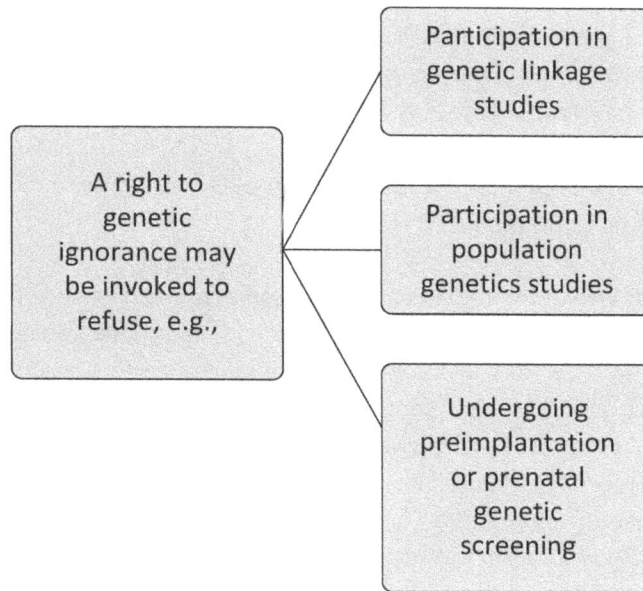

Figure 6.3.1   Genetic Information and the Right to Genetic Ignorance

1. Clients have a right to genetic ignorance, and
2. Given the standard of nondirective genetic counseling, the counselor should abstain from attempting to persuade clients to undergo genetic screening when they competently refuse to do so.

In (1), the right to ignorance is regarded as a liberty that autonomous individuals have in a democratic society. Like other such liberties, this right can be limited only when its exercise may harm others (Takala, 1999). (2) rests on the consensus that nondirective genetic testing is required by respect for patient autonomy. The greatest challenge to (1) and (2) comes from cases where a patient at risk of carrying a gene with a strong disease association plans to raise a family, for an exercise of the patient's right to ignorance in those circumstances may result in the birth of a child at high risk of developing the parent's genetic condition. Refusals to participate in linkage studies fall short of posing a similar challenge, since genetic counselors can attempt to persuade those who claim the right to ignorance for participating in the study by promising that they will not disclose the genetic testing's results to them. Reasonable persuasion need not conflict with nondirective counseling.

Let's then look closely at the prospective-parent scenario. As we have seen, although genetic determinism is false, genetic factors are a component of many diseases and disabilities. Of course, one may have a natural aversion to learning that one is at risk of developing a genetic disease sometime in life. This is a difficult burden to bear and may weigh as a dark foreboding on one's enjoyment of life. But, arguably, if one is at risk of a disorder like Huntington's and plans to have a child, one has a duty to know in advance whether one carries the gene. If one has that duty, then there is no right to genetic ignorance in this scenario. The Children's Welfare Argument now charges

1. If there is a right to genetic ignorance, then it is morally permissible for prospective parents at high risk of genetic disease to refuse genetic testing.
2. Such refusals put their future child at risk of harm.
3. Harming a child is morally impermissible.
4. Therefore, it is morally impermissible for those prospective parents to refuse genetic testing.
5. Therefore, there is no right to genetic ignorance.

This argument assumes that knowingly causing a child to come into existence with a severe hereditary condition amounts to harming it. But if the prospective parents had undergone genetic testing, that child might not have been born at all, so defenders of the right to ignorance find this argument unpersuasive. Among them is Tuija Takala (1999: 292), who further contends that parents have that right because "knowledge cannot be forced upon people." Having a duty to know one's genetic endowment would be contrary to human psychology, and therefore practically impossible.

The Argument from Genetic Ignorance's Foolishness is a rejoinder to this defense of the right to ignorance. It holds that prospective parents at risk of genetic conditions who claim that right will be left with the worse options of undergoing either

- In-vitro fertilization combined with preimplantation genetic diagnosis for the selective transfer of healthy embryos to the uterus, or
- Prenatal screening combined with selective abortion if the fetus carries the gene.

Each of these options is more costly, stressful, and morally problematic than preconception genetic testing of the parents. Therefore, it is foolish to refuse such testing. But this appeal offers only a prudential reason against what's regarded as a moral right to ignorance. If intended as a moral argument, it assumes that parents willing to accept the genetic lottery are doing something morally wrong. This is not evident unless it can be shown that they are harming their future children.

But given what we may call 'Kantian Patient Autonomy,' prospective parents at risk of genetic disease might lack the right to genetic ignorance, and genetic counselors could accordingly be morally obliged to direct them into having genetic testing. Recall that for a Kantian, the duty of respect for patients' autonomy derives from respecting them as persons, which requires the promotion of their autonomous decisionmaking. Rosamond Rhodes (1998) argues that such prospective parents lack the right to genetic ignorance, because without genetic testing their decision to procreate lacks sufficient knowledge and fails therefore to be autonomous. Her objection aims not only at the alleged right to genetic ignorance, but also at the prevalent, nondirective standard of genetic counseling. In the scenario we are considering, however, common morality suggests that any waiver of the prospective parents' right to genetic ignorance would rest more on parental responsibilities to the future child than on the counselor's Kantian obligation of respect for their autonomy.

As a result, Rhodes' objection fails to undermine a *universal* right to genetic ignorance, which unlike an *absolute* right would have exceptions. Furthermore, as we saw above, many question generalizations about harm to future children [...]. Putting that aside, the objection fails to undermine the genetic counselors' view that they have a prima facie duty (i.e., other things being equal) to provide nondirective counseling in light of the need to avoid some moral wrongs of the early 20th-century, 'eugenic' programs. [...]

[...]

Additional References

Pinker, S., "My Genome, My Self," *The New York Times* 1/7/2009. Available online at http://www.nytimes.com/2009/01/11/magazine/11Genome-t.html.

Rhodes, R., "Genetic Links, Family Ties, and Social Bonds: Rights and Responsibilities in the Face of Genetic Knowledge," *Journal of Medicine and Philosophy* 23.1, 1998: 10–30.

Takala, T., "The Right to Genetic Ignorance Confirmed," *Bioethics* 13.3/4, 1999: 288–93.

Review Questions

Directions: Refer to your readings to help answer the questions and prompts below.

1. Check out the Genome Statute and Legislation website. https://www.genome.gov/about-genomics/policy-issues/Genome-Statute-Legislation-Database4.

   Research the laws in your state about genetic testing and genetic therapy. You should be able to locate your state's laws as well as any federal laws. Please summarize any applicable federal or state law.

2. Ask your school's reference librarian for help using a legal search engine. Perform a legal search for any new genetic case law in your state. Do any laws address testing, therapy, discrimination, or genetic genealogy? Do you think that the current laws are fair to criminals whose DNA may be able to be tracked via familial DNA on these large databases?
3. The *"Human Control of Life"* article introduces counselors as "nondirective." Is this the ideal or is it possible to remain neutral in inpatient delivery? Why or why not?
4. Are the three notable stories discussed in the introduction examples of the good use of genetic technology? If you had to write five societal rules about using genetic technology, how would you incorporate autonomy, beneficence, justice, and other principles into your rules?

Chapter 7

Reproductive Technology

Introduction to the Chapter

Complex philosophical ideas arise when reproductive technology meets a moral compass. Questions of personhood, autonomy, access to care, and legislative rights permeate through conception, freezing, termination, rights to use, and surrogate decision-making.

One of the first questions to address is how many presumptive parents can be involved in creating offspring. Should a gestational carrier have the right to terminate a process that could lead to a functioning human being? Does the fetus have the right to stay inside the gestational carrier until it is viable outside the womb? Is the fetus a person at all? This topic has been debated ethically and legally, with much of this stemming from the U.S. Constitution not defining personhood.

The freezing of embryos is an extension of these questions. Are embryos considered persons because of their potential for independent life? What rights do the birth parents have over these embryos? The donor's parents? The gestational carrier? What if the gestational carrier is also the egg donor?

The laws on reproductive technology and surrogacy vary widely from state to state. No current federal law addresses the pressing issues, especially since the *Dobbs v. Jackson Women's Health Organization* (2022) decision overturning Roe v. Wade (1973).

The Centers for Disease Control and Prevention (CDC) follows the related issues; more up-to-date information can be found on its website.

Two historic cases address surrogate rights and the rights to use frozen embryos.

The first well-known case is Baby M. William and Elizabeth Stern hired Mary Beth Whitehead to carry a baby. Whitehead was the gestational carrier and egg donor. Baby M was conceived via artificial insemination with William Stern's sperm. Whitehead had agreed to surrender the baby but changed her mind after Baby M was born. The court granted Whitehead visitation rights to Baby M using the child's legal standard's best interests. This is the standard used for custodial issues in most jurisdictions. This case resulted in the first time a surrogate mother was granted visitation rights. Current surrogacy laws vary by state, with states such as Michigan and Louisiana prohibiting all paid surrogacy and states such as California and Maine allowing compensation for surrogate mothers.

A later case dealt with frozen embryos and a high-profile celebrity divorce. Sofía Vergara's ex-boyfriend, Nick Loeb, sued for possession of the in vitro embryos they created when they were in a relationship. During the fertilization process, they signed documents stating that both parties had to agree for the embryos to be unfrozen and developed. Loeb wanted to implant the embryos into another woman. Vergara sued to stop this. The court held that each party must have the written consent of the other if they want to create a child.

When applying moral theories and principles to reproductive technology:

- Utilitarians believe it is okay to use technology if the benefits outweigh the harms. Surrogacy and cloning are also acceptable unless there is a general disregard for human welfare and human life.
- Kantian ethicists would argue that in vitro fertilization (IVF), surrogacy, and cloning are unacceptable if they treat children as a goal, not as people to be loved and respected.

Learning Outcomes

After reading this chapter, students will:

1. Define and integrate key terms into discussion, writing, assignments, and prompts.
2. Analyze relevant case law and statutes related to reproductive technology.
3. Integrate moral theories and principles into corresponding points to consider that extend from reproductive technology, including unused embryos, freezing gametes, and embryos; wrongful life cases; obligations to actual and potential children; dignity of procreation; presumptive procreative liberty; gamete donation; exploiting motherhood or empowering motherhood; and baby selling.

Key Terms

The following key terms will be introduced and used in this chapter.

- **Artificial Insemination:** the process through which sperm is introduced to an egg without sexual intercourse. Sperm is inserted into the vagina via a catheter.
- **Assisted Reproductive Technology (ART):** a broad term capturing many forms of fertility treatment to achieve a viable pregnancy.
- **Cloning:** the growth of a new organism that is genetically identical to another.
- **Embryo Culture:** the embryo is placed in an artificial nutrient medium following artificial insemination. This allows for controlled embryo growth in the first few days of development.
- **Gamete Intrafallopian Transfer:** the introduction of eggs and sperm into the fallopian tubes.
- **In vitro fertilization (IVF):** when a sperm is introduced to an egg outside the human body. This can typically take place in a lab, where a medical professional takes sperm and injects it into the egg.
- **Surrogacy:** the process in which a woman becomes pregnant for another person or couple.
- **Zygote Intrafallopian Transfer:** introducing a fused egg and sperm, a zygote, into the fallopian tubes. The egg and sperm are fused in a lab.

Introduction to the Readings

The readings that follow focus on a few facets of reproductive technology.

"New Reproductive Technologies," by Gary Seay and Susana Nuccetelli, describes the history and more straightforward cases of IVF therapy. The Nonidentity Problem is explained as prenatal nonexistence versus postnatal nonexistence, or to have never been born versus death. Complex cases of IVF are also described and analyzed.

"Ethical Issues in Reproduction," by Linda Farber Post and Jeffrey Blustein, highlights ethical issues of surrogacy and gestational carriers, including the legal landscape, maternal-fetal issues, and genetic testing/screening.

Selection from "New Reproductive Technologies"

Gary Seay and Susana Nuccetelli

[...]

The Simple Cases

The Simple Case of In-Vitro Fertilization

Some Facts about IVF

Louise Brown, the first IVF or 'test-tube' baby, was born in the UK in 1978 under the care of Cambridge doctors Patrick Steptoe and Robert Edwards. By the mid 1980s, the UK parliament made attempts at regulating this increasingly popular reproductive intervention. It commissioned the Warnock report in 1984, issued the Code of Practice of the Human Fertilisation and Embryology Act in 1990, and founded the Human Fertilisation and Embryology Authority. Updated periodically, the Code of Practice aims at protecting the welfare of future children by mandatory screening of prospective parents. By contrast with the UK, where IVF treatments are regulated and often funded by the NHS, in the US they are unregulated by the federal government and mostly privately financed, at prices driven by the market. This thriving, multimillion-dollar business that accounted for the birth of about 1 million infants since its beginning in the 1980s to 2011 is run by fertility clinics (Calandrillo and Deliganis, 2015). Two associations of physicians who provide IVF (and therefore have a stake in it) act as self-regulators.

As shown by the data in Box 7.1.2, IVF is still a costly, invasive, and ineffective way to pro-create compared to unassisted conception. Since it is mostly privately financed, the relatively small pool of patients who can afford this reproductive assistance chooses providers on the basis of their success rates. Providers compete and are under pressure to boost success rates, which explains familiar failures in their obligations of informed consent and beneficence—such as the transfering of excessive numbers of embryos to the uterus in the hope that at least one will implant and develop to term.

BOX 7.1.2 IVF'S ORIGINS AND OTHER FACTS

- IVF technology originated in veterinary science, producing the first live birth (of a rabbit) in 1959. Since the 1870s, its goal was using lower-quality animals as gestational carriers for IVF embryos of higher-quality animals. Experimentation on humans began in the 1970s.
- In the 1980s, IVF ceased to require surgical retrieval of eggs by laparoscopy. Owing to advances in ultrasound technology, eggs could now be retrieved with a cheaper, quicker, and less invasive procedure: transvaginal ultrasound aspiration. It thus left surgical competitors behind.
- In the US, Elizabeth Jordan Carr became the first US 'test-tube baby' in 1981.
- By the 2000s, after almost 25 years of use, IVF's success rate of live births per initiated cycle was approximately 28% (Greif and Merz, 2007).
- In 2011, 451 fertility clinics reported 163,039 IVF cycles resulting in 47,818 live births and 61,610 neonates. In 2013, although the numbers were slightly higher (467 clinics, 54,323 live births, and 163,209 neonates), IVF continued to account for only 1.5% of all births.
- By 2015, IVF was still funded mostly out-of-pocket. A round cost between $10,000 and $20,000.[1]

The Simple Case

IVF treatments were originally intended for what Singer and Wells (1983) called 'the simple case': married, infertile, heterosexual couples wishing to have genetically related children. However 'simple' those cases may be, they raise a host of moral questions, given people's rights to procreative freedom, the wellbeing of offspring thus conceived, and justice for all involved. Moreover, fertilization outside the woman's body without sexual intercourse by itself represents a radical change in human reproduction that conflicts with the

1. CDC. "ART Success Rates: Latest Data, 2013," http://www.cdc.gov/art/artdata/index.html.

tenets of some cultural and religious traditions. And there are unresolved matters about ownership of the IVF embryos and their moral standing that bear on what is morally permissible to do with them. Other NRTs present related moral questions that we consider in due course. Next, we examine the Problem of Multiples facing both IVF technology and fertility therapy.

[...]

The Nonidentity Problem

The main reply to the Welfare Objection is the so-called Nonidentity Problem. This is the problem that without some NRTs, many children with impairments, whose lives are worth living, would not have existed. When 'harm' is defined as a setback to someone's interests, and a given NRT used to assist a child's conception has caused her an impairment compatible with her having a life worth living, questions arise as to whether the NRT has harmed her. For how could it be in the child's interests not to exist? Clearly, without the NRT that child would not exist, and existing albeit with impairments seems better than not existing at all.

We revisit the Nonindentity Problem [...]. For now, note that not all think it arises. Cynthia Cohen (1996), for example, charges that it confuses prenatal nonexistence (i.e., to have never been born) with postnatal nonexistence (death). Prenatal nonexistence is neither bad nor good, since unlike nonexistence after death, it involves no loss of life's goods.

In our view, the perspective of the impaired offspring matters in evaluating the strengths of the Welfare Objecion and its Nonidentity-Problem reply. Clearly, some severely disabled people do regard their own existence as a harm even when their lives seem above the line of not-worth-living. This is shown by *wrongful-life* actions where plaintiffs typically contend that enabling them to come into existence was an injury. The alleged tort is that a child was born *at all* into a life of suffering which the plaintiff perceives as worse than prenatal nonexistence. Wrongful-life actions are generally dismissed because the courts wish to avoid speculative assessments concerning whether a plaintiff's nonexistence would have been better than her existence with a very low quality of life. Yet if vulnerability to harm is considered from the subjective perspective, then since from the plaintiffs' perspective, causing their existence was a harm, then their cases support the Welfare Objection: impaired children with worth-living lives can sometimes be harmed by being brought into existence.

BOX 7.1.3 NEW REPRODUCTIVE TECHNOLOGIES (NRTS)

Assisted Reproductive Technologies (ARTs):
any NRT that handles both eggs and sperm outside the body.[2]

- In-vitro fertilization (IVF)—fertilization by combination of eggs with sperm in a lab

2. CDC. "What is Assisted Reproductive Technology?" 11/14/2014. http://www.cdc.gov/art/whatis.html.

dish.
- Intracytoplasmic sperm injection (ICSI)—injection of a single sperm into an egg to induce fertilization.

Not in the ART category, as defined above:

- Egg donation—the use of a woman's eggs for creating embryos on behalf of one or more intended parents.
- Surrogacy—arrangement whereby a woman carries a pregnancy on behalf of the intended parents. A surrogate may be the egg donor.
- Intrauterine insemination—assisted placement of semen into a woman's uterus for fertilization.
- Fertility therapy—fertility drug regime to induce egg production.

The Complex Cases

Since the 1980s, social changes and the development of new reproductive interventions have made NRTs available to same sex couples, single reproducers, and postmenopausal (beyond reproductive age) women. Human reproduction assisted by NRTs may involve IVF combined with the use of donated sperm or eggs and surrogate mothers. The expansion of NRTs added ethical challenges to the Problem of Multiples discussed above.

Egg Donation, Gestational Surrogacy, and Postmenopausal Motherhood

IVF was initially used to treat a common type of female infertility that is caused by a fallopian tube blockage preventing the passage of the egg to the sperm or the fertilized egg to the womb. But when the woman's eggs cause infertility, becoming pregnant may then require 'donor' eggs—which in fact are commonly bought by the intended (called also 'social' or 'rearing') parents from an egg-broker agency. When there is no sperm provided by a male partner that could fertilize the woman's eggs, fertilization requires donor sperm, usually bought from a sperm bank. In a scenario where the intended parents use donor eggs and sperm, they are not genetically related to the embryos thus created.

Advances in procreative medicine have also made possible the transfer of IVF embryos into the womb of a surrogate. If implantation occurs, she is the gestational carrier of the embryos. If she provides her own eggs and the pregnancy produces at least one live birth, she is the infant's genetic mother. Surrogates that are only gestational carriers are usually sought when the intended mother is fertile but carrying a pregnancy to term poses a risk to her health. If she uses the services of a surrogate to conceive, she is the infant's intended and genetic mother, but the surrogate is its gestational mother (see Box 7.1.4).

BOX 7.1.4 THREE TYPES OF MOTHERHOOD

- The intended, rearing, or social mother—the woman on behalf of whom the child is conceived.
- The gestational carrier or host—the birth mother.
- The genetic or biological mother—the egg donor.

This and other reproductive scenarios now familiar require procreative interventions that not long ago belonged to the domain of fiction. They include egg donation and gestational surrogacy, reproductive interventions whereby, respectively,

- A woman's eggs are fertilized *in utero* or *in vitro* to create embryos for someone else.
- A so-called gestational mother provides her uterus for carrying a pregnancy to term on behalf of another woman, the intended mother.

With these interventions, the pool of people who may benefit from IVF technology has extended far beyond the simple case to include gay, lesbian, and transgender couples, single individuals, and postmenopausal women. These include women in their 50s and above who wish to bear a child but can no longer use their eggs for fertilization. Traditionally, they were thought to have passed gestational age. Yet today a postmenopausal woman's uterus can be 'primed' with hormone drugs before transferring to her womb for implantation IVF embryos resulting from donor eggs. Since the 1990s, the number of postmenopausal pregnancies has been on the rise, owing in part to advances in cryopreservation of eggs. Although there is some controversy about their chances for successful live births, the evidence suggests that postmenopausal pregnancies do increase the risks of prematurity and low birthweight. They also produce more Caesarean deliveries and maternal complications, such as gestational diabetes and pregnancy-induced hypertension.

For these reasons, countries such as the Netherlands forbid the use of commercial donor eggs after 45. In the US, fertility clinics have an age limit of 50 to 55 and often deny postmenopausal women IVF treatments because of their lower success rates. As discussed below, major moral worries about postmenopausal pregnancies concern the conflict between women's reproductive freedom and beneficence to future children, and the fact that restrictions of NRTs on the basis of age might involve discrimination (Parks, 1999). India allows IVF for any woman who can afford it privately, a policy that became world news when Rajo Devi, 70, gave birth to a girl in 2008. Rajo died eighteen months later from complications of the Caesarean delivery.

Some Facts about Egg Donors and Gestational Carriers

Egg donors are a scarce resource highly prized. Mature eggs and oocytes (the female reproductive cell in the process of developing into an egg) are sought not only for IVF treatments but also for stem cell research. Although some women donate the eggs remaining from IVF rounds altruistically to other women who need them, such donations are insufficient to satisfy current demand. The scarcity of donor eggs in the market is unsurprising in light of the time investment and health risks facing donors. Initially, the woman must pass a battery of mental and physical screenings. Then, she must undergo hormone therapy designed to produce superovulation, and finally, a surgical extraction of the eggs. The risks of complications from the hormone therapy include ovarian hyperstimulation syndrome, which affects 6% of the women and produces varying degrees of discomfort and harm. Heart failure, though rare, has been reported (Gruen, 2007). According to the American Society for Reproductive Medicine (2000), without any such complications, an egg donor spends about 56 hours in the clinic per cycle. Because of demand, egg sale is now a booming market, entirely unregulated in the US. Egg-broker agencies report that potential buyers often look for features in donors that suggest racial and social discrimination (blond hair, blue eyes, tall stature, high SAT scores).

Gestational carriers are also scarce, given the burdens, including physical and mental risks, involved in carrying a pregnancy to term. This market, increasingly global, shows a trend toward 'surrogacy tourism' whereby individuals and couples from the West turn to clinics in the developing world to find surrogates for their embryos at a fee lower than what they would pay in their own countries. Reportedly, the dire financial situations in developing countries sometimes force surrogates into abusive agreements.

Moral Controversies

The above arguments about fertility therapy and the simple case of IVF also bear on the morality of other NRTs. While beneficence and reproductive freedom support their permissibility, the ways they alter human reproduction, handle early life, or treat the women involved argue against it. Here we look closely at the reasons on both sides of this controversy, with an eye to identifying those that pass scrutiny and may be held by reasonable people.

The Benefits Argument

According to this utilitarian argument, NRTs in both simple and complex cases are morally justified since their benefits outweigh their burdens overall. The benefits at issue concern people who, due to involuntary infertility or other reason, are not able to have children with-out such assistance. Once this argument's implicit *principle of utility* is accepted, its soundness depends on evidence about the total balance of NRTs' benefits over burdens for all involved, including prospective parents and children and society as a whole. To defend it, utilitarians may invoke IVF's improved record of success since 1978 and contend that, for other NRTs too, their benefits over time will outweigh costs or risks to women and offspring (Singer and Wells, 1983). In their view, what is needed is not a moral ban but proper regulation to avoid abuses. Yet the Benefits Argument is inconclusive, given the difficulty of calculating benefits over burdens in the long run. For example, should the welfare of orphans be considered? What about credible predictions of future overpopulation and food scarcity?

The Procreative Freedom Appeal

Access to NRTs would also be a moral right given John Robertson's libertarian appeal to procreative freedom (1994: 24). It runs,

1. Decisions that are essential to one's identity and dignity, and to the meaning of one's life, enjoy presumptive primacy.
2. Procreative decisions are so essential.
3. Therefore, procreative decisions enjoy presumptive primacy.

Procreative freedom enjoys "presumptive primacy" because people should be at liberty to make self-regarding reproductive decisions unless there are stronger reasons to the contrary. Harm to others would count as such an overriding reason. Given the presumptive primacy of procreative freedom, individuals requesting NRTs to have children may morally do so provided the technologies will not harm others. While for libertarians procreative decisions can be limited only by harm to others, for utilitarians the limits are set by overall balance of benefits versus burdens. [... S]ome utilitarians also value procreative freedom, defined as a persons' right to decide for themselves whether to have or not to have children. By contrast with libertarians who value it in itself, utilitarians endorse J. S. Mill's view that individual liberty (including procreative freedom) is valuable as a means to happiness.

Whether consequentialist or libertarian, the Procreative Freedom Appeal is consistent with opposition to NRTs with substantial burdens. Neither interpretation entails an obligation of health care providers to honor requests for such reproductive assistance. But does procreative freedom have presumptive primacy? Dissenters include conservative moral theologians who consistently oppose not only NRTs but also contraception and abortion, and feminist theorists who regard NRTs as contrary to women's interests and dignity. We take up their objections in turn, beginning by conservative objections that assume:

1. Any NRT that assists in achieving conception through the conjugal or sexual act of husband and wife is morally permissible.
2. Any NRT that replaces that way of conception is morally forbidden.

The Unnaturalness Objection

Following the Sacred Congregation for the Doctrine of the Faith's *Donum Vitae* (*The Gift of Life*, 1987), conservative Catholic theologians such as John Haas (1998) and William May (2003) object to any NRTs that are incompatible with human conception according to God's plans for nature. In their view, given (1) and (2) above, Nadya Suleman's IVF was forbidden while the McCaugheys' fertility treatment was permissible, even though both NRTs face the Problem of Multiples. Note that condition (2) is quite demanding, since it makes most NRTs morally forbidden. What should infertile people wishing to have children do? May's advice is to accept their fate and adopt if they are a married couple.

The *Unnaturalness Objection* to most NRTs draws a bright moral line between natural and unnatural NRTs, based on whether they accord with God's plans for nature or do not. But the existence of such a bright line is questionable, even within religiously grounded bioethics. For surely IVF is too expensive and risky to become a standard way to conceive. But 'nonstandard' does not mean 'unnatural' in the sense of 'contrary to God's plan for nature.' In fact, the meaning of 'natural' as invoked in this objection is unclear. It cannot be *what occurs in nature*, without technical or institutional intervention, since *natural* reproduction does not require the married couple's sexual act. Suppose it is *whatever avoids interference with God's plans for nature*. Then, as we saw in connection with the Sanctity-of-Life doctrine in Chapter 11, that definition presupposes some religious beliefs. As a result, it is likely to be divisive since it involves beliefs that not everyone shares about God and His role in the natural order. But put this problem aside. Why think that some NRTs do interfere with God's plans? It cannot be because they are innovations. Otherwise *all* scientific progress would interfere with God's plan and be impermissible.

On the other hand, suppose the traditional family manifests the natural order because departures from it can result in psychological harm to the children. In surrogacy, for example, learning that a social parent is not also a genetic parent might be psychologically stressful for the offspring. If the parents keep secrecy instead, that might erode trust within the family. Under this interpretation, the Unnaturalness Objection becomes a version of the Children's Welfare argument discussed above, which has the advantage of recognizing the Problem of Multiples equally facing scenarios such as *the McCaugheys* and *Nadya Suleman*.

Embryo Mishandling

The objection to NRTs from Embryo Mishandling targets specifically IVF treatments because they typically:

1. Produce far more embryos than would be safe to transfer to the uterus.
2. Let some embryos die (those at high risk of carrying impairments).
3. Store the remaining embryos (in the US, indefinitely), to be used later by the intended parents or donated to other parents or researchers.

The objector finds all three morally problematic. IVF treatments involve (1) because creating one embryo at a time would undermine their already low success rates. But (1) leads to the problem of what to do with any remaining embryos. And how defective must a gene be to morally justify (2)? (3) requires freezing the embryos, which thereby enter a state of suspended animation (neither alive nor dead). Is that morally permissible? Transferring *all* embryos to the uterus would avoid (2) and (3), and is sometimes defended on religious grounds. But it risks pregnancies with multiples.

IVF enthusiasts reply that, at only a 30% survival chance, most embryos are naturally aborted in *un*assisted conception, and "no one suggests that natural conception is, for this reason, wrong, or that it *would* be wrong if the probability of surviving were significantly lower than it is" (McMahan, 2007: 34). Yet unlike IVF, these natural abortions may be justified by *double effect*, as an unintended side effect of procreation.

A different line of reply first acknowledges that the objection would succeed if embryos had the moral standing of, for example, *paradigm persons* like us. It would then be impermissible to create more embryos than needed, destroy some, and freeze others indefinitely. But having paradigm-person standing requires certain psychological capacities that a 5- or 6-day-old embryo clearly lacks. This perhaps explains why society has generally accepted IVF. In any event, the controversy now turns on the moral standing of embryos, an unsettled issue discussed in Chapter 10.

The Feminist Critique

Some feminists charge that NRTs

1. Undermine women's dignity and power.

2. Exploit and commodify women.

Either (1) or (2) is a reason for the moral wrongness of NRTs. Support for (1) comes from the fact that these technologies, developed and administered mostly by men, give them control over conception and birth. Men have a history of negligence in the medical care of women. Traditionally, assistance in natural conception was in the hands of midwives, but in the 19th century male doctors gradually replaced midwives. Childbirth became a 'medical condition' to be treated in hospitals, with a consequent rise in mortality and morbidity rates, owing in part to iatrogenic infections acquired in the new setting (Warren, 1988). In addition to endangering women in this way, the medicalization of pregnancy and childbirth disempowered women by giving control of their childbearing to men. NRTs extended this disempowering to the fertility clinic. Furthermore, IVF's origin in veterinary science adds injury to women's dignity.

In addition, reproduction is now a high-profit business where women's eggs, wombs, and indeed reproductive capacity are traded as commodities. The fertility clinic encourages pregnancies 'by catalog order,' whereby mostly white, well-off prospective parents select donors and surrogates according to values that reflect societal biases. Egg donation and surrogacy are particularly problematic because they commonly involve selling eggs and renting wombs respectively, thus introducing market values into pregnancy and childbirth. Since women are treated as mere means, NRTs undermine their interests as a group (Anderson, 1990; Raymond, 1989).

Moreover, women seeking NRTs cannot give informed consent because of the pressure of

Natalism
The prejudice that people should procreate

Natalism, a widespread societal expectation that is particularly demanding for women, conflicts with procreative freedom. If natalism determines decisions to seek assistance with NRT, consent to it lacks voluntariness. Consent is undermined too when women enter surrogacy and egg donation contracts because of their financial needs. Donors and surrogates may also suffer exploitaition by more wealthy individuals seeking their services.

But not all agree with this feminist critique. To Mary Anne Warren (1988), NRTs can boost women's reproductive autonomy, thus advancing their interests. But it should be regulated to require, for example, quotas of female medical professionals at fertility clinics. To Lori Gruen (2007), commodification is compatible with respect for women's dignity. By contrast with buying organs, payment for eggs (or wombs) compares to compensation for athletic or scientific achievements—neither of which undermines the athletes' or scientists' dignity. Furthermore, whether surrogates and egg donors are exploited depends on proper regulation of contracts and the meaning of 'exploitation.' As ordinarily understood, 'explotation' need not apply to these women any more than to wage laborers. This reply, however, ignores the difficulties in regulating a trade marked by global economic inequality between the surrogates and egg donors in the developing world and the more wealthy Western individuals seeking their services.

[...]

Additional References

Anderson, E., "Is Women's Labor a Commodity?" *Philosophy & Public Affairs* 19.1, 1990: 71–92.

Calandrillo, S. P. and C. V. Deliganis, "In Vitro Fertilization and the Law: How Legal and Regulatory Neglect Compromised a Medical Breakthrough," *Arizona Law Review* 57.2, 2015: 311–42.

Cohen, C., "Give Me Children or I Shall Die!" *Hastings Center Report* 26.2, 1996: 19–27.

Greif, K. F. and Jon F. Merz, *Current Controversies in the Biological Sciences: Case Studies of Policy Challenges from New Technologies*. Cambridge: MIT Press, 2007.

Gruen, L., "Oocytes for Sale?" *Metaphilosophy* 38, 2–3, 2007: 285–308.

Haas, J. M., "Begotten Not Made: A Catholic View of Reproductive Technology," *United States Conference of Catholic Bishops*, 1998. Available online at http://www.usccb.org/issues-and-action/human-life-and-dignity/reproductive-technology/begotten-not-made-a-catholic-view-of-reproductive-technology.cfm.

McMahan, J., "Killing Embryos for Stem Cell Research," *Metaphilosophy* 38.2/3, 2007: 170–89.

May, W. E., "Begetting vs. Making Babies," in *Human Dignity and Reproductive Technology*, pp. 81–92. Lanham, Maryland: University Press of America, 2003.

Parks, J., "On the Use of IVF by Post-Menopausal Women," *Hypatia* 14.1, 1999: 77–96.

Raymond, J., "Reproductive Technologies, Radical Feminism, and Socialist Liberalism," *Journal of Reproductive and Genetic Engineering* 2.2, 1989: 133–42.

Robertson, J. A., *Children of Choice: Freedom and the New Reproductive Liberties*. Princeton: Princeton University Press, 1994.

Singer, P. and D. Wells, "In Vitro Fertilisation: The Major Issues," *Journal of Medical Ethics* 9.4, 1983: 192–5.

Warren, M. A., "IVF and Women's Interests: An Analysis of Feminist Concerns," *Bioethics* 2.1, 1988: 37–57.

Selection from "Ethical Issues in Reproduction"

Linda Farber Post and Jeffrey Blustein

[...]

Surrogacy and Gestational Carriers

Baby M was born to Mary Beth Whitehead, conceived with her own oocytes and sperm from William Stern, the husband of Elizabeth Stern, the intended child-rearing parents. The Sterns and Ms. Whitehead entered into a contract according to which Ms. Whitehead would relinquish her parental rights in favor of Mrs. Stern upon the birth of the child. However, she decided to keep the child, so the Sterns sued to be recognized as the child's legal parents. In an important decision by the New Jersey Superior Court, the contract was ruled invalid according to public policy, Ms. Whitehead was recognized as the child's legal mother, and family court was ordered to determine whether Ms. Whitehead, as mother, and Mr. Stern, as father, should have legal custody of the child, according to the traditional "best interests of the child standard." Ultimately, Mr. Stern was awarded custody of Baby M, Mrs. Stern legally adopted her, and Ms. Whitehead was given visitation rights.

Are there legitimate reasons to prevent people from becoming or hiring surrogates or gestational carriers? Is the practice so dangerous, risky, or contrary to the public good that it should be banned? What ethical values are promoted by permitting the practice?

First a word of clarification. A *gestational carrier* is a woman who carries to term a child conceived with the gametes of a couple to whom she relinquishes the child upon delivery. As such, she is a parent only in the gestational, rather than the genetic, sense. A *surrogate*, by contrast, provides her own oocytes, fertilized with sperm from the man in another couple to whom she relinquishes the child upon delivery. Her contribution is both gestational and genetic. Mary Beth Whitehead was a surrogate.

Surrogacy is far more accepted in the United States than in most countries; however, there is no national consensus on how to deal with it even here. As of 2014, 17 states have laws permitting surrogacy, some with restrictions; 6 states prohibit enforcement of surrogacy contracts; and in 21 states, there is neither a law nor a published case regarding surrogacy (Lewin 2014).

The ethical arguments that support allowing women to serve as surrogates or gestational carriers are rooted in several values: autonomy, beneficence, and reproductive freedom. According to the autonomy argument, women should be free to make decisions about their own bodies, including waiving their parental rights before the birth of children they help conceive or carry. The beneficence argument emphasizes the good that surrogates and gestational carriers can provide couples whose desire for a child with all or part of their genetic makeup has been impeded by the woman's infertility or inability to carry a pregnancy to term. Surrogacy also enhances a woman's reproductive freedom to have a child to whom she is genetically related.

Despite these benefits, there are many reasons to be cautious about surrogacy and gestational carrier arrangements. Relinquishing a child whom one has carried to term can be emotionally traumatic for the carrier, as happened in the Baby M case. An additional concern is that women may agree to serve as surrogates because they see this as an opportunity to improve their economic situations and, as a consequence, the inducement of financial compensation is potentially exploitative. According to 2008 statistics, the mean compensation for a gestational carrier in the United States was approximately $20,000 (Brezina and Zhao 2012). Financial compensation for the delivery of a baby also seems to be tantamount to baby selling, which is both immoral and against public policy. These concerns, while worth taking seriously, can be addressed and should not justify complete prohibition of the practice of surrogacy. The concern about the emotional cost to the surrogate or carrier can be addressed to some extent by pre-conception counseling and requiring a waiting period before the surrogate relinquishes her parental rights; exploitation is less a worry if financial compensation is limited to payment for medical expenses associated with or incurred during pregnancy and, because this remuneration is not for the delivery or relinquishing of a baby, it is less likely to be considered baby selling (Steinbock 1988). Nevertheless, because surrogate and gestational carrier arrangements depart so radically from traditional social norms of parenthood, the risks of objectification of women remain (Tieu 2009; Atwood 1986).

Disputes involving surrogates and gestational carriers may sometimes come to the attention of your ethics committee and you may be able to provide useful guidance to the parties involved. The questions that loom large in an ethics analysis are whether the surrogate or gestational carrier is being exploited; what emotional and psychological risks she faces; what the impact of surrogacy on the families of both the surrogate and the receiving parents is likely to be; and whether permitting surrogacy constitutes endorsement of buying and selling babies.

Termination of Pregnancy

Marlise Munoz, 33 years old, was 14 weeks pregnant when her husband found her unconscious on the bathroom floor. Rushed to the hospital, she was found to have suffered a massive pulmonary embolism and was declared brain dead. The declaration was final and uncontested by either the hospital or the patient's family. Mr. Munoz requested that, in keeping with what his wife would have wanted, the mechanical supports maintaining her organ function be removed. The hospital responded that state law required that she be kept on "life support"[1] until sufficient fetal development created a reasonable chance of survival upon delivery, which would require that Mrs. Munoz's body remain connected to mechanical supports for at least an additional eight weeks. Mr. Munoz insisted that, in deference to his late wife's wishes, the hospital disconnect the mechanical supports immediately, even though he recognized that this would prevent the development and delivery of a viable baby (Ecker 2014).

What rights do the mother and the father have in this situation? What steps should be taken to preserve and support the fetus? Should the mother's body be kept on mechanical supports solely to allow a live birth?

The Legal Landscape

Roe v. Wade is the landmark 1973 U.S. Supreme Court case that legalized abortion and one of the most important legal cases in the field of bioethics. The ruling established that a right to privacy under the due process clause of the Fourteenth Amendment of the U.S. Constitution extends to a woman's decision to terminate a pregnancy. But the ruling also balanced this right against two legitimate state interests in its regulation: protecting the potentiality of life and protecting the health of the mother. The Court held that these interests become stronger over the course of the pregnancy, and it employed a trimester approach to make this more precise: for the first two trimesters, the decision is substantially that of the pregnant woman and her doctor; in the third trimester, the state may proscribe abortion in order to protect nascent human life. In a 1992 case, *Planned Parenthood of Southern Pennsylvania v. Casey*, the Court reaffirmed the essential holding of *Roe* but replaced the trimester framework with the "undue burden" standard intended to protect women from unreasonable barriers to abortion. A fuller discussion of the leading Supreme Court cases related to abortion appears in part IV.

Roe v. Wade prompted a national debate on the legality and morality of abortion that continues to this day, dividing the country into so-called pro-choice and pro-life camps. Whether *Roe v. Wade* will survive the many challenges to its constitutionality remains uncertain in light of the conservative bent of the current Supreme Court.

Meanwhile, however, a number of states, as well as the U.S. Congress, have attempted to make the exercise of the right to abortion more difficult for pregnant women. As of this writing, Oklahoma, Texas, and North Carolina require that pregnant women undergo and view fetal ultrasounds, along with graphic explanations of their significance (Rocha 2012). In North Dakota, providers are required to provide information about the gestational age and development of the fetus, show them a fetal sonogram, and say that, if the

---

1. *Life support* in this context is misleading, since it suggests that Mrs. Munoz's life was being maintained by technological assistance, whereas, in fact, she was legally and medically dead. [...]

woman terminates the pregnancy, she will be "ending the life of a separate human being with whom [she has] an enduring relationship." In West Virginia, women considering abortion are required to undergo a vaginal sonogram, even in cases of rape. Some states require that women be told that the list of risks to the procedure includes depression, suicide, and infertility. In 2003, a Republican-controlled Congress passed the controversial Partial Birth Abortion Ban Act, which the pro-life camp defended as protecting the rights of the unborn and the pro-choice camp rejected on the ground that it constituted an unjustified infringement of the woman's right to abortion. The act was ruled constitutional by the Supreme Court in 2007 in *Gonzalez v. Carhart*. [...]

Ethical Issues

More has been written about abortion than any other bioethical issue and, despite the vast literature, it is a matter that continues to generate passionate and polarizing debate. Beginning in 1971 with the landmark article, "A Defense of Abortion," by the philosopher Judith Jarvis Thomson and continuing without interruption until today, articles and books have exhaustively explored every facet of the issue. The most general way of stating the ethical problem of abortion is by asking what makes it right or wrong to voluntarily terminate a pregnancy. This divides into two sub-questions: (1) what is the moral status of the fetus? and (2) why does a pregnant woman have the right to terminate her pregnancy? The issue of moral status is important because those who have moral status deserve the protection of moral norms, that is, principles and rules that state obligations and rights. Determining the moral status of a fetus or embryo does not settle the question of what may ethically be done to it, for moral status can come in degrees, but even beings with comparatively little moral status deserve moral consideration.

Several answers to when the embryo or fetus acquires moral status have been proposed. One suggestion is that moral status is acquired at conception, even before an embryo, technically speaking, has developed. Another is that the fetus acquires moral status when pathways develop to transfer pain signals from pain sensors to the brain, around 26 weeks or 6 months. Various other developmental milestones have been proposed as marking the advent of moral status, but these are not straightforward empirical determinations. Each suggested milestone has to be defended on moral grounds. To no one's surprise, consensus remains and likely will remain elusive.

Commonly accepted justifiable grounds for abortion, on which there is wide but not universal agreement, are rape, incest, and threat to the life of the mother. More controversial reasons include the mother's maturity, threat to the mother's psychological health, conflict with the mother's other life goals, and lack of support system and financial resources. Selective reduction, in which one or more embryos in a multiple pregnancy are aborted to enhance the likelihood that the remaining embryo(s) will thrive, is problematic because of the painful and difficult selection it requires. Selective abortion of fetuses with disabling conditions has generated particular controversy. According to the disability rights critique, prenatal diagnosis followed by abortion of fetuses with disabling conditions is morally problematic for a number of reasons: it expresses negative or discriminatory attitudes not only about the disabling traits themselves, but about those who have them; it also signals intolerance of diversity in both the family and society at large (Parens and Asch 2000), ultimately altering for the worse what it means to be a parent.

The pregnancy termination case of Marlise Munoz no doubt generates conflicting opinions among individuals depending on their views regarding the ethical permissibility of abortion and the reasons that might legitimate it. Questions to be asked when doing an ethics analysis include the following: What moral significance does the preservation of fetal life have? Is it one factor among others or is it the overriding consideration? What is the fetal prognosis if the pregnancy is maintained for another eight weeks and delivered? Would the mother want her body to be supported mechanically so that her baby could be delivered? What rights does the father have? Should the hospital attempt to override the father's decision to terminate mechanical supports? The goal of your ethics committee deliberations should be to draw attention to these various moral considerations and to try to come to some conclusions about their respective weights.

Maternal-Fetal Issues

Janet Jones was 32 weeks pregnant when clinical signs began to indicate that all was not right with her pregnancy. Fetal monitoring revealed a decrease in fetal heart rate that could indicate inadequate blood flow through the placenta. She was followed closely by her obstetrician during this time and, when the fetus's decelerations worsened, her doctor recommended delivering the baby by caesarean section before things got worse. Janet, however, refused. She did not believe her fetus was in serious difficulty and, in any case, she had spent her entire pregnancy preparing for natural childbirth and wanted to deliver her baby that way. Her obstetrician, Dr. DiSalvo, and other members of the obstetrical staff tried to convince her of the need for a C-section, but she continued to refuse and, as fetal condition worsened, they became increasingly worried. They felt a responsibility to do whatever they could to deliver her baby alive before it suffered irreversible brain damage. Finally Dr. DiSalvo warned Janet that if she continued to reject his advice, he would have no choice but to get a court order to perform a C-section over her objection. The rest of the obstetrical staff, though bothered by this threat, supported his stand.

According to *Roe v. Wade*, pregnant women in the United States have a constitutional right to terminate an unwanted pregnancy at least during the first two trimesters, which is not inconsistent with their moral obligation to do whatever is necessary to ensure the success of a desired pregnancy. Women who intend to carry their pregnancy to term are advised to take care of their own health for their sake and for the sake of their future child. But, the ethics and legality of abortion are separate matters from the moral responsibilities of women who choose to carry a pregnancy to term and deliver a child. These are obligations that pregnant women have *now* to the *child-who-will-be-born*. Thus, pregnant women are advised not to drink or smoke, not to take illicit drugs, and to avoid exposing themselves to environments that present a risk to the health of the developing fetus.

Women are also expected to agree to medical interventions, such as caesarean section, that their doctors believe are in the best interests of their to-be-born child. The important distinction between a moral and a legal obligation is that, while these intuitively obvious measures can be seen as *moral* obligations, it is a further question whether they should be translated into *legal* obligations (Post 1997). As a general matter, a woman's right to privacy and self-determination cannot be legally conditioned on the well-being of her future child, but neither should she be relieved of the moral obligations to the child she intends to bring into the world.

Yet, restrictions on a pregnant woman's right of self-determination have taken several forms. Women have been ordered by courts to undergo emergency cesarean sections; incarcerated until delivery if they have taken illegal drugs while pregnant; and punished after delivery for engaging in behaviors during pregnancy that, in the opinion of doctors and courts, endangered the fetus. These actions have been justified by states modifying their child abuse and neglect laws to define a "child" as any being from conception on, thereby expanding their *parens patriae* authority to include fetal protection. These measures depart significantly from the customary legal position that personhood within the meaning of the Fourteenth Amendment occurs when a live birth takes place. Only at that point may the state, under its protective powers, intervene on behalf of the neonate, who now has independent and legally protectable rights (Post 1997). The seriousness of these responses to alleged maternal irresponsibility, as well as their punitive, coercive, and, often, arbitrary nature, shows how much rides on others' assessments of maternal conduct and how important it is to proceed cautiously in making them.

There are reasons to be wary of such interventions. First, obstetricians, like all physicians, are not infallible. Many of their past convictions about diet, ideal weight gain, and exercise during pregnancy are now considered obsolete. Moreover, doctors may disagree with their colleagues, as well as with their patients, about what promotes maternal and fetal health. Second, even granting the soundness of the medical advice, as noted above there is a difference between a moral obligation to do or avoid doing something and an obligation that is legally enforceable. Additional arguments, over and above the existence of the moral obligation itself, are needed to justify the use of state authority to curtail a pregnant woman's autonomy and infringe on her liberty.

Especially important in relation to maternal-fetal issues, there are pragmatic as well as moral reasons not to resort to the heavy-handed strategies described above. First, punitive and coercive responses to alleged maternal misconduct threaten to drive pregnant women away from prenatal care, with potentially worse results for the future child than if non-punitive approaches were adopted. Second, there is no bright line that demarcates punishable from non-punishable conduct. If the goal is to discourage irresponsible maternal behavior, why stop at smoking, alcohol, and illicit drugs? What about failure to have regular prenatal check-ups or take prenatal vitamins? If nothing else, this slide along the continuum of undesirable behaviors is increasingly unenforceable. From the standpoint of the future child's well-being, it is generally better to treat the pregnant woman and her fetus not as two separate entities in conflict with each other, but as a single biological and social unit with common interests (Post 1997; Rothman 1986).

There are cases, however, in which a pregnant woman's right against non-consensual bodily invasion may be limited by the overwhelming likelihood of significant and preventable harm to the future child (Chervenak and McCullough 1991). The most common example is refusal of a cesarean section where the harm to the fetus from refusing the surgery is clear-cut, imminent, and potentially devastating. What makes these cases especially difficult for caregivers is that, with surgery, this almost-baby can be saved. The case of Janet Jones may be an example of this type. In some cases, court orders have been obtained to authorize the contested intervention [...].

Given the well-settled right of capable patients to refuse unwanted treatment, [...] this radical departure from legal and ethical precedent has ominous implications. It may have the counterproductive effect of discouraging pregnant women from seeking prenatal care out of fear that they might be forced to undergo unwanted surgery for the sake of their fetus. [...R]efusal of recommended treatment does not, by itself, confirm decisional incapacity. Yet, in these situations, surgery over the patient's objection is sometimes justified by the presumption of incapacity, the logic being that no rational woman would deliberately put her future child at risk. As "A Defense of Abortion" so brilliantly illustrates, it is hard to imagine analogous actions of non-consensual bodily invasion, especially for the sake of another, occurring in any other patient population or clinical setting. An obstetric case that raises the possibility of court-ordered caesarian section might come to the attention of your ethics committee and your careful analysis of the relevant rights, interests, and obligations will be crucial to its resolution.

Prenatal/Newborn Genetic Testing and Genomic Newborn Screening

The increasing ability to detect actual or potential medical problems enables parents and care professionals to intervene in ways that have profound health benefits. To appreciate the ethical implications, however, it is necessary to distinguish two types of assessment: *testing* and *screening*. Prenatal genetic testing is offered to individual prospective parents, generally on the basis of family history, to identify a specific genetic variant or mutation in their offspring. Genetic testing of newborns may be offered on the same familial basis or because suggestive symptoms have already appeared. Currently, this testing is undertaken only for identifiable *early-onset* conditions, the early diagnosis of which can lead to interventions that have therapeutic value. Newborn testing for *late-onset* conditions or for medical conditions for which there is no cure or other type of medical benefit is ethically problematic and may be objectionable because the child may be able to live a normal life for many years before the onset of disease. Also problematic is prenatal genetic testing for the purpose of identifying fetuses with disabilities or minor medical conditions, although this might be defended as an exercise of reproductive freedom. In a more speculative and ethically contentious vein because of its eugenic overtones, there is the use of prenatal genetic testing to create so-called designer babies by identifying genes that are not associated with medical conditions but with desirable traits, such as superior intelligence and memory.

The aim of newborn screening is different. As currently practiced, screening is intended to identify newborns from a particular population who could be helped if their heightened risk of a specific disease were recognized. Parents could then be offered follow-up genetic testing or some type of therapeutic recommendation.

In contrast, whole genome screening (WGS) of newborns, which examines the entire genome, raises ethical and social issues that targeted newborn genetic testing does not. It is now technically feasible to analyze a newborn's entire genome to reveal her genetic variations. One concern, however, is cost: WGS is currently prohibitively expensive for general use. More important, the clinical utility of newborn genomic screening is questionable, given the current state of scientific knowledge. Unlike the relationship between genetic variation and monogenetic diseases, the relationship between genetic variation and polygenetic disorders, which comprise the majority of human genetic diseases, is still not well understood, making it difficult to interpret and, therefore, make diagnostic, prognostic, or therapeutic use of this information.

As to ethical issues, although there is some overlap between those raised by newborn testing and screening programs and genomic newborn screening, the latter raises distinct problems because of the wide net it casts. WGS can provide information on many genetic variants whose significance is not understood and that may not be linked to disease or significant impairment. Or they may be linked to late-onset conditions, such as Alzheimer's disease, or to conditions, such as Huntington disease, for which there is no cure or ameliorative intervention. The danger is that parents anticipating medical problems in their basically healthy children might subject them to interventions that are unnecessary, burdensome, and even damaging. In addition, the psychological impact of this information on young people could be extremely traumatic and disruptive to their lives.

To be sure, genetic testing of newborns raises some of the same ethical issues. There are questions about what the consent process should be and who should be able to provide consent, the impact of the test results on children and families, safeguarding the privacy of the genetic information revealed, and preventing discriminatory repercussions in employment or insurability. But genomic newborn screening magnifies the double-edged implications, potentially providing vast amounts of useful or unnecessary information to health professionals and families, as well as the risk of creating a "medicalized society" (Almond 2006). On the positive side, newborn genomic screening could offer important diagnostic, prognostic, and therapeutic tools, potentially leading to disease prevention, early intervention, and the development of more effective medicines that are tailor-made to a child's specific medical condition.

An additional concern is the effect that the availability of WGS may have on notions of good parenting and parents' procreative decision making. Given the widely advertised possible benefits genomic information might provide, parents may be susceptible to the notion that they have a duty as good and responsible parents to take advantage of this type of screening (Donley, Hull, and Berkman 2012). The corresponding duty is that of the genetics professionals who, in addition to providing accurate information, also provide explanation, interpretation, and counseling. From an ethics perspective, analysis should focus on the potential benefit-burden-harm ratio; the interests and vulnerabilities of the child and the parents; and the obligations of health care professionals to provide information, support, and guidance in making decisions with profound and lasting implications.

References

Almond B. 2006. Genetic profiling of newborns: Ethical and social issues. *Nature Reviews/Genetics* 7:67–71.

Atwood M. 1986. *The Handmaid's Tale*. Boston: Houghton Mifflin Company.

Baily MA, Murray T. 2008. Ethics, evidence, and cost in newborn screening. *Hastings Center Report* 30(3):23–31.

Brezina PR, Zhao Y. 2012. The ethical, legal, and social issues impacted by modern assisted reproductive technologies. *Obstetrics and Gynecology International*: 1–7.

Chervenak FA, McCullough LB. 1991. Justified limits on refusing intervention. *Hastings Center Report* 21(2):12–18.

Donley G, Hull SC, Berkman BE. 2012. Prenatal whole genome sequencing: Just because we can, should we? *Hastings Center Report* 42(4):28–40.

Ecker JL. 2014. Death in pregnancy: An American tragedy. *New England Journal of Medicine* 370(10):889–91.

Post LF. 1997. Bioethical considerations of maternal-fetal issues. *Fordham Urban Law Journal* 24(4):757–75.

Lewin, T. 2014. Surrogates and couples face a maze of state laws, state by state. *The New York Times*, September 14, p. A1.

Rocha J. 2012. Autonomous abortions: The inhibiting of women's autonomy through legal ultrasound requirements. *Kennedy Institute of Ethics Journal* 22(1):35–58.

Rothman BK. 1986. When a pregnant woman endangers her fetus. *Hastings Center Report* 16(1):24–25.

Steinbock B. 1988. Surrogate motherhood as prenatal adoption. *Journal of Law, Medicine & Health Care* 16(1):44–50.

Tieu MM. 2009. Altruistic surrogacy: The necessary objectification of surrogate mothers. *Journal of Medical Ethics* 35(3):171–75.

Review Questions

Directions: Refer to your readings to help respond to the questions and prompts below.

1. Research the laws on reproductive technology, gamete freezing, embryo freezing, and surrogacy in your state. What is legal or banned? Has this changed over time, or is this original legislation?
2. Is it ever possible for legislation to move faster than science? How can society predict advances in science or the legal issues that will develop?
3. Does this technology undermine the role of women in procreation? Some argue that women and motherhood are reduced to "wombs for rent." Considering that many people cannot afford the high cost of ART, does this further marginalize impoverished women who may turn to surrogacy for money?
4. Natalism is the idea that people should procreate. Is society buying organs or wombs when surrogacy and egg donation are used? Or, is it true reproductive freedom to use your body and organs as you see fit?

References

Dobbs v. Jackson Women's Health Organization, 597 U.S. 215 (2022)
Roe v. Wade, 410 U.S. 113 (1973)

Chapter 8

Abortion

Introduction to the Chapter

In 2022, fifty years after the landmark decision *Roe v. Wade*, the U.S. Supreme Court issued its decision in *Dobbs v. Jackson Women's Health Organization* by overturning a woman's right to an abortion. Abortion is the most contentious issue in the United States. It changes votes, decides elections, and divides other affiliations.

As with all other bioethical issues, individuals are entitled to their beliefs. These are individual morals. Laws are different. Laws are the rules prescribed by a government that apply to its members. Ethics, however, is the application of rules provided by outside codes of conduct. It is not a person's individual choice or the law of a nation. It is a reasoned, logical analysis of an issue.

Health care providers are entitled to their own beliefs and individual morals. However, they must also follow the governing laws of their jurisdiction. When those two conflict, providers may sign a conscience clause allowing practitioners to exempt themselves from complying with a law they find morally or religiously objectionable. Ethically, all providers must pay close attention to applicable laws and seek to sign a conscience clause if their employment would require them to perform procedures, such as abortion, that they morally object to.

Abortion laws vary in every state. Be sure to know the current law in your jurisdiction. Be sure to consider your feelings, personally and professionally, and seek to sign a conscience clause, if necessary.

Three main U.S. Supreme Court cases address abortion.

Roe v. Wade (1973) held that the due process clause of the 14th Amendment is violated when state statutes criminalize abortion except to save the mother's life. The Texas courts used a trimester approach in their holding, stating that an abortion was left to the woman and her physician during the first trimester. Then, a state could regulate abortion during the second trimester for the health of the mother. After viability, abortion could be prohibited unless it is to save the mother's life.

Planned Parenthood of Southeastern Pennsylvania v. Robert P. Casey (1992) is an example of stare decisis, Latin for "let the decision stand." It reaffirmed the holding of *Roe v. Wade* that a woman has a right to choose an abortion before viability but changed to the undue burden test instead of the trimester framework. The state may not interfere with a woman's choice to have an abortion before viability without undue interference from the state. The state can restrict abortions after viability because the state has a legitimate interest in protecting health and safety. The 14th Amendment protects liberties, and it is not an undue burden to require informed consent, parental consent, or a waiting period.

Dobbs v. Jackson Women's Health Organization (2022) reversed *Roe v. Wade* and *Planned Parenthood v. Casey*. There is no constitutional right to an abortion. Accordingly, abortion laws were up to the state government, serving legitimate state interests such as respect for life, health, and integrity of medicine and avoiding discrimination.

When applying moral theories and principles to abortion:

- Utilitarians agree that reproductive technology, cloning, surrogacy, and other procedures are acceptable if well-regulated.
- Kantian ethics would argue that abortion rights depend on whether the unborn is a person. The status of personhood implies worth. If not, the right of a woman to self-defense takes priority.
- Natural law theorists include Roman Catholics, who hold that the unborn is a person from the time of conception, with rights equal to the mother. Any type of direct killing is wrong, including to save the life of the mother.

Learning Outcomes

After reading this chapter, students will:

1. Define and integrate key terms into discussion, writing, assignments, and prompts.
2. Analyze relevant case law and statutes related to reproductive technology.
3. Integrate moral theories and principles into corresponding points to consider that extend from abortion, including privacy, 14th Amendment, due process, equal protection, potentiality, prenatal testing, sex selection, minor or significant disabilities, woman's right to self-defense, compelling state interest, trimester approach, undue burden, and health and safety of a woman.

Key Terms

The following key terms will be introduced and used in this chapter.

- **Abortion:** termination or expulsion of a pregnancy by removal of tissue, products of conception, embryo, fetus, or placenta from the uterus of the carrier.
- **Conscience Clause:** a legal document that allows a practitioner to exempt themselves from complying with a law they find morally or religiously objectionable.
- **Induced Abortion:** intentional ending of a pregnancy.
- **Spontaneous Abortion or Miscarriage:** death or expulsion of a pregnancy before an embryo or fetus can survive outside the uterus independently.
- **Therapeutic Abortion:** medically indicated abortion.

- **Viability:** ability to live, develop, and successfully exist; capability and capacity to live.

Introduction to the Readings

The readings that follow highlight some aspects of abortion.

"Personhood in the Abortion Debate," by Gary Seay and Susana Nuccetelli, describes who qualifies as a moral person depending on the definition of a person by looking at psychological capacities, psychological-property criterion, and human-property criterion.

"Abortion in the Hard Cases," by Gary Seay and Susana Nuccetelli, delves into the problematic cases of abortion for fetal defects, such as congenital disorders, wrongful birth, and wrongful life cases. Abortion for sex selection is also analyzed.

Selection from "Personhood in the Abortion Debate"

Gary Seay and Susana Nuccetelli

[...]

Personhood

The Ambiguity of 'Person'

Who qualifies as a moral person depends in part on what 'person' means. Consider,

1. The bones found in the cave were of a *person*, not of a tiger.
2. No computer developed so far can compete with a *person*.
3. The prisoners should not be killed, because they are *persons*.

In (1), 'person' means *human being* in the sense of *being of the species Homo sapiens*. This concept is purely *descriptive*, not moral, since whether something is a human being is a matter of species membership, to be settled by genetic testing. (2) illustrates a more common descriptive concept of 'person,' whereby beings that have some complex psychological capacities such as the ability to reason are persons. As you can see in the capacities listed in Box 8.1.1, some social capacities are also considered crucial to being a person in a descriptive sense. Paradigm persons need not have all such capacities, or may have them only to some degree. But persons typically have some, and possession of a cluster of them is *sufficient* for being a person.

BOX 8.1.1 PSYCHOLOGICAL CAPACITIES TYPICAL OF PERSONS

A person typically

- Has preferences, conscious desires, feelings, thoughts, a sense of time, nonmomentary interests that involve a unification of desires over time, etc.
- Is able to remember its own past actions and mental states, envisage a future for itself, experience pleasure and pain, take moral considerations into account in choosing between possible actions, interact socially with others, communicate with others, and/or undergo change in a reasonably nonchaotic fashion.
- Is self-conscious, capable of rational thought, and/or capable of rational deliberation.

Yet there is disagreement about the short list of psychological or social capacities that should be in that cluster, and about to what degree a being must have them to be a person. In spite of such disagreements, it is clear that possession of some such capacities to a significant degree gives a being personhood. Furthermore, having personhood in this sense also gives a being the full moral standing[...], which implies that killing a person is (all things being equal) a grave moral wrong. In the language of rights, persons are said to have a right to life. Example (3) above, where the personhood of the prisoners is offered as a reason for the wrongness of killing them, illustrates 'person' in this moral sense.

The above examples illustrate the ambiguity of the word/concept 'person,' whose meaning may vary from sentence to sentence. In those examples, it is used to express one or more of these properties:

1. Being a human being
2. Having some psychological/social capacities typical of persons
3. Having full moral standing

The relation between these properties is a complex matter to be taken up in this [reading]. For now, note that (1) through (3) are not exclusive: paradigm persons have all three at once. 'Person' in its most common, descriptive meaning refers to things that satisfy (2), which is sufficient for possession of (3). But given the conservative Sanctity-of-Life doctrine[...], beings that have (1) have (3) too, whether or not they also have (2)—for example, permanently unconscious patients and human fetuses. But not all agree. In *Marlise Muñoz*, her fetus had (1), but did it have also (3)? For those defending the hospital's decision, it did. But those sympathetic with the husband may contend that fetuses are not persons under the most common ordinary meaning of that word which is associated with possession of (2). If fetuses lack (3), allowing them to die or even inducing their death by abortion may be morally permissible.

Criteria of Personhood

Anything that is a person, then, enjoys full moral standing. Having certain psychological or social capacities is one among other criteria of personhood offered to determine *which* beings enjoy that standing. Criteria of personhood may offer *necessary and sufficient*, or only sufficient, conditions for having full moral standing. Of the two, criteria offering only sufficient conditions are more modest and therefore likely to succeed. For 'person' may be among the concepts resistant to definition by necessary and sufficient conditions. Compare 'sister': once you have determined that, to qualify for sisterhood, someone must be both a female and a sibling, you can sort out sisters and nonsisters. Neither being female nor being a sibling is sufficient in itself for being a sister, but each is necessary. And the two together are sufficient: anyone who fulfills both conditions is a sister. Sometimes, as in this case, it is a combination of two or more necessary conditions taken jointly that determines membership of a class. Other times it is one condition that is at once both necessary and sufficient. For example, being a figure with exactly three internal angles is necessary and sufficient for being a triangle.

But there is a long history of failed attempts at finding necessary and sufficient conditions for being a person. Good candidates are the two meanings of 'person' exemplified above: having certain complex psychological or social capacities, and belonging to the species *Homo sapiens*. Yet a closer look suggests that neither condition, by itself, amounts to a necessary and sufficient condition for being a person. Let's illustrate the problem by means of some candidates for the psychological capacity necessary and sufficient for personhood. If the capacity is thinking critically, then infants are not persons, and neither are adults with severe mental impairments or dementia, which conflicts with commonsense intuitions about them. Or consider having a complex language. Now humans who, because of a congenital disorder or injury, permanently lack linguistic abilities aren't persons, which is also implausible. And if the conditions are relaxed, so as to consist only in having sentience (the capacity to feel pain and pleasure), then lizards, mice, and cats end up being persons. The failure to identify adequate necessary and sufficient conditions of personhood favors a modest criterion offering only sufficient conditions, something we'll assume for the criteria coming next.

BOX 8.1.2 CRITERIA OF PERSONHOOD

Ambitious Criteria—Aim at identifying necessary and sufficient conditions for being a person, such that

- Without them no one is a person, and
- They are enough all by themselves to make something a person.

Modest Criteria—Aim at identifying the psychological capacities that are sufficient for falling under the ordinary concept 'person.'

Psychological-Property Criteria

These criteria of personhood take the possession of some psychological/social capacities to be sufficient for personhood, something consistent with the ordinary meaning of 'person.' But *which* complex psychological capacities are sufficient for being a person in that ordinary sense of 'person' and to what degree? Although so far there is no agreed upon psychological-property criterion, many agree with philosopher John Locke (1632–1704): self-consciousness, rational thought, a sense of time, and memory are sufficient for personhood. In his view, any being with the capacities for desiring to remain alive and for recognizing itself as itself and as the same being at different times and places is a person.

Bioethicist David DeGrazia (2007: 178–9), aware that that there is no consensus among Lockeans about a precise list of complex forms of consciousness "typical" of persons, argues that an adequate cluster of sufficient conditions for personhood includes autonomy, rationality, self-awareness, linguistic competence, sociability, and moral agency. Possession of *enough* of these is sufficient for being a person. At the same time, there are borderline cases of human beings who are neither persons nor nonpersons—for example, fetuses, anencephalic newborns, and patients in PVS or with severe dementia. But the proposed cluster determinately applies to paradigm persons, defined as "normal human beings who are beyond infancy and toddler years" (p. 178). Typical of persons is being "psychologically complex, linguistically competent, and highly social" (p. 177). If possession of such features determines personhood, it follows that any nonhumans with comparable psychological features are persons too. Thus, in this view personhood extends beyond our species to apply to, for example, extinct hominid species, fictional characters, and perhaps the Great Apes and other higher mammals.

DeGrazia thus offers a modest approach to criteria of personhood that appears unaffected by the present lack of consensus among scholars about which specific psychological capacities are sufficient for personhood, and to what degree. But its modesty comes at the price of a low performance in the problematic cases of interest to bioethics. Consider the abortion debate, in which it matters whether the human fetus has the standing of a person with a right to life. Since the fetus has none of the psychological properties deemed sufficient for personhood, the view leaves undetermined whether fetuses are persons. After all, they might acquire their personhood via a different cluster of capacities (recall that in this view the proposed capacities are only sufficient, not necessary). Furthermore, since the same could be said for individuals who permanently lack cognitive capacity, this criterion is unlikely to be of much help with the moral quandaries [...] in connection with brain death and disorders of consciousness.

The Human-Property Criterion

This criterion relies solely on species membership, holding that

> Mere membership of the species *Homo sapiens* is sufficient to be a person.

Since the human-property criterion does not invoke possession of psychological capacities as sufficient for personhood, it seems more determinate than psychological-property criteria. After all, whether a being belongs to *Homo sapiens* can be clearly established by DNA testing. But a closer look reveals some indeterminacy, since drawing clear boundaries among certain species is difficult in nature. For example, it is an unsettled matter in evolutionary biology whether the Neanderthals belonged to a distinct species *Homo genus* or were a subspecies of *Homo sapiens*. This criterion cannot, then, tell whether the Neanderthals had full moral status. And since there is now abundant evidence of their interbreeding with *Homo sapiens*, it is also indeterminate about whether the resulting offspring were persons. Even if the vagueness of 'person' may account for these complications, a problem remains. For, given the human-property criterion, humans who are ordinarily thought to lack the full moral standing of paradigm persons would have it—for example, anencephalic babies and permanently unconscious patients. Any criterion with such consequences runs into over-inclusiveness, a problem considered next.

[...]

Additional Reference

DeGrazia, D., "Human-Animal Chimeras: Human Dignity, Moral Status, and Species Prejudice," in Gruen, Grabel, and Singer 2007, pp. 168–87.

Selection from "Abortion in the Hard Cases"

Gary Seay and Susana Nuccetelli

[...]

Two Hard Cases for Abortion Critics

Abortion to Save the Mother's Life or Health

In some circumstances, a pregnancy may endanger a woman's health or even life. Consider this case:

> *Savita Halappanavar*, a 31-year-old Indian dentist who had a practice in Ireland, was seventeen weeks pregnant when she suffered a miscarriage in October 2012. She repeatedly asked doctors at University Hospital, Galway, for an abortion, but, although they conceded that the fetus was not viable, they refused to perform one because fetal heartbeat was present. As a result of her untreated miscarriage, Mrs. Halappanavar contracted septicemia leading to multiple organ failure and died. News of her death brought an outcry from both sides in the abortion debate. Many people in Ireland called for amending the law, even when a 1992 Supreme Court ruling already allowed

exceptions to the abortion ban where "a pregnant woman's life was at risk because of pregnancy, including the risk of suicide." In 2013 a new bill was signed into law by President Michael Higgins authorizing abortion whenever necessary to save the woman's life or when she is in danger of taking her own life (its most contested provision). The Catholic Church, whose doctrine is influential in Ireland, opposed the bill.

Abortion for women in this condition seems permissible, given the different moral standings of mother and fetus [...], and the health care providers' obligations of beneficence (i.e., to prevent serious harm to the woman) and respect for autonomy (when she has made a valid request for an abortion). But particularly relevant to the case is the woman's right to self-defense when abortion is the only way of preventing serious harm to her. According to a principle underlying this claim, an aggressor's threat of death or serious bodily harm can justify the use of deadly force in response if there is no other way to deflect the attack. In Ms. Halappanavar's case, the 'aggressor' was the miscarried fetus.

But for critics who consider abortion an absolute wrong, the fetus is a person with a right to life, and in cases where its natural development threatens the woman's life or health, it is an innocent threat, so that the use of deadly force is morally forbidden. The Natural Law tradition, for example, distinguishes innocent from guilty threats whose propensity to cause serious harm renders them culpable and gives the targeted potential victim a moral right to defend herself in ways proportionate to the threat.

Even so, [...] the *Principle of Double Effect* can help Natural Law theorists to vindicate common morality's intuition that an abortion to save the mother's health or life is morally permissible. It would be so provided

- The death of the fetus is the only alternative available,
- It is not a mere means to the good end (to save the mother), and
- It is a foreseen but unintended consequence of the medical effort to save her life.

Yet as illustrated by John Finnis (1994), this reasoning fails to justify some cases of abortion to save the mother's life or health that seem morally permissible. Finnis justifies abortion for ectopic pregnancy, where the aggressor is a normal fetus that has implanted in a fallopian tube (threatening a lethal hemorrhage), provided the intention is to resolve this medical condition and there is no alternative. At the same time, for Finnis, abortion when the pregnancy poses a risk to a woman with a weak heart is impermissible, because here the termination is intended and a means to the good end. The intention is to kill the fetus to save the mother's life. He also thinks impermissible abortion to save a suicidal mother, because there are other treatment options—something not always true as a matter of medical fact. In any event, these sharply differing verdicts are a problem for Natural Law abortion critics, since no acceptable moral view should issue different moral verdicts in relevantly similar situations. Furthermore, in cases involving a pregnancy that endangers a woman's life, making a decision about the moral permissibility of an abortion should not drive parents and health care providers to double-effect reasoning and its often obscure speculation about intentions, means, and ends.

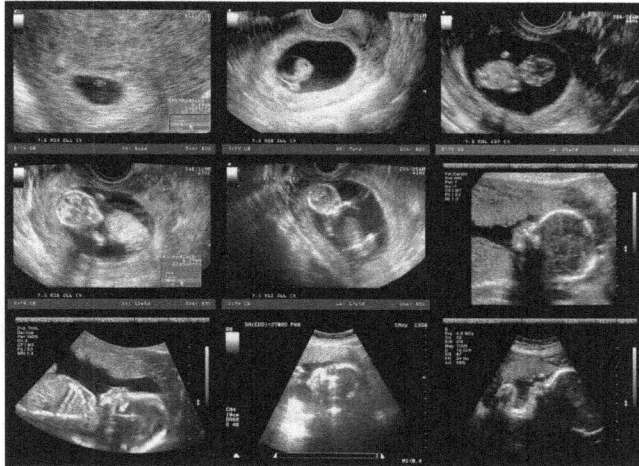

Image 8.2.1

©iStockPhoto/Linda Epstein

Abortion for Fetal Defects

The life prospects of neonates born with some disorders detectable during pregnancy can be very grim. But new forms of medical intervention and therapies available during pregnancy, such as corrective intrauterine surgery, have lowered the number of affected neonates. Also contributing to this tendency is progress in prenatal screening and diagnostic testing, which has increased the number of terminations of pregnancy for fetal defects. Abortions for fetal defects and to save the mother's life or health are therapeutic abortions. Before considering why abortions for fetal defects are a hard case for abortion critics, let's first have a quick look at some disorders detectable *in utero* that commonly lead to such abortions.

Some Facts about Congenital Disorders

Congenital disorders or anomalies are health impairments *present at birth*. Some produce long-term disabilities that impact not only the infants and their families, but also the health care system and society at large. They range from mild to severe. According to the World Health Organization (see also Figure 8.2.1), in 2014 approximately one neonate in 33 had a congenital disorder, totaling 3.2 million neonates globally. Together with conditions such as preterm complications and neonatal infections, they accounted for 2.7 million infant deaths in 2010.

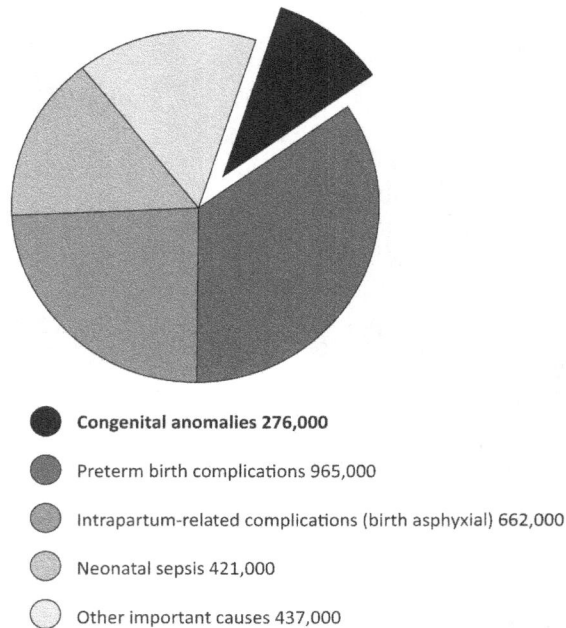

Congenital anomalies 276,000

Preterm birth complications 965,000

Intrapartum-related complications (birth asphyxial) 662,000

Neonatal sepsis 421,000

Other important causes 437,000

Figure 8.2.1   Global Neonatal Deaths in 2013

Disorders such as neural tube defects and Down syndrome can now be detected during pregnancy. When this happens, the expectation often is a therapeutic abortion. In order to see why parents and health care givers then face a difficult decision, let's have a quick look at these disorders. Anencephaly and spina bifida are neural tube defects originated during the first month of gestation, when the fetus's neural tube forms and must close to allow the development of the brain and skull in the upper part, the spinal cord and vertebrae in the lower part. Anencephaly results from the neural tube's failure to close completely in the upper part. Born without portions of the brain, anencephalic babies are not only blind and deaf, but can never be conscious. If they have a working brain stem, they may retain spontaneous functions such as breathing and heartbeat, and have reflex responses to touch. Most of them are stillborn, and those born alive generally die within hours or days of birth. There is neither a treatment to improve their poor prognosis nor a known cause for the onset of the disorder during fetal development (though maternal malnourishment is thought to play a part). In spina bifida, the neural tube enveloping the spinal cord fails to close properly during the first month of fetal development. This typically causes cognitive and developmental impairments, incontinence of bowel and bladder and a number of physical disabilities, including restrictions in mobility and paralysis of the lower limbs in varying degrees. The severity of impairments varies, with myelomeningocele presenting the most serious. According to the US National Library of Medicine, myelomeningocele affects one out of 4,000 infants in the US.[1]

Another type of congenital disorder is Down syndrome, which results from an extra chromosome or 'trisomy' for chromosome 21 (hence its alternative name, 'Trisomy 21'). It is characterized not only by mental

1. US National Library of Medicine. "Myelomeningocele," 11/3/2015. https://medlineplus.gov/ency/article/001558.htm.

impairment ranging from mild to severe, but also by deficits such as hearing loss, difficulties in verbal expression, and higher risks of congenital heart disorders, leukemia, and gastrointestinal anomalies. [...P]arental fears of social stigma, negative implications for the psychological development of siblings, and the burdens of caring for an infant with Down syndrome were reasons fueling some controversial decisions to forgo life-saving treatment, which in turn prompted deep changes in legal and moral reasoning about end-of-life measures for such newborns. Today Down syndrome can be detected prenatally through screening and diagnostic tests. When the condition is diagnosed, about 90% of fetuses are aborted.[2]

Abortion for Fetal Defects Is Permissible

Reasons supporting abortion for fetal defects are generally utilitarian. Consider a scenario in which a routine prenatal screening of a pregnant woman reveals that her fetus may have severe impairments—something later confirmed by diagnostic tests. The future infant will be blind and deaf, as well as quadriplegic and in pain whenever touched. It will also almost certainly have severe mental impairment. Utilitarian considerations suggest that bringing such an impaired individual into the world would increase the total amount of pain, both physical and psychological, and since a world with *less pain* is a *better* world, it would follow that the abortion is not only permissible but mandatory. Caring and fairness towards the future disabled child and its family support the same conclusion, for it would be unfair for the infant herself to have to endure a life of only suffering—as it would be also for those who would have to bear most of the burden of her care.

Fueling these arguments is the view that severe impairments are harms for those who have them and for their families, held by disabled persons and their parents who have acted as plaintiffs in lawsuits known as wrongful-birth or wrongful-life actions against health care providers. In a wrongful-birth action, the plaintiffs, usually the parents and/or child, allege that the birth of an impaired child could have been prevented by avoiding conception or terminating a pregnancy, had the providers not been negligent. Such negligence may consist of a failure to inform prospective parents about their likelihood of having an impaired child, or to conduct proper prenatal screening and testing. Either way, the result is an injurious deprivation of parental choice, as exemplified by this case.

> In *Berman v Allan* two obstetricians faced legal charges for neglecting to inform Ms. Berman about the availability of screening and diagnostic tests for Down syndrome, which her baby had. The court awarded the Bermans compensation under the tort of wrongful birth, whereby the injury is the parents' deprivation of a choice. But it rejected the Bermans' wrongful-life action filed on behalf of their child. In an action of this sort, the injury consists, not in interfering with parental choice, but in enabling a severely disabled child to come into existence.

Here the court found the physicians culpable for wrongful birth but rejected the Bermans' contention that the case involved wrongful life. In wrongful-life litigation, the cause of action is the tort that, due to medical malpractice, a child was born into a life of suffering rather than not having being born at all. Such lawsuits

---

2. Mark L. Schrad, "Does Down Syndrome Justify Abortion," *New York Times*, 9/4/2015.

are generally dismissed because the courts don't wish to engage in speculative philosophical assessments of whether a child's nonexistence is better than her existence with a very low quality of life.

Abortion for Fetal Defects Is Forbidden

Critics of abortion may insist on the wrongness of the practice for fetal defects, because of the uncertainty of judgments about the quality of life of a future child when fetal defects are detected during pregnancy. Consider myelomeningocele, the most severe type of spina bifida. Anecdotal and survey evidence from adults with myelomeningocele suggests that these patients' quality of life is not always as poor as some think (Davis, 1983; Barry, 2010).

Similar reasons can be offered against abortion for Down syndrome. In 2014, Richard Dawkins, a celebrated evolutionary biologist at Oxford, endorsed such abortions in his Twitter response to a woman who wondered what to do if she were to learn that her fetus had Down syndrome. "Abort it and try again," tweeted Dawkins. "It would be immoral to bring it into the world if you have the choice. ..." But to BBC journalist Caroline White, whose son has Down syndrome, Dawkins's remarks were offensive. She argued that Dawkins's view was probably formed at a "time when disabled people and people with Down's were labeled and then hidden away, never given the chance to integrate, reach their full potential or form meaningful relationships with their wider community." White invokes anecdotal evidence from her son against such prejudicial assumptions about the quality of life of people with Down syndrome. More generally, the strategy can be used against the utilitarian argument for abortion for fetal defects based on the poor quality of life of people with certain disabilities. But since both sides make quality-of-life judgments, their arguments seem inconclusive.

An argument against abortion for fetal defects that avoids such judgments is Christopher Kaczor's (2011: 180). It notes that no one would seriously argue that a 6-year-old child should be killed because he is partially paralyzed. But then, given that the development of a human being is continuous from conception, it follows that killing a 6-month-old fetus with the same disability—indeed *any* disabled fetus—is equally wrong. However, what is permissible for a 6-month-old fetus need not be permissible in the same way for a 6-year-old child. [...T]hat children develop out of fetuses does not entail that what applies to children applies equally to fetuses. After all, children and fetuses need not have comparable psychological capacities and interests. Those who take these considerations to bear on moral standing can insist that, although it is morally wrong to kill a 6-year-old child because he is partially paralyzed, it might not be morally wrong to abort a 6-month old fetus because it has a congenital disorder. Therefore, this argument too fails to provide conclusive reasons against common-morality's intuition that abortion for fetal defects is morally permissible.

Two Hard Cases for Abortion Defenders

Abortion for Sex Selection

Now that the sex of a fetus can be discovered by prenatal testing, parental decisions to terminate a pregnancy are sometimes affected by the desire for a child of a certain sex. Fetuses of the 'wrong' sex are simply aborted. The practice falls into the category of

Sex-selective abortion (SSA)

Any elective abortion used as a method of birth control to produce an offspring of the desired sex.

Since SSA is a post-conception method, it raises special moral issues for abortion defenders. Some of these issues also affect preconception methods [...]. They involve feminist concerns about medical interventions that in practice favor the birth of male children, given the data from both developed and developing countries (especially in China, Armenia, and Azerbaijan).

The SSA problem for defenders of abortion arises for those who think that, in the first two trimesters of pregnancy, abortion is morally permissible *for whatever reason*. When the destruction of a fetus because of its sex occurs during that period, they must find it justified whatever the parents' motivation. But common morality has it that SSA's motivation renders the practice morally wrong. Thus, these abortion defenders must either explain away that intuition or change their views on abortion.

To explain away the intuition they may either:

1. Deny that SSA is morally wrong by justifying the practice in certain contexts, for example, when the family already has two female children and wants a boy this time.
2. Hold that SSA is wrong, but for reasons that have nothing to do with abortion.

[...] Our concern here is (2), which takes SSA's wrongness to derive from some bad consequences likely to result from the practice. One such consequence is sex ratio imbalance, already a problem in countries where SSA systematically pursues male offspring. In China today there are approximately 121 boys to every 100 girls. If this trend continues, that could be a harmful development, since men will find it more difficult to find mates of the opposite sex, and prostitution and human trafficking rates may then rise significantly. Another harmful consequence of SSA is that, since the aborted fetuses in some countries are nearly always female, SSA might implicitly devalue women. The abortion defender can invoke these bad outcomes to concur on the wrongness of SSA, even if the aborted fetuses are not persons and have only minimal moral standing or none at all.

Given these replies, one could be a defender of abortion and yet argue that SSA amounts to sexism or throws the ratio of women to men in a society out of balance in a potentially harmful way. But such imbalance and prejudice could be corrected through public policy. Furthermore, they merely suggest that SSA is prudentially wrong, without addressing its moral aspect. Abortion defenders still need to explain away the intuition that SSA seems morally wrong given the motivation behind the practice.

Late-Term Abortion

If moral standing increases with fetal development, the loss of a developed fetus is worse than the loss of an early fetus or an embryo. The onset of consciousness is a turning point that occurs between weeks 25 and 32 of gestation, when an electroencephalograph can detect organized electrical activity in the cerebral cortex. Owing in part to this fact about human development, and also to the rising influence of religious conservatism in public policy, many have called for strict state regulation of abortion after week 20, with some possible exceptions for woman endangerment or fetal defects. But it is not these exceptions that raise a late-term abortion problem for abortion defenders. Rather, it is the moral permissibility of late-term abortions sought for reasons substantially similar to those offered on behalf of abortion in the typical case.

[...]

Additional References

Barry, S., "Quality of Life and Myelomeningocele: An Ethical and Evidence-Based Analysis of the Groningen Protocol," *Pediatric Neurosurgery* 46, 2010: 409–14.

Davis, A., "Right to Life of the Handicapped," *Journal of Medical Ethics* 9, 1983: 181.

Kaczor, C., *The Ethics of Abortion: Women's Rights, Human Life, and the Question of Justice.* New York: Routledge, 2011.

Review Questions

Directions: Refer to your readings to help answer the questions and prompts below.

1. The *Dobbs* case originated when Jackson Women's Health Organization, Mississippi's only abortion clinic at the time, sued the Mississippi State Department of Health, naming Thomas E. Dobbs, the state health officer. A 2018 Mississippi law banned abortions after the first 15 weeks of pregnancy, challenging the holding of *Planned Parenthood v. Casey* (1992), which prevented states from banning abortion before fetal viability, about 24 weeks. The Mississippi law was based on a model advanced explicitly by a Christian-based legal organization that intentionally sought to challenge *Roe*. It proved successful. The basis of *Roe* and *Casey* was that the Due Process Clause of the 14th Amendment to the U.S. Constitution protected a woman's right to an abortion. What other laws are currently protected by due process? What other laws are now considered privacy rights?

2. The articles discuss many ways to define and determine personhood. How would you define personhood as a provider, using science and law? Is this different from your definition of an individual? Is there anything the articles should have considered in their writings?

3. When reviewing case law, it is necessary to "time travel" back to the period during which the case was decided. It aids understanding to see the entirety of the decision. Research the events, societal norms, and other considerations for the years the abortion case law was decided. What does this tell us about the law, or does the law tell us about the period in which the case was decided?

Constitutional tests were used to decide the three major Supreme Court cases about abortion, such as compelling state interest and profound interest. Different approaches were also used to evaluate the facts and law, such as the trimester approach, health and safety of the woman, undue burden, and viability. Research these terms and draft definitions in your own words. How do they contradict each other? How are they similar?

References

Dobbs v. Jackson Women's Health Organization, 597 U.S. 215 (2022)
Planned Parenthood of Southeastern Pa v. Casey, 505 U.S. 833 (1992)
Roe v. Wade, 410 U.S. 113 (1973)

Chapter 9

Death and Dying

Introduction to the Chapter

Hurricane Katrina raged into New Orleans as a Category 5 storm in 2005. Record-setting winds and rains battered the city, breaking levees and causing historic flooding. Katrina's devastation was unprecedented. Approximately 90,000 square miles were destroyed, and an estimated 2,000 lives were lost.

New Orleans's Charity Hospital became the epicenter of controversy over the evacuation, triage, and failed disaster planning. Generators flooded, causing power outages and resulting in patients being manually ventilated. Temperatures inside the facility rose to over 100 degrees. Food and water supplies ran out. Rescue attempts fell short. Sick patients, their families, and staff suffered for days. At least 55 patients perished before they could be evacuated. It was later discovered that 10 patients were given lethal doses of medicine without their consent, despite their desire to live. Dr. Anna Pou allegedly provided these doses to 10 patients before the last of the hospital staff evacuated. She claimed she was afraid to leave sick and suffering patients without care when there were no plans for rescue. Many viewed Dr. Pou's decision as murder, while others saw it as euthanasia or assisted suicide.

As medical interventions have advanced, physician-assisted suicide and euthanasia have become exceedingly controversial. The point of medical futility, or when science/medicine has no viable treatment options or cure, means patients and families face heart-wrenching decisions. While most recognize the need for comfort care, many dispute what that is. *Euthanasia* is a Greek word meaning "good death," and thus, the term itself has come to embody painless relief from suffering. The concept of dying a good death rests in the exercise of autonomy, beneficence, and mercy.

A multitude of case law codifies the current legal landscape. Two of the most prominent are *Quinlan* and *Cruzan*.

Matter of Quinlan Supreme Court of New Jersey (1976) this case not considered a suicide or homicide case, and thus, no criminal or no civil liability attaches when a patient does not have a meaningful hope of recovery. The state does not have an interest in maintaining a life that remains, long term, in a persistent vegetative state. The right of privacy to determine the removal of mechanical assistance belongs to the patient and their guardian. That guardianship shall be determined by the trial judge. The doctors should consult with the guardian, the patient's next of kin, and the hospital ethics committee.

Cruzan v. Director, Missouri Department of Health (1990) held that the state is interested in protecting human life and cannot accept the patient's family members substituting their judgment about withdrawing life-sustaining treatment. The court must have clear and convincing proof of an incompetent patient's wishes, like in a living will.

Other prominent legal cases are *Vacco v. Quill (1997), Washington v. Glucksberg (1997), the Terri Schiavo cases, and Nancy Klein.* Each of these addresses additional matters concerning homicide, malpractice, autonomous choice, refusal of treatment, and proxies.

When applying moral theories and principles to the topic of death and dying:

- Rule utilitarians typically believe that the slippery slope argument of allowing sanctioned deaths would tip society towards dreadful outcomes.
- Kantian ethics believe human beings should be cared for because of their intrinsic worth as a person and would not support suicide.
- Natural law theorists condone any euthanasia, although they acknowledge the difference between killing and ending suffering.

Learning Outcomes

After reading this chapter, students will:

1. Define and integrate key terms into discussion, writing, assignments, and prompts.
2. Analyze relevant case law and statutes to predict future trends.
3. Integrate moral theories and principles into corresponding points to consider that extend from death and dying, including integrating, determining, and defining life and death; the American Medical Association's opinion on physician assisted suicide; autonomy, mercy, and harm; suicide pacts; infant euthanasia; doctor suicide and vulnerable groups; death and dignity; self-determination; duty to die; family involvement in end of life decisions; ; and alternatives to brain death.

Key Terms

The following key terms will be introduced and used in this chapter.

- **Active Euthanasia:** the act of ending a person's life by intentionally injecting a lethal agent.
- **Euthanasia**: the act of ending a person's life by intentionally stopping intolerable suffering using a painless method. It is the concept of dying a good death based on exercising autonomy, beneficence, and mercy.
- **Involuntary euthanasia:** the act of ending a person's life without their consent because the person wants to live. This is considered murder.

- **Medical Futility:** science/medicine has no viable treatment options or cure.
- **Nonvoluntary Euthanasia:** the act of ending a person's life without their consent and clearly expressed wish to die.
- **Passive euthanasia:** the act of ending a person's life by allowing a patient to die of natural causes after the withdrawal of life-saving or life-supporting care, motivated by the best interest of the patient.
- **Physician-Assisted Suicide (PAS): when** a physician provides a lethal dose of medications to a competent patient to voluntarily self-administer and cause their own death.
- **Voluntary Euthanasia:** the act of ending a competent person's life with their consent and clearly expressed wish to die.

Introduction to the Readings

The readings that follow focus on a few facets of Death and Dying.

"When Life Supports Are Futile or Refused," by Gary Seay and Susana Nuccetelli, examines the difference between a biological life and a biographical life. The focus is on quality of life and when futile life-sustaining treatment should be removed to hasten death, if ever. The landmark cases listed above are discussed with a focus on disagreements with futility judgments and how to resolve them.

"Medically Assisted Death," by Gary Seay and Susana Nuccetelli, discusses PAS and euthanasia. It details objections from justice, nonmaleficence, and Oregon's Death With Dignity Act. Suicide tourism, tight-to-die arguments, and appeals to integrity and trust as forbidding physician-assisted dying complete a good summary of the various beliefs.

"End–of–Life Measures for Severely Compromised Newborns," by Gary Seay and Susana Nuccetelli, discusses severely compromised infants and the Groningen Protocol. Five conditions must be met for morally and legally permissible euthanasia. End-of-life measures appeal to psychological personhood, and reasons supporting and opposing end-of-life measures for the severely compromised are explained.

Selection from "When Life Supports are Futile or Refused"

Gary Seay and Susana Nuccetelli

[...]

The Moral Grounds of Medical Futility

The Biological versus Psychological Life Argument

When there is disagreement over what is best for a patient, the dispute may hinge on how best to maximize the patient's wellbeing in a compromised condition. But this challenge may arise in a vast array of different forms with different diseases, injuries, and disorders, and at all possible levels of severity. To see what is at stake, it may help to begin with a worst-case scenario. Consider the case where a patient has irreversibly lost all capacity for consciousness. The quality of life when someone becomes permanently unconscious is so poor that it is not at all clear how LST could benefit that patient. James Rachels (1986) famously defended the claim that a patient in PVS has a biological *but not* a biographical life. People in that condition lack the psychological capacities necessary for being the subject of a life, such as self-awareness and memories. Without these, the patient remains a living, human body, with no biographical life. Since the rule against hastening death, and indeed killing, applies only to persons who have a biographical life, so the argument goes, forgoing LST for a patient in PVS is therefore permissible. Jeff McMahan (2002) would agree. For him, these patients are alive only as human organisms but not as persons whose lives demand moral and legal protection. Only *minded* organisms with the capacity for consciousness qualify as persons.

In either version of the argument, these patients' exceedingly poor quality of life justifies hastening their death by forgoing futile LST. Quality of life does matter, after all, for end-of-life decisions—something acknowledged by the Law Lords in *Bland* when they deemed life no longer in Tony's interest. But the argument is vulnerable to important objections. First, from the *fact* that a patient like Tony permanently lacks consciousness, the *normative* conclusion that it is permissible to hasten his death by forgoing LST does not follow. As we saw earlier, it is not clear that judgments of value can be validly inferred from statements of fact. Moreover, not all agree with the moral decisionmaking role this argument gives to *having interests*. Among those who do agree, some think that even the dead can have residual interests that could be undermined by, for example, false claims about their past. That explains why certain behaviors toward them seem morally forbidden (Foster, 2013). In light of these criticisms, as it stands, the argument falls short of supporting its conclusion.

The Appeals to Justice and Beneficence

The health care professionals' duties of justice and beneficence provide stronger grounds for forgoing futile treatments. First, since medical resources are limited, if an intervention is foreseeably futile, then providing it amounts to wasting medical resources that could have been used to help others. And that is unjust to the patients who might have benefitted from it. Furthermore, futile interventions may give false hope to patients whose terminal condition is not yet obvious and who might thereby be deprived of a last chance to put their affairs in order. Such patients might also fall into despair when they see their hopes suddenly crushed. Another reason against futile interventions is that they might make some patients more uncomfortable or less lucid at the end of life, thereby preventing them from enjoying good moments with friends and family. Given the duty of beneficence, health care providers must prevent such harms. Therefore, justice and beneficence make obligatory the avoidance of futile interventions.

Disagreements about Futility Judgments

A patient or surrogate may disagree with the health care providers' judgment that a treatment will do no good, or its burdens outweigh the benefits. Such conflicts are less likely to arise with judgments involving quantitative futility. [...P]atients' requests for treatment lack the force of refusals. Although beneficence is a fundamental duty of health care providers, they need not provide treatment deemed futile, even life supports. This follows from their right of professional autonomy and their special epistemic (knowledge-based) authority. Owing to their professional experience and scientific expertise, their assessment of a treatment's likely benefits carries a special warrant of credibility.

Conflicts more often concern judgments about the qualitative futility of a treatment for a patient, and may involve the patient or surrogate, health care providers, and the courts. These conflicts rest not on different predictions about likely outcomes, but on differing views about whether those outcomes are valuable.

As we saw in the above cases, the doctor disagreed with a guardian appointed by a lower court in *Bland*, the patient's parents with the state of Missouri in *Cruzan*, the hospital with the parents in *Quinlan*, and the patient with the hospital in *Nancy B*. While some of these parties considered life supports medically appropriate for the patient, others regarded it as (qualitatively) futile. In each of the cases, the decision would turn on an assessment of whether the treatment's outcome could be a benefit for the patient in making his or her life better overall. Such assessments are necessarily value-laden, for they depend on what the decisionmaker regards as a beneficial outcome to be sought or a harm to be avoided.

The last recourse in conflict resolution concerning futility assessments is the courts, which represent the state's interests in protecting the patient. Their rulings tend to invoke legal doctrines developed out of landmark cases such as those considered here: from *Quinlan* the principle of substituted judgment, from *Cruzan* the emphasis on patient self-determination and evidenciary standards for advance directives, and from *Bland* the best-interest standard so influential in British courts, to name but a few of the proxy decision-making procedures [...]. Conflicts, however, are more often resolved without judicial intervention by dialogue among affected parties, input from institutional ethics committees, and reference to the health providers' policies concerning futile treatment, which increasingly try to strike a balance between consideration of health outcomes and respect for patient autonomy.

[...]

Additional References

Foster, C., *Medical Law: A Very Short Introduction*. Oxford: Oxford University Press, 2013.
McMahan, J., *The Ethics of Killing: Problems at the Margins of Life*. Oxford: Oxford University Press, 2002.
Rachels, J., *The End of Life: Euthanasia and Morality*. Oxford: Oxford University Press, 1986.

Selection from "Medically Assisted Death"

Gary Seay and Susana Nuccetelli

[...]

Physician-Assisted Suicide

Physician-Assisted Suicide and Voluntary Active Euthanasia

The so-called right-to-die movement has had more success in decriminalizing regulated forms of PAS than VAE. The rationale for this tendency is twofold:

1. PAS is more clearly a voluntary act, at least in the sense that it is the patient who, as a competent and informed moral agent, chooses to self-administer the lethal agent.
2. PAS involves no direct act of killing by health care professionals, who need not even be in the room when the patient self-administers the lethal agent.

Health care professionals who are willing to assist in terminations of life also regard (1) and (2) as advantages of PAS over active euthanasia, partly because they are typically wary of causing a patient's death intentionally and directly. But not all agree with this rationale or with the movement to legalize PAS.

The Objection from Justice

According to this objection, a policy of providing only PAS is unfair to patients who want assistance in dying but are unable to administer a lethal agent to themselves because they are, for example, in late stages of Alzheimer's or completely paralyzed. Consider,

> *Tony Nicklinson*, a 58-year-old Briton afflicted with Locked-in Syndrome, wasn't terminally ill. He might have had many years of life ahead of him. But, as a reporter from the BBC put it, he was "in terminal despair." As a result of irreparable brain damage from a catastrophic stroke he suffered during a business trip, Nicklinson was totally paralyzed and mute, yet he remained conscious. He could still move his eyes, and he communicated by blinking or nodding to letters shown to him on a board. By this means, he instructed his attorneys to seek two declarations from the High Court: (1) that it would be lawful for a doctor to assist him in ending his life, and (2) that the current law for assisted death in the UK infringed on his right to a private life protected by the European Convention for Human Rights, art. 8. A panel of High Court judges rejected his request, and a few days later, on August 21, 2012, Nicklinson, who had been refusing food and water, died from untreated pneumonia. On appeal pursued by his wife, in 2014 the Supreme Court reasserted that a revision of the British ban on assisted suicide was not for the courts to make, but for Parliament.

Where only PAS is lawful, some disabled patients like Nicklinson lack the right to assisted death that other patients have. This state of affairs amounts to discrimination and is therefore unjust. Refusal of food and fluids is the only recourse available to them if they find life unacceptable. Furthermore, if ending one's life amounts to a right guaranteed by the Fourteenth Amendment to the US Constitution, as some have claimed (Dworkin et al., 1998), then US jurisdictions where only PAS is lawful violate that right.

The Objection from Nonmaleficence

This objection, if sound, supports a ban not only on PAS but also on VAE. It contends that, since death is not in a person's best interest, the health care providers' assistance in dying is forbidden by their duty of nonmaleficence. Supporters of the objection are likely to remind us of the notorious assistance in dying provided during the 1990s by *Dr. Jack Kevorkian*, a retired Michigan pathologist who made a career of helping people to die. Nicknamed "Dr. Death" by the tabloid press, Dr. Kevorkian devised suicide machines with which patients could self-administer lethal drugs or carbon monoxide. According to some accounts, at least 93 deaths were assisted by Dr. Kevorkian between 1990 and 1998. Of that number, however, it appears that only 17 deaths involved terminally ill patients. Many of Kevorkian's patients, though terrified of future mental deterioration and a foreseen death, were not even in pain. Moreover, they were often people Kevorkian barely knew, so he was hardly in a position to judge the necessity of the drastic step each was about to take. Many bioethicists, though sympathetic to the right-to-die movement, wrote him off as a publicity-seeking crank. Kevorkian was ostracized by the medical profession, and his license to practice eventually revoked. Indicted several times on charges of assisting a suicide and other offenses, he continually eluded conviction. But his audacity ultimately brought his downfall in a notorious case:

> *Thomas Youk* was suffering from amyotrophic lateral sclerosis (ALS), a progressive, degenerative neurological disorder. In 1998 Dr. Kevorkian videotaped himself administering voluntary active euthanasia to Youk by lethal injection. Afterwards, he allowed the tape to be broadcast on the CBS News program *60 Minutes*, daring the authorities to arrest him. The Michigan district attorney was all too happy to oblige him, and soon Dr. Kevorkian found himself sentenced to ten years in prison for second-degree murder. He served eight before being released on parole in 2007.

But prevention of Kevorkian-style recklessness that threatens harm to patients can perhaps be achieved without a total ban on PAS. For one thing, Kevorkian's activities were unregulated. Proponents of lawful PAS have no problem in condemning them while insisting that such abuses are less likely to occur if strictly regulated PAS is available when continued life has ceased to be a benefit. After looking at Oregon's model of regulated PAS, we consider another problem for the Objection from Nonmaleficence: 'suicide tourism,' a growing phenomenon suggesting that a total ban on PAS only encourages patients to seek it away from home, in places where regulations might make Kevorkian-style scenarios unlikely.

Oregon's Death with Dignity Act

There is a relatively recent trend in the United States toward legalizing regulated PAS. Originally approved by voters by a margin of 51.31% in 1994, Measure 16, Oregon's Death with Dignity Act, made Oregon the first state with a statute that allows qualifying terminally ill adults to obtain prescriptions for lethal drugs. Challenged by a group of doctors and patients, a Court of Appeals ruled against the plaintiffs in 1997, and in 2006 the US Supreme Court voted 6-to-3 to uphold the statute, leaving individual states free to enact similar laws. Some did exactly that: Washington in 2008, Vermont in 2013, and California in 2015. In 2008–09, a court decision in the state of Montana had the effect of providing immunity for physicians who practiced regulated PAS, though no statute specifically legalized PAS.

In all these states, safeguards for the practice mirror those of the Oregon Death with Dignity Act, which states, among other conditions, that qualifying patients must

1. Be at least 18 years old, resident of Oregon, and able to make and communicate autonomous decisions,
2. Have a terminal illness that, as certified by at least two doctors, will likely lead to death within six months, and
3. Make two oral and one written request for PAS to the physician.

For doctors, the Act stipulates that participation in PAS is optional. The attending physician must be licensed in the state, must inform the patient of alternatives including palliative care, and must ask the patient to notify next-of-kin. If either of the doctors evaluating an application judges the patient incompetent, they must refer her for a psychological exam. When all conditions are met, there is a 48-hour waiting period before the patient can pick up the prescribed drugs at a pharmacy. Only she can administer them.

Not all requests for PAS meeting the Act's conditions are actually granted: only approximately one out of six (Ganzini et al., 2001). Of those granted, only one out of ten actually results in suicide—which suggests that PAS in Oregon is a measure of last resort. Furthermore, although over the years more patients have made use of PAS (e.g., 38 in 2002, 21 in 2001, 27 in 1999, and 16 in 1998), there is no reason to think that the practice is expanding in a worrisome direction. Nor are there reasons to think that PAS is more requested by minorities, women, and the elderly or poor. Merrick (2005: 234) reports that in 2002, the patients whose deaths resulted from PAS, compared with those who died of other causes, were younger (69 median age), and more likely to have cancer (84%) and to be enrolled in hospice programs (92%). More men used PAS than women. Except for one patient, all others had health insurance—which suggests that financial pressure was not conditioning their decisions. According to the Oregon Department of Human Services 2003, only a few patients reported pain as a reason for requesting PAS. Main reasons were the loss of autonomy, including control over bodily functions, and decreasing ability to participate in enjoyable activities. On the whole, commentators are generally agreed that the practice of PAS in Oregon has not fallen outside of established safeguards in ways that justify concern (Okie, 2005; Merrick, 2005; Lewy, 2010; Sumner, 2011). Furthermore, the support for the practice by Oregonians suggests that it has not undermined their trust in health care professionals.

Among the objections, two concern the need for legalizing VAE too: the Appeal to Justice mentioned above, and an Objection from Failed Attempted Suicides which can cause patients great harm. If PAS is the only legal form of medical assistance in dying, physicians cannot legally help those patients. Others argue that the Oregon Act is too permissive and prone to abuses, since in the end it is for the attending physician to determine whether a case meets the safeguards, and there need be no previous relationship between physician and patient. So patients can shop around for a physician sympathetic to their request. In addition, there is no requirement that the second opinion be that of a specialist in the patient's condition (Foley and Hendin, 2002; Keown, 2002). These criticisms can be addressed by sharpening the terms of the Act. More radical are objections PAS faces together with VAE. We'll consider these after first looking at a growing phenomenon that argues for legalizing at least PAS.

Suicide Tourism

Beneficence provides another argument for PAS: namely, preventing harm to patients who travel abroad to obtain it because it is unlawful where they live. Patients from, among other jurisdictions, Britain, Australia, the USA, and until recently, Canada, engage in suicide tourism. Let's look closely at the UK phenomenon. The ban on suicide in Britain was lifted by the 1961 Suicide Act, which also made aiding and abetting a suicide unlawful. This provision, however, is not without rationale, for the state also has a duty to protect vulnerable individuals from being persuaded or coerced into committing suicide. Such crimes, though rare, do sometimes occur. For example, in 2011 detection work by a crime-aficionado and retired teacher landed William Melchert-Dinkel, a Minnesota nurse, in prison, convicted of assistance in two suicides. He apparently used the Internet for pro-suicide 'counseling' of vulnerable individuals, effectively persuading at least two to commit suicide.

Under this legislation, *any* assistance in a suicide—even from compassionate motives—amounts to secondary participation in crime punishable by up to fourteen years in prison (section 2.1). Many terminally ill patients facing much suffering or loss of autonomy consequently fear to seek assistance from friends or loved ones in terminating their lives. Anyone providing such assistance would risk prosecution—as would anyone accompanying a loved one to obtain legal PAS abroad. *The Guardian* reports that, according to data from the Director of Public Prosecutions (2009), at least 90 people in the UK did so between October 2002 and 2008, risking prosecution upon return. Two terminally ill Britons every month go to Switzerland for PAS, and 20 people commit suicide at home for reasons related to a terminal illness.[1] In 2008 the parents and a friend of 23-year-old *Daniel James* were subject to police investigation for facilitating his trip to Switzerland for an assisted suicide. In the end, prosecution was declared "not in the public interest."

Yet it is one thing to be spared prosecution and quite another to have immunity from it. Until the landmark victory considered next, patients wishing to pursue PAS abroad faced considerable uncertainty about possible prosecutorial measures against those who accompany them.

> *Debbie Purdy*, afflicted with multiple sclerosis (MS), challenged the Director of Public Prosecutions in court to reveal prosecutorial policy in England and Wales regarding those who, with compassionate intent, facilitate a PAS abroad. She was not asking for immunity for her husband if he were to accompany her to Switzerland, but for clarification about the extent of help not liable to prosecution. In her view, prosecutorial unclarity violated her right to privacy protected by the European Convention for Human Rights, art. 8. On appeal, in 2009 the Law Lords ruled that unclarity in the application of the Suicide Act did indeed amount to an interference with respect for her privacy and family life.

Ms. Purdy's successful litigation amounted to a turning point in the UK law on assisted suicide. But when MS finally made her condition "unacceptable," she was far too weak to travel to Switzerland. She died at a hospice in Britain in 2014 from self-imposed starvation.

Physician-Assisted Dying: For and Against

Physician-Assisted Dying Is Morally Permissible

Beneficence-Based Arguments

It seems morally permissible, and even obligatory, for medical professionals to provide aid in dying—for example, when a terminally ill patient's pain is no longer controllable by analgesia and she requests it. A virtue ethics version of this Argument from Mercy invokes compassion as an essential virtue for medical professionals (Sumner, 2011). Understood as consequentialist, the argument invokes beneficence, the principle that they should always seek the best interest of their patients and keep them from uncompensated harms. Suffering is bad *as such*, especially when uncompensated by benefits. True, death is also bad. But in some

---

1. Mark Tran, "Assisted Suicide Campaigner Debbie Purdy Dies Aged 51," *The Guardian*, 12/29/2014.

cases more harm is prevented by helping a patient die quickly and painlessly than by prolonging a life of unbearable suffering. Another consequentialist argument for PAD also rests on beneficence. The Appeal to Nonabandonment reminds us of the physicians' duty not to leave their patients without medical care, which sometimes requires providing aid during the dying process.

Given these arguments, PAD may be morally defensible even in the form of nonvoluntary active euthanasia. At this point, however, a critic may object that, with modern medicine's array of analgesics and the development of highly skilled palliative care, no one need die in agony. Yet the fact remains that in some cases, pain cannot be controlled. Moreover, suffering includes other things besides pain—air-hunger, for instance, and nausea and seizures, as well as psychological syndromes less controllable than physical pain.

For other critics, the Appeal to Mercy entails that assistance in dying is a moral duty in medicine, which seems implausible. For one thing, no country or state that permits regulated assisted death has made participation by health care providers a professional duty. Providers are at liberty to participate in PAD, but not obligated to do so. Proponents of the Argument from Mercy may simply dig in their heels and hold fast to their basic position that helping qualified patients die as quickly and painlessly as possible is a professional *moral* duty, whatever the law may say.

An Autonomy-Based Argument

A different line of argument for PAD invokes the principle of autonomy to support the so-called right to die, understood as part of each person's right to control what happens to her own body. Given the right to die, patients should be able to control whenever possible the circumstances of their deaths, which involves the ability to choose a death that conforms to their own standard of dignity. In addition, they should be permitted to decide for themselves how much suffering is enough. This right-to-die argument runs

1. If the principle of autonomy is plausible, then patients have a right to die.
2. The principle of autonomy is plausible.
3. Therefore, patients have a right to die.

This basic argument takes different forms in litigation about PAD. Here is one:

> *Diane Pretty*, 42, feared that her motor neuron disease would cause her death by choking and asphyxia, as often happens in the final stage of that disorder. In 2001 she sought immunity from prosecution for her husband if he were to aid in her suicide, thus challenging the UK 1961 Suicide Act. Her defense rested on her right to privacy, protected by the European Convention for Human Rights, art. 8. After a defeat in the trial court and eventually also in the House of Lords, she appealed to the European Court, arguing that the British courts had abridged her human rights by refusing her request. The European Court dismissed her claim. Ten days later, in May 2002, Mrs. Pretty died by asphyxia in precisely the way she had most feared.

Diane Pretty's argument, like other right-to-die arguments, suggested that third parties are morally *permitted* to assist in someone's death under certain circumstances. But [...] autonomy is a negative right requiring noninterference. A patient's right to assistance in dying, if it exists, is a positive right. As such, it does not create a positive obligation of others to assist. Indeed, the courts have systematically rejected the notion that there is a duty to aid in someone's death. On the other hand, refusals of treatment are negative rights, which do create duties of noninterference, given the patient's right to privacy and bodily integrity.

The upshot is that, although competent patients have a right to make autonomous decisions about the time and manner of their deaths, relatives are under no moral obligation to provide assistance. Similarly, health care providers are at liberty to withhold assistance whenever there is a conflict with their own professional rights to autonomy and integrity. Compare capital punishment: even if some states, given their laws, can legally execute condemned prisoners, and even if physicians in those states are permitted to assist in administering the lethal injections and pronouncing the prisoner dead, they are not *obligated* to assist in either. Thus, a properly understood right-to-die argument supports the claim that PAD is morally permissible, which avoids the consequentialist arguments' problematic implication that providing it is among the physician's moral obligations.

Physician-Assisted Dying Is Morally Forbidden

A common objection to PAD rests on the Sanctity-of-Life doctrine. But from our evaluation of that doctrine [...] we can infer that only the conservative version must forbid PAD on moral grounds. The liberal version can accommodate the patients' right to death. We have argued that the conservative Sanctity-of-Life doctrine makes controversial assumptions. Here we consider other objections to PAD.

The Appeals to Integrity and Trust

The Appeal to Integrity charges that physician-assisted dying conflicts with an essential commitment of medical professionals: the absolute ban on intentionally killing patients. Medicine, like other professions, is not merely a set of technical proficiencies but involves devotion to an ideal. For teachers, that ideal is truth and wisdom, for attorneys and jurists it is justice, and for physicians it is healing—broadly construed as to include the conservation and extension of health and life whenever possible. This ideal gives rise to duties that are specific to medicine, including the duty not to kill one's patients.

But this argument faces the objection that medicine might have more than one essential purpose: a significant part of medicine today has very little to do with healing (Seay, 2005). For example, elective plastic surgery and fertility treatments aim not at healing and the conservation of life, but at the improvement of people's quality of life as perceived by them. Furthermore, there are cases in which the duty of nonmaleficence will itself be dependent on respect for autonomy, since what counts as harm sometimes depends on what the patient values.

The Appeal to Trust invokes a devotion to healing and the avoidance of harm, together with the consequent refusal to intentionally kill, that have been the distinguishing marks of Hippocratic medicine since antiquity. The trust that patients must feel toward their physicians if healing is to be possible would be undermined by permitting assisted death. Critics, however, object that although patients generally value their lives and expect medical professionals to value them too, there are exceptions. In some end-of-life situations, patients might instead expect health care professionals to honor their autonomous choice for death with dignity or for relief of suffering through a quicker death. In any such case, although a physician is not obligated to administer a lethal agent, a willingness to do so might, in the patient's eyes, be evidence of her trustworthiness. Furthermore, the Appeal to Trust rests on a prediction about PAD's negative effects on the patient–health care professional relationship. In connection with the next argument, we consider whether that prediction corresponds with the facts from societies that allow PAD.

The Slippery-Slope Argument

Different versions of this argument against PAD contend that the practice would ultimately have very bad consequences. Among possible bad consequences are sliding into permitting involuntary euthanasia, undermining efforts to provide adequate palliative and hospice care at life's end, and discriminating against women, the elderly, the cognitively impaired, the poor, the disabled, and other vulnerable individuals. Fueling the argument is the risk of abuse that might occur if, for example, women seek assisted death in large numbers to spare their families the burden of caring for them. The argument commits a *fallacy* when the 'sliding' to a bad consequence is in fact unlikely to occur, for it provides *no good reason* to think that it will occur.

Proponents of assisted death may reply that the predicted mistakes and abuses of the practice can be minimized with proper safeguards. For PAS, Oregon's safeguards include that the patient must be afflicted with an extremely debilitating, irreversible condition, have a hopeless prognosis, and have made, consistently over time, a competent, well-informed request for assistance in dying. For euthanasia, *informed consent* or reliable ways of determining the patient's preferences is required in the Netherlands. Thus an assessment of the Slippery-Slope Argument needs to consider evidence from these jurisdictions about how the safeguards are working. Only then we can determine whether risk of abuse is a serious threat.

The Dutch Experience

In the Netherlands, for example, PAS and VAE have been legal since the 1980s—first, decriminalized by prosecutorial policies and then by the 2002 Termination of Life on Request and Assisted Suicide Review Procedures Act. Safeguards for VAE require that:

1. There are no reasonable alternatives.
2. The qualifying patient
    a. Has made a clear, voluntary, and well-considered request for assisted death,
    b. Is in a hopeless condition that causes unbearable suffering, and
    c. Is informed about that condition and prospects.
3. The euthanizing doctor
    a. Has consulted with another independent physician, and
    b. Has terminated the patient's life with due medical care and attention.

It must be noted that terminations of life without explicit request by patients have occurred, but their numbers are diminishing: 0.8% in 1990, 0.7% in 1995, 0.7% in 2001, and 0.4% in 2005 (Rietjens et al., 2009). There have also been nonvoluntary euthanasia cases. In half of these, doctors invoked patients' previous wishes and in all cases consulted the patient's family. Other areas of concern involve (1) pediatric patients and patients with mental suffering, both eligible for physician-assisted death under certain conditions, and

(2) assisted deaths that are not reported as such by physicians. Not surprisingly, critics and defenders of the Dutch policy interpret the data on these problems differently. But according to recent analysis of the data (Sumner, 2011; Lewy, 2010), there appears to be no evidence that decriminalization has had negative effects on palliative and hospice care. And there is no evidence that PAD is sliding on other slippery slopes.

In Belgium, where VAE with safeguards has been legal since 2002, the evidence points to improvement in palliative and hospice care, which observers interpret as a sign that a patient's request for assistance in dying is not prompted by the lack of proper alternatives. In addition, some recent qualitative studies of physicians' responses to patients' requests for termination of life indicate that only a small number of general practitioners, on whom the practice of VAE rests in Belgium, are actually willing to administer it. In most cases, they make attempts at persuading the patient to pursue other options, including terminal sedation in extreme cases. As a result, at least so far, there seems to be no tendency to slide into expanding the scope of assisted death (Sercu et al., 2012), with the exception of the Child Euthanasia Bill signed into law in 2014. This legislation grants terminally ill children of any age who are in "great pain" the right to request euthanasia provided they also make conscious repeated requests to die, have the parents' and medical team's consent, and there is no treatment to alleviate their distress. Opinion polls showed that the bill had broad support by the public. But it was opposed by Catholic leaders and many pediatricians, who argued that it would put vulnerable children at risk. Similar legislation exists in the Netherlands for children over twelve years old.

Regarding the claim that decriminalization of assisted death would put vulnerable people at risk—such as women, the mentally impaired, the physically disabled, the poor, and ethnic and racial minorities—the evidence is inconclusive. Some argue that abuses are more likely to occur when assisted dying is left unregulated, citing the case of Dr. Kevorkian, who assisted in the deaths of many more women than men. As we saw, in Oregon, periodic studies do not point to a disproportionate number of women or other vulnerable people undergoing assisted death. Even so, potential for mistakes and abuses cannot be ruled out a priori. The possibility of these remains an open question to be settled by further empirical data.

[...]

Additional References

Dworkin, G., R. G. Frey, and S. Bok, eds., *Euthanasia and Physician-Assisted Suicide.* Cambridge: Cambridge University Press, 1998.

Foley, K. and H. Hendin, "The Oregon Experiment," in *The Case against Assisted Suicide: For the Right to End of Life Care*, pp. 114–74. Baltimore: Johns Hopkins University Press, 2002.

Ganzini, L., H. D. Nelson, M. A. Lee, D. F. Kraemer, T. A. Schmidt, and M. A. Delorit, "Oregon Physicians' Attitudes about and Experience with End-of-Life Care since Passage of the Oregon Death with Dignity Act," *Journal of the American Medical Association* 285.18, 2001: 2363–9.

Keown, J., *Euthanasia, Ethics, and Public Policy: An Argument against Legalisation.* Cambridge: Cambridge University Press, 2002.

Merrick, J. C., "Death and Dying: The American Experience," in Blank and Merrick 2005, pp. 219–42.

Okie, S., "Physician-Assisted Suicide—Oregon and Beyond," *New England Journal of Medicine* 352, 2005: 1627–30.

R (on the application of Purdy) v *Director of Public Prosecutions*, UKHL 45 (2009).

Rietjens, J. A. C. et al., "Using Drugs to End Life Without an Explicit Request of the Patient," *Death Studies* 31, 2007: 205–21.

Seay, G., "Euthanasia and Physicians' Moral Duties," *Journal of Medicine and Philosophy* 30, 2005: 1–17.

Sercu, M., P. Pype, T. Christiaens, M. Grypdonck, A. Derese, and M. Deveugle, "Are General Practitioners Prepared to End Life on Request in a Country Where Euthanasia is Legalized?" *Journal of Medical Ethics* 38.5, 2012: 274–80.

Sumner, L. W., *Assisted Death: A Study in Ethics and Law.* Oxford: Oxford University Press, 2011.

Selection from "End-of-Life Measures for Severely Compromised Newborns"

Gary Seay and Susana Nuccetelli

[...]

Neonatal Euthanasia

Reasons for letting a severely compromised infant die also support medically assisted neonatal euthanasia, or the deliberate ending of a newborn's life as quickly and painlessly as possible. A notable exception to the general unlawfulness of neonatal euthanasia is the Netherlands, where in 2005, after much debate about the right thing to do with newborns who are suffering badly with no realistic chance of relief, pediatricians adopted a regulation for neonatal euthanasia, the Groningen Protocol (GP). It was first published in the *New England Journal of Medicine*, after having been administered for seven years to some new-borns with myelomeningocele (MMC), the most serious form of spina bifida. It considers euthanasia morally and legally permissible provided five conditions are met:

1. The diagnosis and prognosis is certain,
2. The newborn is in hopeless and unbearable suffering,
3. There is a confirming second opinion by an independent doctor,
4. Both parents give informed consent, and

5. The procedure meets medical standards.

Dr. A. Verhagen and other pediatricians at Groningen developed the GP in response to a particularly painful, terminal case of neonatal epidermolysis bullosa, in which an infant's skin becomes detached from its body. Although euthanasia was then illegal, the GP was envisioned as a set of guidelines for future cases and as a way of making the administration of neonatal euthanasia more open and transparent. Its explicit goals are providing merciful assistance in dying for infants who:

- Cannot possibly survive, even with life-sustaining treatment (LST)—e.g., preemies with very undeveloped kidneys or lungs;
- Have only a small chance of survival and a virtual certainty of a very poor quality of life if they do survive—e.g., neonates with catastrophic hypoxic damage to the brain or other vital organs; and
- Though not LST-dependent, will likely have "a very poor quality of life."

These recommendations have since drawn considerable attention in the pediatric literature, largely as a proposal hotly contested on moral grounds. They have been endorsed by some physicians (mostly in the Netherlands) but emphatically rejected by others. By the time the GP was published in 2005, 22 Dutch newborns, all with MMC, had been given euthanasia on the grounds that their condition guaranteed a hopeless prognosis (Verhagen and Sauer, 2005). However, in other countries, although forgoing LST for newborns is sometimes permissible, euthanasia for them never is.

Utilitarians on Neonatal Euthanasia
End-of-Life measures (EoL) for these newborns include forgoing life supports and euthanasia. The former measures, which include withholding and withdrawing life supports, are commonly considered permissible as instances of letting die, whereby nature takes its course. But the latter measure, which amounts to actively killing them, rarely is. Utilitarians generally reject the killing/letting die distinction, holding that there is no moral difference between intentionally killing a compromised neonate and letting it die (Rachels, 1986; Kuhse and Singer, 1985). In fact, other things being equal, hastening an infant's death may be unjustified morally while actively inducing its death (neonatal euthanasia) may be justified. After all, letting it die prolongs the neonate's process of dying, causing it more pain and greater burdens for parents, health care providers, and society. A quicker killing as painless as possible is then morally preferable. Keep in mind that the reasons for either EoL are the same: futility, mercy, and the argument considered next.

The Appeal to Psychological Personhood
The fact that newborns with profound mental impairments may lack the psychological capacities necessary for being persons is a reason for the moral permissibility of neonatal euthanasia (and other EoLs). The argument is

1. It is sometimes permissible to kill beings that are not persons.
2. Some medically compromised infants will never be persons.

3. Therefore, it is sometimes permissible to kill those newborns.

In order to avoid discriminating against disabled children, proponents of this argument need support for premise (2). Without it, the argument is reminiscent of the reasoning that sanctioned slavery, racial discrimination, even genocide. In all of these, victims were declared 'nonpersons.' But, given a standard view on personhood, having certain psychological capacities is necessary for having the moral standing of persons, even when they disagree about *which* are sufficient. The facts about infants with profound mental impairments, together with that standard view on personhood, supports premise (2). Yet it is unsettled which capacities are necessary and sufficient for personhood. And not everybody agrees with that view. [...F]or other theorists it is instead membership of *Homo sapiens* that determines which beings are persons. Thus this Appeal to Psychological Personhood has no force with those who reject its premise (2).

The Analogy to Abortion for Fetal Defects

This argument contends that if abortion at the limits of viability (about 24 weeks of pregnancy) is permissible, ending the life of a compromised neonate also is. Consider neonates born at 23 weeks: they have a gestational age and life prospects similar to some fetuses aborted at 23 weeks for their defects. The only difference between them is location, which cannot make a moral difference. Yet the proposed analogy seems weak because actions that are permissible for human fetuses need not be permissible for newborns. For example, location does make a difference in the law, which (usually) counts only newborns as persons, not fetuses.

Reasons against Neonatal Euthanasia

The main objection to neonatal euthanasia runs along the lines of the above objection to forgoing life supports for preemies. It holds that medicine cannot always accurately predict the future quality of life of a severely compromised newborn. Consider infants with the most serious type of spina bifida (MMC), all eligible for euthanasia under the GP. According to critics, "MMC in and of itself is not a terminal illness when treated actively, and it is becoming evident that the majority of these patients, even those severely affected, will survive to develop into dignified adults who are satisfied with their lives. ... The criteria outlined for patient selection in the GP are not supported by long-term quality-of-life evidence pertaining to patients with MMC" (Barry, 2010: 414). Advances in prenatal and palliative care, it seems, now afford to these patients a quality of life that is not as poor as described by neonatal euthanasia's advocates. Although focused on euthanasia for neonates with MMC, this objection generalizes. For, the first 22 patients given euthanasia under the GP all had MMC. If predictions about such patients' future quality of life are often mistaken, that would undermine justification for neonatal euthanasia.

This criticism should not be confused with the objection that legalized neonatal euthanasia is inevitably a slippery slope into lawlessness and the indiscriminate application of the procedure in inappropriate cases. The Dutch experience shows no evidence of these. On another version of this objection, neonatal euthanasia would undermine the ethics of medicine and sow distrust of health care providers. But data collected in the Netherlands (Verhagen, 2013) after the GP became accepted also fail to support this objection.

[Reading] Summary

This [reading] focused on newborns at high risk of death or severe long-term disability. Uncertainty about what is medically best for these infants emerged as a crucial element of the moral quandaries faced by parents and health care providers. In the US, the prevailing standard for decisionmaking had long been parental choice, but with the Baby Doe regulations of the early 1980s became the infant's best interests. Even so, the presumption in favor of honoring reasonable treatment decisions made by the parents (including nontreatment) persists.

Today the groups of infants severely compromised at birth include a great number of premature and low birthweight neonates. The evidence about their grim prospects, together with the uncertainty about each infant's chances of growing up to be healthy—or to have disabilities compatible with a satisfying life—presents parents and health care providers with difficult moral choices. These include whether the medically compromised newborn should receive (1) critical care, (2) only palliative care, or (3) neonatal euthanasia. Protocols consistent with (1) and (2) are used around the world. Regulated (3) is legal only in the Netherlands since 2005. Figure 9.3.1 summarizes main moral arguments for and against end-of-life measures consisting in forgoing life supports or euthanasia. Main objections to the provision of critical care rely on consequentialist considerations of futility and mercy, together with the view that infants with profound cognitive impairments are not persons. Although such objections also favor (3), their strength is called into question by the uncertainty of predictions about the future quality of life of some compromised infants.

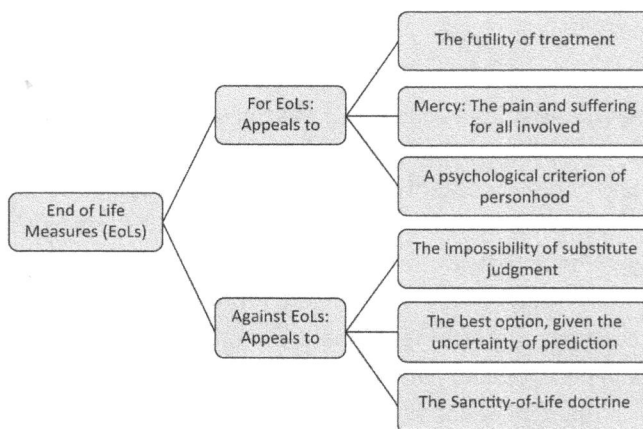

Figure 9.3.1   Arguments for and against End-of-Life Measures (EoLs) for Severely Compromised Newborns

[...]

Additional References

Barry, S., "Quality of Life and Myelomeningocele: An Ethical and Evidence-Based Analysis of the Groningen Protocol," *Pediatric Neurosurgery* 46, 2010: 409–14.

Rachels, J., *The End of Life: Euthanasia and Morality*. Oxford: Oxford University Press, 1986.

Verhagen, E., "The Groningen Protocol for Newborn Euthanasia: Which Way Did the Slippery Slope Tilt?" *Journal of Medical Ethics* 39.5, 2013: 293–5.

Review Questions

Directions: Refer to your readings to help respond to the questions and prompts below.

1. When can a wrong action, such as intentionally ending a life, produce good consequences?
2. How does the premise of "no harm" apply to the different forms of euthanasia, PAS, or neonatal euthanasia? Does this violate or support the moral principles of mercy, beneficence, or autonomy?
3. An interesting provision of the law is called a conscience clause. How would a conscience clause work in cases where a health care provider is asked to assist with a procedure, such as euthanasia, that they object to?
4. If *Vacco* or *Glucksberg* had been decided differently by the courts, how would this affect current laws? How could this affect suicide tourism?
5. Compare and contrast Oregon's Death With Dignity Act and the Groningen Protocol. Are either of these documents more aligned with the Dutch Experience? Would any of this guidance impact the decisions made at Charity Hospital? Why or why not?

References

Cruzan v. Director, Missouri Dep't of Health, 497 U.S. 261 (1990)
In re Quinlan, 355 A.2d 647 (NJ. 1976)

Chapter 10

Access to Care

Introduction to the Chapter

Access to health care is a complex issue. It has amassed attention and debate despite the United States having one of the most advanced systems of medical innovation. The challenge is meeting the needs of individuals and communities.

Health insurance is one of the significant problems. Millions of Americans do not have health insurance, or their health insurance policies do not offer adequate coverage. Even for those who can afford a policy, copayments, deductibles, and out-of-pocket expenses prevent people from seeking care. People may also not be eligible for public programs like Medicaid or Medicare.

Another barrier to health care is geographic limitations. Long travel distances and a lack of public transportation compound the problem. Plus, it can be challenging for those struggling financially to take even more time off work to travel distances and arrange costly childcare for appointments. This is exacerbated by rural, underserved areas experiencing a shortage of providers, facilities, and services, especially in primary care and mental health.

This makes access even more difficult for marginalized populations. Minorities, immigrants, LGBTQ+ individuals, uninsured or underinsured, and homeless populations face even more significant access issues. Structural barriers like administrative difficulties, language barriers, and cultural insensitivity are social determinants of access.

These complexities are further emphasized by the fact that the United States has no legal right to health care. The one exception is under the Emergency Medical Treatment and Labor Act (EMTALA). It provides the right to treatment and stabilization in emergencies. Humanitarians assert that sick and suffering patients should always have access to care. It is additionally arguable that people be treated similarly, resources be made available, and services be prioritized.

Society must consider the fair and equal distribution of care, benefits, risks, and costs so that all patients are treated similarly. The COVID-19 pandemic brought every issue of access and allocation of care issues to the forefront of daily life. The lack of hospital beds, ventilators, vaccines, and treatment cost lives. The failure of strategic disaster planning and the shortage of trained providers with years of higher education forced society to reevaluate processes.

A critical U.S. Supreme Court case about public health is *Jacobson v. Massachusetts* (1905). The Court held that health boards can protect the public by mandating or requiring vaccines. It is a valid exercise of police power and does not violate the Constitution to protect the commonwealth.

This ruling is important because it provides the legal basis for establishing that individual freedoms can be limited for the common good. Public health outweighs personal choice.

When applying major moral theories to access and allocation of health care:

- Utilitarians would view access to care as prioritizing patients who would most benefit from treatment while using the most appropriate care. This view wants something that will produce the greatest good for the most significant number.
- Kantian ethics provides that an action is acceptable if its intention is good. The core idea is that human beings are not mere objects. Persons are worthy of respect and should be treated as such. They believe in universal health care because a just society provides access to health care to all its members.
- Natural law theorists would find that medical interventions must be beneficial to the health and well-being of the patient. For example, abortion is morally permissible if it is done to protect the mother.

Learning Outcomes

After reading this chapter, students will:

1. Define and integrate key terms into discussion, writing, assignments, and prompts.
2. Analyze relevant case law and statutes to predict future trends.
3. Integrate moral theories and principles into corresponding points to consider that extend from access to care, including dividing up health care resources, tight to health care, ethics of rationing, care for a killer, black market in organ transplants, exotic medical lifesaving therapy allocation, QALY to determine quality of life; and federal and state policies.

Key Terms

The following key terms will be introduced and used in this chapter.

- **Duty to Treat:** the obligation to provide care and meet patient needs, regardless of condition or circumstance.
- **Emergency Medical Treatment and Labor Act (EMTALA):** this 1996 law requires emergency departments to provide medical screening and examination to anyone seeking treatment, no matter their legal status, citizenship, and ability to pay. Patients' emergency medical conditions must be stabilized.
- **Justice and Health Care:** a fair and equitable distribution of quality health resources; this includes dismantling the effects of racism, poverty, and barriers to access and working towards sustainable

policies.

- **Patient Protection and Affordable Care Act:** law that provides numerous rights and protections, making health care coverage fair, understandable, and affordable.
- **Right to Health Care:** access to timely, quality, and affordable health care services regardless of social, economic, or political status; race; religion; gender; or sexual orientation. This also includes the freedom to control one's health and body and be free from interference. The United States right to health care.
- **Scarce Resource Allocation:** deciding how to distribute limited resources among competing demands or uses, including medicine, machines, equipment, staff, and the building of stakeholder policies.
- **Universal Health Care:** all people can access full-service health care they need and can afford.

Introduction to the Readings

The following readings focus on access and allocation of health care resources.

"Social Ethics of Medicine: Allocation Resources, Health Insurance, Transplantation, and Human Subjects Research," by Robert M. Veatch and Laura K. Guidry-Grimes, examines how resources should be distributed, including arguments about rationing. It discusses both subjective and objective Hippocratic utility, evaluating patient welfare versus outcomes. Social utility and justice are defined, and ethical issues, such as the right to health care, are detailed. The final section of the article discusses organ transplantation. It highlights procurement allocation based on social utility and justice.

"Resource Conservation," by Cristina Richie, is about the difference between health care needs and wants about medical prioritization. Are some procedures a model of therapy or enhancement?

Selection from "Social Ethics of Medicine: Allocating Resources, Health Insurance, Transplantation, and Human Subjects Research"

Robert M. Veatch and Laura K. Guidry-Grimes

[...]

Allocation of Healthcare Resources

The area of bioethics that poses social ethical questions most dramatically is the allocation of healthcare resources. In the era of escalating healthcare costs, managed care, and global budgets for healthcare, the most controversial ethical issue is how scarce resources should be allocated (American Medical Association, Council on Ethical and Judicial Affairs, 1995; Anderlik, 2001; Daniels and Sabin, 2008; Menzel, 2007; Newdick, 2005; President's Commission, 1983; Ubel, 2000).

The Demand for Healthcare Services

In the United States in 2016, we spent about $3.3 trillion on healthcare.[1] That is more than $10,348 per person and 17.9 percent of the gross domestic product. In spite of the fact that this is double the median of comparable countries and 27.7 percent higher than the next highest country (Switzerland) (Sawyer and Cox, 2008), the health of Americans is in a sorry state. It ranks 43rd in the world in life expectancy at birth[2] and 56th in infant mortality.[3] What is not recognized is that the continual recitation of aggregate social indicators such as life expectancy and infant mortality implies that maximizing aggregate health is the morally legitimate goal. In 2009, over 50 million Americans had no health insurance (DeNavas-Walt et al., 2010, p. 23). By 2016, as the Affordable Care Act began to take effect, the number had dropped to 28 million (Barnett and Berchick, 2017), but increased by 3.2 million people in 2017 as the Trump administration tightened access (Bump, 2018). Still others were covered only part of the year or were woefully underinsured. There are dreadful differences in health based on income, education, and race. Enormous international differences exist as well.

The Inevitability of Rationing

Some people argue that we do not need to ration healthcare. If we just diverted resources from foolishness and waste elsewhere, enough would be available for healthcare. At this point, one can plug in his or her favorite budget target: the defense department, junkets for members of Congress, tobacco subsidies, highway construction, and the like. This may be a good argument when we talk to people outside of healthcare, but still it is not realistic. The cost of doing everything we would like to do in medicine for everyone who would like to receive it exceeds the gross domestic product. And that is without considering obligations to others in less wealthy parts of the world. Rationing is inevitable. There will always be more demands for healthcare services (some of which are only marginally helpful) than there are resources. In such a world, rationing is morally necessary. Even if we recognize that there are enough funds to provide a decent minimum for everyone (and then some), every health plan must exclude some services—not only luxuries and useless treatments, but also marginal tests and procedures for some patients who have high-priority needs.[4] Let's try to get at the moral logic of this rationing, what is often expressed as a movement for cost containment.
[...]

Ethical Responses to the Pressures for Cost Containment

The different ethical principles discussed in this volume offer very different ethical responses to the dilemma of pressures for cost containment. [...]

Ethical Principles at the Level of the Individual

The Subjective Form of Hippocratic (Patient-Benefiting) Utility
The original form of the Hippocratic Oath would have each physician treat for myocardial infarction (MI) by

striving to benefit the patient according to the physician's judgment. That, of course, is exactly what these physicians, including the atypical physician who insisted on unusually long lengths of stay for his patient, were trying to do. The outlier physician's long hospital stays were what was called for by subjective Hippocratic utility. That physician believed the long hospital stays were best, even though colleagues would disagree.

The graph in Figure 10.1.1 is a schematic representation of the cardiology resource problem. It can function as a general model of clinician investment of resources in patient care. The length of stay, which is represented on the horizontal axis, is an approximation of resources invested.[8] On the vertical axis, the aggregate (i.e., accumulated) net medical good done is represented. The curve shows that early units of investment are more efficient than later ones. They do more good than later units, which is another way of saying the early days in the hospital do more good than the later ones. If one keeps investing in more and more days, eventually no more good will be done; the curve becomes flat. A patient who is kept in the hospital even longer may actually begin to experience a net harm. Iatrogenic infection and other hospital-caused harms lead the curve to turn down, indicating that the aggregate good done for the patient may actually decrease.

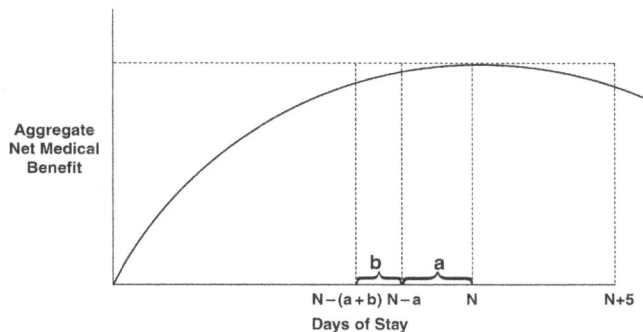

Figure 10.1.1   Aggregate Net Benefit as a Function of Days of Stay

The Objective Form of Hippocratic (Patient-Benefiting) Utility

Shifting from the goal of patient welfare assessed subjectively by the individual clinician to a more objective measure of effects through peer review and outcomes research may, by eliminating useless medical treatment, actually increase the net good done for the patient, while as a side-effect conserving resources. Imposing peer review constraints on the outlier who is the intensive utilizer of days of stay will drive days of stay back to the consensus of colleagues.

This length of stay, symbolized by point N in Figure 10.1.1, approximates objective net medical benefit. Driving care back to this level by peer review is primarily motivated out of the modified Hippocratic concern of objectively promoting the patient's welfare, but resources are saved as a side-effect. (Of course, peer review may also identify some under-utilizers of treatment resources. Aggressive, patient-welfare-oriented peer review will increase expense in those cases. The net savings will be the reductions in overtreatment minus adjustments for under-treatment.) The concern is still patient-centered; it focuses on patient welfare. With Hippocratic utility, cost containment is a fringe benefit.

[...]

Social Utility

Both those committed to social utility and those committed to justice would back down the curve in Figure 10.1.1, moving to the left from the maximal amount of good that could be done (point N) for the MI patients. They would even move to the left of all the beneficial care that the patient desired (point $N - a$). They would do so in different ways, however. Social utilitarians would eliminate expenditures as long as the marginal resource would do more good spent somewhere else. Backing down the curve, they would stop at the point at which the marginal resource spent on MI patients would do more good than if it were spent in any other way. Mathematically, if the highest point on the vertical axis (point N) is designated as B_{max}, they would move from that point to the left until the slope of the curve for MI patients was as steep or steeper than what the slope would be on any other curve representing expenditures for any other purpose. This is the driving idea behind cost–benefit analyses. Social utilitarians strive to identify alternative benefits that could have been obtained from each dollar spent on marginal health resources.

The Oregon Health Services Commission was doing precisely this when it did an initial ranking of possible uses of its Medicaid dollars. It attempted to identify the most efficient uses and ranked them highest. At least at the time, inefficient uses tended to be of two kinds: services for patients who would very likely do well even without them (e.g., the later days of stay for MI patients) and services for patients who were so ill that the services had almost no chance of helping (such as end-stage AIDS patients). When the commissioners and others looked at the list, however, they found the initial results morally unacceptable. Some patients who were, according to their data, inefficient to treat nevertheless seemed to have moral claims, claims that are best characterized as claims of justice.

Justice

In the case of the allocation of limited funds for MI patients, those committed to the principle of justice—at least those who interpret justice to require allocating on the basis of need—would back down the curve in Figure 10.1.1 to the point at which the MI patients would be as poorly off or worse off than any other patients. As long as there were other patients in the system worse off, they would divert the funds. If the DRG system were properly designed and its goal were to target resources for the worst off, the reimbursement would be arranged precisely to accomplish that goal. A perfect reimbursement would exist, according to one who would give justice the first priority, if the $7100 was exactly the amount needed to keep the MI patients from being worse off than anyone else.

If the cardiology department operates on a global budget (i.e., if it allocates its total income among its total group of patients), this would still leave the problem of how to allocate among its patients. If the department allocated its resources solely on the basis of the principle of justice, it would pay attention only to who is the worst off. It would not consider how the funds could be used most efficiently, which would be the concern of the social utilitarians.

Many people believe that both justice and social utility are relevant to the allocation decision, so that some reconciling of social utility and justice is called for.

[...]

Ethical Issues

The legislation is designed to increase greatly the number of people insured while making people pay their fair share of the costs. The ethical controversy starts in the disputes about what counts as one's fair share (Annas, 2010; Brody, 2010; Murray, 2010). The private free market in insurance would be one in which insurers can exclude those who are ill or predictably will have high expected health costs, and young, healthy people with very low healthcare costs would either be charged very low amounts for their insurance or opt out entirely from insurance, posing serious issues. Those born with serious, expensive genetic illness would never be able to pay for their insurance at market rates and the healthy would be uninsured or pay very small amounts.

The Right to Healthcare

This raises the moral issue of whether all humans can, in some sense, be said to have a "right" to healthcare. Certainly, they cannot have a right to all the healthcare they could possibly desire. This would include luxury services (cosmetic surgery) and procedures so expensive that the system could not survive. Likewise, it seems they could not have a right to services not proven effective or at least to services demonstrated not to accomplish the outcome they seek (gold spikes for cancer).

The issue is whether humans have any basic right to obtain certain healthcare services and, if so, who has the correlative obligation to provide them. The services would have to meet criteria that are related to the ability of a society to provide resources and would surely be limited to a core of services that meet criteria of effectiveness and cost-effectiveness. Some would argue against a right to even these basic services on the grounds that society simply has no such responsibility (Sade, 1971). Others, however, offer at least three grounds upon which everyone would have a right to such services and that a society has an obligation to provide them.

(1) Healthcare and Society's Interest

First, at least some healthcare, including some basic health services, may be in the interests of the members of society. Treatment of infectious diseases may benefit others as well as the patient. Not only will society save money; the health of others may require that infectious diseases be treated to avoid illness and death of others. Other services may benefit society in the long run by reducing social costs and eliminating the need for more complex medical services. It may simply be good, self-interested action to provide these services to everyone.

(2) Healthcare as a Social Good

Second, some may view healthcare as a "social good" that has been made possible by society and that therefore everyone has a right of access. The knowledge that makes medicine possible is produced socially. Public funds and private charities generate knowledge in such a way that it would be impossible to say that only those who choose to have insurance have a right to them. Everyone who pays taxes or otherwise contributes to the functioning of social institutions is in some sense partly responsible for the production of medical knowledge. Likewise, physicians and other healthcare professionals receive education that, even in private schools, is heavily subsidized by the government and charities. No physician can claim he or she created the skills of the professional without public support. If members of the society are part of the creation of medical knowledge, they have some right to access to the benefits it produces.

(3) Healthcare as a Matter of Justice

A third ground on which people might be said to have a right to a basic level of healthcare services is more fundamental. The principle of justice, interpreted as most modern commentators would interpret it, requires that social practices be arranged so as to benefit everyone and especially the worst off among us. Thus, according to advocates for social justice, a basic social institution such as healthcare that limited its benefits to those who can afford to pay will have failed to respond to a fundamental moral claim of the members of the society least able to protect themselves. That is probably the fundamental moral basis for the over-whelming majority of more developed countries and many less developed ones committing to some form of near-universal access to basic healthcare. Albeit limited by the resources available to the society, almost all societies provide that access.

Mandatory Coverage

The single most controversial element of the Affordable Care Act has been the requirement that almost everyone have insurance or pay a penalty. For individuals the charge is less than the cost of insurance ($695), but this offends some with libertarian inclinations. For employers the risk is a fee if employees avail them-selves of the subsidy to buy insurance they need because of the absence of the employer's coverage. The principle of autonomy, some would say, is violated by this quasi-mandatory participation. As of this writing, these fees are eliminated beginning in 2019.

Those who reject mandatory participation need to face the fact that many other forms of social insur-ance are mandatory in American society: Everyone is taxed to provide "mandatory" fire protection; everyone with an automobile is required to buy insurance. Other social goods such as education, the armed forces, public transportation, and the social security system include mandatory participation in funding. Even those who have moral objections (say to the military) must pay their share of taxes. To the extent that healthcare is a social good like highways and fire protection, it is argued that everyone must pay a fair share in order for the society to function.

Even if healthcare is not social in these ways, as a practical matter it would be very difficult for society to restrict access to those who have proper insurance. Consider someone picked up unconscious on the street by emergency medical personnel. If insurance is optional and only those with insurance or ability to pay get hospital services, it would be almost impossible for emergency medical technicians (EMTs) and emergency room (ER) personnel to know whom to treat. As a practical matter, society should have a rule that every-one gets treated and should pay their fair share for such services. Likewise, children and mentally incapable adults should receive basic medical services. In fact, the law requires that parents provide such services and pay appropriately for them. Without mandatory coverage (or some sort of bond to cover costs), those inca-pable to decide about their own care could not get treatments that the law has determined they deserve. As a practical matter, mentally incapable persons must be covered, and society needs to make arrangements to cover those capable to choose to reject insurance, at least for infectious diseases, emergency services, and services needed to keep people healthy enough to fulfill their duties to family members and others upon whom they are dependent and their duties as citizens.

The Multiple Lists Problem

This raises a final problem with universal or nearly universal health insurance, what can be called the *multiple lists problem*. It seems clear that, if there is to be near-universal coverage, it has to be limited to some list of covered services. Luxury services, very expensive services that produce only marginal benefits, and experimental services surely will not be included in the basic tier. Many assume that this means there should be a standard list of "medically necessary" services to which everyone should be entitled.

The problem with that is that no medical service is "medically necessary" if one is willing to bear the consequences of omitting it. Moreover, different medical services are considered critical to different people. For some, abortion or aggressive attempts at life preservation are crucial. For others these interventions may be useless or even immoral. Less well understood is the fact that literally every medical intervention decision requires an evaluation of whether the expected benefits are worth the burdens, side-effects, and other costs. The necessity of an intervention is a function of how much the expected outcome is valued in comparison with the negatives it brings.

Thus, different people would choose quite different lists of services as part of the "basic tier" of insured health services. If everyone gets the same standard package of services, the ones who design the list will benefit most; those culturally most distant from the designers (those who have different beliefs and values) will get less. They may not see any value in a covered service and therefore reject it even if it is fully covered, or they may see only slight value, but be forced into a position in which their insurance premiums are used for relatively unattractive services while those they really want (such as alternative medicine) are excluded. Moreover, the people who are in a position to design levels of coverage will come from a socioeconomic position that will not match that of many people who need coverage, and these different positions can lead to diverging health priorities. An evidence-based and thoughtful coverage plan should take into account social determinants of health[10] as well, but expanded reimbursements might not correlate with increased access when there is a dearth of healthcare resources in certain areas (which goes to show how very complex these problems are in establishing a just healthcare system).

This suggests that any single package of health services connected to universal or near-universal insurance will benefit some more than others. If everyone must pay but some are expected to get more benefits than others because of their unique values, something is unfair. The alternative would be to let groups supporting a range of alternative values design insurance packages that could compete in the marketplace. Each would have to cover certain services (ER treatments, infectious disease treatments, and care for children and other mentally incapable individuals). Each would also have to cover conditions for which risk is well known in advance in order to avoid those who know they are low risk choosing plans without that item being covered, thus leaving those known to be a risk as the only ones choosing the packages with the covered service. (Consider that only young black people and others of child-bearing age with sickle-cell trait would be the ones selecting insurance plans that cover sickle-cell disease because others would know they never would need that coverage.) It may be that, even with universal or near-universal insurance such as is promised with the Affordable Health Care Act, multiple plans will have to be offered, each with its own unique bundle of healthcare services provided, and that all of those offered would cover conditions requiring treatment to protect the public as well as those to which the risk is well-known and predictable in advance. Giving everyone an entitlement to a fixed dollar premium with which they could shop from a list of plans with different coverages might be the only fair way to make sure that all cultural tastes are served. Unfortunately, continuing to link health insurance primarily to employment means that, at most, a small number of choices will be available.

It is very early in the U.S. development of nearly universal health insurance (even if systems in other countries are more mature). There will surely be many ethical controversies as well as practical problems as the plan is rolled out over the next decade.

Organ Transplantation

A third area in which bioethics is necessarily social is organ transplantation. (For more detailed discussions, see Task Force on Organ Transplantation, 1986; Shelton and Balint, 2001; Swazey and Fox, 2009; World Health Organization, 2010; Veatch and Ross, 2015.) The ethics of transplantation generally involves three issues: the fundamental morality of transplanting body parts, the ethics of organ procurement, and the ethics of allocation. All of these involve social moral controversies.

Is Performing Transplants "Playing God"?

The first moral issue is whether transplanting human body parts from one being to another is tampering with the human's basic nature in ways that go beyond what is acceptable human conduct. The controversy is exacerbated when the organs come from nonhuman animals. Some people consider organ transplant not only psychologically repulsive, but morally and religiously questionable as well. Nevertheless, the major Western religious traditions all are supportive of organ transplant, even transplants involving the heart—the traditional, romantic "seat of the soul." [...]

Procurement of Organs

Procuring organs for transplant has been a more mundane, but no less controversial, issue. Procurement raises even more directly the question of the relation of the individual to society. Some commentators have held that human organs of the deceased cannot possibly be of any use to the dead person and should automatically become the property of the state to be used for good social purposes, including not only transplant, but research, education, and other medical therapies. Some countries have now legislated that organs can be taken without expressed consent provided the individual or family have not registered an explicit objection (an opt-out model). This has been called "routine salvaging" (Dukeminier and Sanders, 1968). It is the law in some Latin, Scandinavian, and Asian countries. The United States, Australia, Japan, and several other countries, however, have remained committed to the opt-in model of donation of organs.[11] They rely on the belief that the individual has rights against the state, and these rights extend to control of the corpse. Organs may, therefore, be procured only with the expressed consent of the person from which they are taken (or that person's representative). This view reflects the individualism of liberal Western political philosophy. The principles of informed consent, and the related respect-for-persons principles of fidelity to commitments and truth telling, control the procurement of organs in these countries.

Because there is a chronic, severe shortage of transplantable organs from suitable deceased donors, more and more organs are being procured from living donors. Although in theory unpaired, life-preserving organs such as the heart or liver could be procured, such procurement would amount to killing the donor and is not seriously contemplated by most people. Procuring a single kidney, however, is feasible and increasingly common. Also, a part of a liver (a liver lobe) can be procured and transplanted. Since liver tissue regenerates, the long-term consequences are normally manageable.

Living donors of kidneys and liver lobes are almost always close family members or friends capable of consenting to the procurement. Occasionally, an altruistic person volunteers to donate to a stranger, in which case the organ is usually allocated using the algorithm for distributing organs to those on the waiting list for deceased donor organs. These donors (sometimes called "non-directed" donors) must be screened for mental and physical issues and, at least in the United States, by law no money or other valuable consideration can be exchanged. Ethical controversy has arisen over whether unrelated donors (either friends or strangers) are morally acceptable and, more recently, over whether donor–recipient pairs could exchange organs to make the system more efficient.

For example, because kidneys must be blood-compatible, people of O-blood type can only receive organs from an O-blood organ donor. A family member with O-blood could give a kidney to a loved one with some other blood type, but those who are not O-blood type normally cannot give a kidney to an O-blood recipient. One option would be for the non-O family member to give a kidney to the deceased donor waiting list to be allocated according to the normal protocol in exchange for which the next suitable O-kidney from a deceased donor could go to the person in the family of the living donor.

This adds a kidney and shortens the overall waiting time of those on the list because two people (one extra person) are removed from the list. The problem, however, is that the people of O-blood type higher on the list than the one whose family contributed the kidney are passed over and actually have the waiting time increased. Since they were the hardest to transplant, they already had the longest waiting times. This means that the worst off (the ones with the predictably longest wait times) do even worse, even though the group on the wait list does better on average. A defender of maximizing social utility finds this outcome acceptable, but the defender of the moral principle of justice who interprets the principle as requiring fairness will have moral objection (Zenios et al., 2001).

The problem is even more complicated in the case of swaps or exchanges involving two or more living donors (Montgomery et al., 2006). A person of O-blood type willing to donate to a stranger could, instead of donating to the wait list, provide that kidney to someone with O-blood who has a family member or friend willing to donate, but who has an incompatible blood type, say, someone of type A. The A-blood kidney could then be given to a recipient with A-or AB-blood who has a donor available who is incompatible for reasons other than blood type (e.g., a size difference) thus creating a "chain" of donations. If that donor happened to be of O-blood, the chain could start all over. Otherwise the final kidney in the chain could go to someone on the waiting list who has no available donor.

Two ethical problems arise. First, some people find the exchange inherently offensive because it means receiving a stranger's kidney rather than a family member's. Presumably, such people would have the right to refuse to participate, waiting instead for a deceased donor even though it might take much longer. Second, without the exchange, the original donor's O-blood kidney would have gone to the waiting list, meeting the need of the hardest-to-treat group of patients. With an exchange such as the chain described, the final kidney will likely not be usable by the hardest-to-treat group on the waiting list. Thus, the fairness problem re-emerges.

Organ Allocation

Some of the most dramatic and contested social ethical issues arise today over the ethics of allocating scarce organs for transplant. In late 2018 there were more than 114,000 people waiting for organs in the United States. The supply is inevitably scarce and will be at least until artificial organs or animal organ sources become more routine.

When there is an inevitably short supply of a resource, the social ethics of resource allocation becomes crucial. What has been said earlier in this [reading] made clear that, if a libertarian, free-market allocation is unacceptable, two principles will govern allocation: social utility and justice.

CASE 27

ALLOCATING LIVERS: LOCAL VERSUS REGIONAL PRIORITY

The liver is an organ crucial for life. People with severe liver disease need a transplant to survive. There is no treatment alternative as there is with kidneys. About 13,500 people in the United States are on the waiting list for livers. In 2017, over 1200 people died waiting for a liver. Recently, a national public policy controversy over the allocation of livers has posed a stark choice. When a liver is procured from a recently deceased person, that liver can be used locally or can be transported to a more distant transplant center. Serious disagreement exists over whether livers should be kept locally or moved to patients who are further away but with more urgent need. For each patient needing a liver transplant, a statistic called a MELD (Model for End-stage Liver Disease) score can be calculated. It predicts patient death within three months and can be used to determine which patients on the waiting list have the greatest urgency for a transplant. After excluding those who are already too ill to be listed for a transplant, livers are generally given to the person with the most urgent need. The controversy is over whether this system should first be applied only to the patients living near to where the organ was procured or should go to patients with higher MELD scores nationally or regionally.

The federal government's Department of Health and Human Services was concerned that some local areas had more very sick candidates for liver transplant than others. This meant that the current policy of using livers first locally led to relatively well-off patients getting livers when much sicker patients in other areas did not get transplanted. The concern was that equally sick patients were getting treated differently in different areas. The government issued a rule requiring the United Network for Organ Sharing

(UNOS) to develop a policy that would treat patients more fairly (U.S. Department of Health and Human Services, 1999).

The UNOS—the national body charged with obtaining and allocating organs—favored keeping livers locally. Defenders of a local priority pointed to several factors including the advantage of a shorter time before transplant so that organs would deteriorate less, a concern that transporting organs to treat sicker patients might produce worse outcomes, and a belief that people would be more willing to donate organs if they were used locally. The ethical issue was whether fairness requires transporting organs to those areas with the sickest patients or the added advantages of using organs locally justifies the unequal access.

Social Utility

An ethic of allocation driven solely by the principle of maximizing social utility would, in this case, favor a priority for local allocation of livers. At least three benefits support that conclusion: getting organs in better condition, treating patients with predicted better outcomes, and possibly getting more organs. Everyone would agree that it makes no sense to transport organs such a great distance that they become useless. Thus, most people oppose a national sharing of livers. The inequalities of access can be addressed adequately if livers are shared within each of the 15 regions of the country created by the UNOS. But regional sharing poses at least some risk of deterioration of the organs and good social utilitarians—those committed to maximizing the aggregate social benefit—would insist on the shortest possible time between procurement and transplant. They would also insist that the livers go to the patients who can get the most benefit. Often in medicine those might be the sickest patients, but in the case of liver transplant, the sickest—the patients closest to death based on the MELD scores—would not do as well as healthier patients. Finally, they would insist on using organs in such a way that people were most inclined to donate. If a local use would encourage donation (a point that some have doubted), then they would opt for local use even if it meant that the most needy patients did not get the organs. Many at UNOS, including many of the physicians in the UNOS leadership, favor utility maximizing; that is, using organs in such a way that the most possible good is done, even if that meant unequal access (Heiney, 2000).

Justice

Those committed to the importance of the principle of justice in allocating scarce resources—including many of the nonphysicians involved in organ allocation—are not automatically swayed by the data showing that more years of graft survival could result from local allocation. They claim that, especially with a public program such as organ transplantation, all persons should have an equal right to the benefits of the program regardless of their geographical location. For kidney allocation, they tend to favor adjustments in the organ allocation formula to provide more equal access by adding weight to factors such as time on the waiting list, blood type, and a marker for previous exposure to foreign tissue that decreases the chance of finding a suitable organ. For livers they favor allocation to those most likely to die without transplant even if these patients may not do as well.

Balancing Social Utility and Justice

The resolution of this dispute will depend on how we should resolve conflict among competing ethical principles [...]. The tensions between the public officials at the Department of Health and Human Services—the ones concerned about justice or fairness—and the UNOS officials—the ones concerned about maximizing social utility—reflect the underlying dispute about two very different ethical approaches. Not being able to resolve the question of which principle deserves priority, they reached a compromise. They negotiated a policy of giving some weight in the allocation to considerations of medical utility (such as a priority in allocating livers to patients with acute fulminating liver failure) and some weight to considerations of justice, measured mainly by MELD scores. Likewise, in allocating kidneys, some weight is given to predictors of good outcome (HLA match, patient age, and sensitivity to foreign tissue) and some is given to fairness and more equal access (expressed in terms of time on the waiting list). The UNOS Ethics Committee is formally committed to the importance of both ethical principles (UNOS, 2010).

[...]

Bibliography

American Medical Association. "Principles of Medical Ethics of the American Medical Association." *Journal of the American Medical Association* 164 (1957): 1119–1120.

American Medical Association. *Current Opinions of the Judicial Council of the American Medical Association.* Chicago: American Medical Association, 1981.

Barnett, Jessica C., and Edward R. Berchick. "Health Insurance Coverage in the United States: 2016." *United States Census Bureau Report Number P60-260*, September 17, 2017. www.census.gov/library/publications/2017/demo/p60-260.html, accessed August 18, 2019.

Bump, Philip. "3.2 Million More People Were Uninsured at the End of 2017 than at the End of 2016." *Washington Post*, January 16, 2018. www.washingtonpost.com/news/politics/wp/2018/01/16/3-2-million-more-people-were-uninsured-at-the-end-of-2017-than-at-the-end-of-2016/?utm_term=.96ad18895ad1, accessed August 18, 2019.

DeNavas-Walt, Carmen, Bernadette D. Proctor, and Jessica C. Smith. *U.S. Census Bureau, Current Population Reports, P60–238, Income, Poverty, and Health Insurance Coverage in the United States: 2009.* Washington, DC: U.S. Government Printing Office, 2010.

Sawyer, Bradley, and Cynthia Cox. "How Does Health Spending in the U.S. Compare to Other Countries?" *Peterson-Kaiser Health System Tracker*, February 13, 2008. www.healthsystemtracker.org/chart-collection/health-spending-u-s-compare-countries/#item-relative-size-wealth-u-s-spends-disproportionate-amount-health, accessed August 18, 2019.

Veatch, Robert M. "Case Study: Risk Taking in Cancer Chemotherapy." *IRB*, August–September 1979: 4–6.

Social Ethical Theory

Bentham, Jeremy. *An Introduction to the Principles of Morals and Legislation*, ed. J.H. Burns, and H.L.A. Hart, intro. F. Rosen. New York: Oxford University Press, 1996 [1789].

Engelhardt, H. Tristram. *The Foundations of Bioethics*, 2nd ed. New York: Oxford University Press, 1996.

Lebacqz, Karen. *Six Theories of Justice: Perspectives from Philosophical and Theological Ethics.* Minneapolis, MN: Augsburg, 1986.

Mill, John Stuart. *Utilitarianism.* Indianapolis, IN: Hackett, 2001 [1863].

Rawls, John. *A Theory of Justice.* Cambridge, MA: Harvard University Press, 1971.

Veatch, Robert M. *The Foundations of Justice: Why the Retarded and the Rest of Us Have Claims to Equality.* New York: Oxford University Press, 1986b.

Allocation of Scarce Medical Resources

American Medical Association, Council on Ethical and Judicial Affairs. "Ethical Considerations in the Allocation of Organs and Other Scarce Medical Resources Among Patients." *Archives of Internal Medicine* 155, No. 1 (1995): 29–40.

Anderlik, Mary R. *The Ethics of Managed Care: A Pragmatic Approach.* Bloomington, IN: Indiana University Press, 2001.

Baker, Robert, and Martin Strosberg. "Triage and Equality: An Historical Reassessment of Utilitarian Analyses of Triage." *Kennedy Institute of Ethics Journal* 2 (1992): 103–123.

Daniels, Norman, and James E. Sabin. *Setting Limits Fairly: Learning to Share Resources for Health*, 2nd ed. Oxford and New York: Oxford University Press, 2008.

Kaplan, R.M., and J.W. Bush. "Health-Related Quality of Life Measurement for Evaluation Research and Policy Analysis." *Health Psychology* 11 (1982): 61–80.

Menzel, Paul. "Allocation of Scarce Resources." In *The Blackwell Guide to Medical Ethics*, ed. Rosamond Rhodes, Leslie P. Francis, and Anita Silvers. Malden, MA: Blackwell, 2007, pp. 305–322.

Neuhauser, Duncan, and Ann M. Lewicki. "What Do We Gain from the Sixth Stool Guaiac?" *New England Journal of Medicine* 293, No. 5 (1975): 226–228.

Newdick, Christopher. *Who Should We Treat? Rights, Rationing, and Resources in the NHS*, 2nd ed. Oxford and New York: Oxford University Press, 2005.

Oregon Health Services Commission. *Prioritization of Health Services: A Report to the Governor and Legislature*. Oregon: Oregon Health Services Commission, 1991.

President's Commission for the Study of Ethical Problems in Medicine and Biomedical and Behavioral Research. *Securing Access to Health Care*, Vol. 1. Washington, DC: U.S. Government Printing Office, 1983.

Strosberg, Martin A., Joshua M. Weiner, and Robert Baker, with I. Alan Fein. *Rationing America's Medical Care: The Oregon Plan and Beyond*. Washington, DC: Brookings Institution, 1992.

Ubel, Peter. *Pricing Life: Why It's Time for Health Care Rationing*. Cambridge, MA: MIT Press, 2000.

Veatch, Robert M. "Voluntary Risks to Health: The Ethical Issues." *Journal of the American Medical Association* 243 (1980): 50–55.

Veatch, Robert M. "Autonomy's Temporary Triumph." *The Hastings Center Report* 14, No. 5 (1984): 38–40.

Veatch, Robert M. "DRGs and the Ethical Reallocation of Resources." *Hastings Center Report* 16, No. 3 (1986a): 32–40.

Health Insurance

Annas, George J. "The Real Pro-life Stance—Health Care Reform and Abortion Funding." *New England Journal of Medicine* 362, No. 16 (2010): e56.

Brody, Howard. "Medicine's Ethical Responsibility for Health Care Reform—the Top Five List." *New England Journal of Medicine* 362, No. 4 (2010): 283–285.

Murray, Thomas H. "American Values and Health Care Reform." *New England Journal of Medicine* 362, No. 4 (2010): 285–287.

Sade, Robert M. "Medical Care as a Right: A Refutation." *New England Journal of Medicine* 285 (1971): 1288–1292.

U.S. House of Representatives. *Compilation of Patient Protection And Affordable Care Act [As Amended Through May 1, 2010] Including Patient Protection and Affordable Care Act Health-related Portions of the Health Care and Education Reconciliation Act of 2010*. Washington, DC: U.S. Government, 2010. Available at: http://housedocs.house.gov/energycommerce/ppacacon.pdf, accessed August 18, 2019.

Organ Transplantation

Dukeminier, Jesse, and David Sanders. "Organ Transplantation: A Proposal for Routine Salvaging of Cadaver Organs." *New England Journal of Medicine* 279 (1968): 413–419.

Heiney, Douglas A. *Memorandum: Proposed Liver Allocation Policy Development Plan for Public Comment*. Richmond, VA: UNOS, 2000.

Montgomery, Robert A., Sommer E. Gentry, William H. Marks, Daniel S. Warren, Janet Hiller, Julie Houp, Andrea A. Zachary, J. Keith Melancon, Warren R. Maley, Hamid Rabb, Christopher Simpkins, and Dorry L. Segev. "Domino Paired Kidney Donation: A Strategy to Make Best Use of Live Non-directed Donation." *Lancet* 368, No. 9533 (2006): 419–421.

Moss, Alvin H., and Mark Siegler. "Should Alcoholics Compete Equally for Liver Transplantation?" *Journal of the American Medical Association* 265 (1991): 1295–1298.

Shelton, Wayne, and John Balint. *The Ethics of Organ Transplantation*. New York: JAI, 2001.

Swazey, Judith P., and Renée C. Fox. "Ethical Issues in Organ Transplantation in the United States." In *The Cambridge World History of Medical Ethics*, ed. Robert B. Baker and Laurence B. McCullough. New York: Cambridge University Press, 2009, pp. 678–683.

Task Force on Organ Transplantation. *Organ Transplantation: Issues and Recommendations*. Washington, DC: United States Department of Health and Human Services, 1986.

UNOS. "Ethical Principles to be Considered in the Allocation of Human Organs" (Approved by the OPTN/UNOS Board of Directors on June 22, 2010).

U.S. Department of Health and Human Services, Health Resources and Services Administration. "Organ Procurement and Transplantation Network; Final Rule." *Federal Register* 42, CFR Part 121 (1999): 5650–5661.

Veatch, Robert M., and Lainie F. Ross. *Transplantation Ethics*, 2nd ed. Washington, DC: Georgetown University Press, 2015.

World Health Organization. *WHO Guiding Principles on Human Cell, Tissue and Organ Transplantation*. Geneva: World Health Organization, 2010.

Research Involving Human Subjects

Brody, Baruch. *The Ethics of Biomedical Research: An International Perspective*. New York: Oxford University Press, 1998.

Carse, Alisa L., and Margaret Olivia Little. "Exploitation and the Enterprise of Medical Research." In *Exploitation and Developing Countries: The Ethics of Clinical Research*, ed. Jennifer Hawkins and Ezekiel J. Emanuel. Princeton, NJ: Princeton University Press, 2008, pp. 206–245.

Katz, Jay. *Experimentation with Human Beings*. New York: Russell Sage Foundation, 1972.

Lederer, Susan E. "The Ethics of Experimenting on Human Subjects." In *The Cambridge World History of Medical Ethics*, ed. Robert B. Baker and Laurence B. McCullough. New York: Cambridge University Press, 2009, pp. 558–565.

Levine, Robert J. *Ethics and Regulation of Clinical Research*, 2nd ed. New Haven, CT: Yale University Press, 1988.

Lyerly, Anne Drapkin, Margaret Olivia Little, and Ruth Faden. "The Second Wave: Toward Responsible Inclusion of Pregnant Women in Research." *International Journal of Feminist Approaches to Bioethics* 1, No. 2 (2008): 5–22.

Moreno, Jonathan D. *Undue Risk: Secret State Experiments on Humans*. New York: W. H. Freeman and Company, 2000.

National Commission for the Protection of Human Subjects of Biomedical and Behavioral Research. *The Belmont Report: Ethical Principles and Guidelines for the Protection of Human Subjects of Research*. Washington, DC: U.S. Government Printing Office, 1978.

Price, David, ed. *Organ and Tissue Transplantation*. Aldershot, Hampshire and Burlington, VT: Ashgate, 2006.

Veatch, Robert M. *The Patient as Partner: A Theory of Human-Experimentation Ethics*. Bloomington, IN: Indiana University Press, 1987.

Zenios, Stefanos A., E. Steve Woodle, and Lainie Friedman Ross. "Primum Non Nocere: Avoiding Harm to Vulnerable Wait List Candidates in an Indirect Kidney Exchange." *Transplantation* 72, No. 4 (2001): 648–654.

Selection from "Resource Conservation"

Cristina Richie

[...]

Identifying Health-Care Need or Health-Care Want through Two Paradigms

Undoubtedly, drawing the line between health-care needs and wants will be a complex exercise. There will not always be a clear demarcation. Some objections to medical prioritization based on health-care need are made in a spirit of selfishness and anxiety for material luxuries: that is, the apprehension around limiting or refusing opportunities for medical consumerism. Other objections to Green Bioethics might come from the "merchants of doubt": climate change deniers.[1] Both protestations are irrational. There is almost no way that logic can change the mind of someone dogmatically set on consumption despite scientific data, so these arguments will not be addressed. However, other objections to medical prioritization come from those who foresee logistical issues with the dichotomy of health-care need and health-care want themselves. This is a valid concern.

An appropriate resistance to speaking in terms of "health-care need" or "health-care want" comes from the recognition that there are situations where medical developments, techniques, or procedures do not clearly fit into the category of health-care need or health-care want. For example, prosthetics and wheelchairs may not seem to be a health-care need, because not every person requires them. However, since mobility is often a prerequisite for obtaining other human needs like food and water, basic wheelchairs and simple prosthetics for the mobility-impaired are health-care needs.

Contextualization plays into perceptions of health-care needs and wants as well. What may be extraordinary technology in developing countries (e.g., respirators for critically ill newborns) is generally not extraordinary in developed countries. Economic availability, health-insurance coverage or out-of-pocket expense, consumer desire, age, sex, and ability can factor into unclear cases of health-care need. Unclear cases of health-care need—such as breast implants after mastectomy (not reconstruction of pectoral muscles), synthetic growth hormones for diminutive children, pharmaceuticals for "attention deficit disorder," and amniocentesis—require attention because improper categorization endangers access to health-care needs while also risking the provision of unnecessary and resource-draining health-care wants.

To counter this humanitarian and ecological minefield, two paradigms can address situations where medical developments, techniques, or procedures are not immediately apparent as a health-care need or a health-care want. The first paradigm originates from biomedical ethics and examines the contested demarcation between medical function and medical enhancement. Within biomedical ethics, function correlates with health-care need, while enhancement correlates with health-care want. The second paradigm emerges from ecology and examines the distinction between quality of life and standard of living. Under the ecological paradigm, quality of life indicates health-care need, but standard of living indicates a health-care want.

Green Bioethics thus draws on biomedical and environmental ethics from two different but complementary points making the very amorphous concepts of "health-care needs" and "health-care wants" more concrete. These paradigms recognize medical developments, techniques, and procedures as a continuum.

Function vs. Enhancement: The Contribution of Biomedical Ethics

The first way to differentiate between health-care need and health-care want utilizes the biomedical model of therapy or function, and enhancement. As a foil to enhancement, which is generally regarded as medically unnecessary, bioethicists have worked with the category of "therapy," which is generally deemed to be within the goals of medicine. Andrea Vicini notes,

> Frequently, in bioethical discourse, the discussions on technological incorporation have been formulated in terms of the distinction between therapy and enhancement. As this dyad goes, at least in most cases, therapies should not raise ethical concerns, because they aim at promoting healing and, as such, human flourishing. Enhancement, on the contrary, requires more careful discernment.[2]

The discussion surrounding these terms traces back several decades. In 1998, Erik Parens proposed the distinction between enhancement and therapy.[3] Later, in 1999, Gerald P. McKenny favored the use of the terms "therapeutic" and "nontherapeutic" over "enhancement" and "therapy."[4] By 2014, Michael Hauskeller contended that the distinction between enhancement and therapy had been dissolved because the public perception is that enhancement *is* a type of therapy.[5] Biomedical ethics, however, retains the distinction.

Enhancement itself is difficult to define, but it generally denotes a baseline functioning, which is then added to. Bioethical concerns about enhancing medical developments, techniques, or procedures often originate from an anthropological concern for maintaining a human identity.[6] Other ethical considerations are related to justice, access, and of course, potential for abuse. For Green Bioethics, the ethical content of therapy or enhancement is located in resource use.

While enhancement has commonly been paired with therapy, Green Bioethics differentiates between enhancement and *function* for several reasons. Function is more precise, and therefore less subject to misinterpretation, than "therapy." Function has a specific, achievable goal with a clear terminus for medical intervention—that is, bringing a person to a level necessary to obtain human needs, in a way appropriate to age and other limitations of the individual.[7] In contrast, therapy may involve a prolonged period of treatment without end. Function resonates with Howell and Sale's third goal of medicine: "return[ing] a patient to a state of normal wellbeing and function,"[8] thus retracing established ground in health-care ethics. Therapy often has a faddish or trivial connotation to it (e.g., hydrotherapy, aromatherapy). Although the term function cannot escape ableist critiques, neither can therapy.[9] Thus, function will be used.

Medical function does not have to be perfect, but as Daniel Callahan writes, "decent."[10] While even the term "decent" is open to interpretation, it is pithy enough to convey a general sense of use, without digressing into long qualifications at each turn. In determining the difference between enhancement and function, several considerations should be made.

Function or enhancement must account for the unique abilities of each individual. The goals of medicine are not meant to homogenize everyone into one mold of "ability," but rather work with what Jean-Jacques Rousseau considers "natural inequalities."[11] Each person is a mixture of endowed, natural (i.e., biological, genetic) characteristics, capabilities, and developed strengths. A young girl might have an aptitude for speed, but she can also become a fast runner through training and determination. Of course, people are also limited in various ways, and certain physical abilities will be out of range for some. A paraplegic could not become a fast runner through training at this time in medical history, although she might be an Olympic wheelchair-race athlete. A functional or enhancing medical development, technique, or procedure must be assessed relative to each person's baseline.

Function or enhancement is also relative to people in other stages of life. Age-related conditions demand special attention. Middle adulthood modifies the body. "Low testosterone," "infertility," "slow metabolism," and "menopause" are defined as physical deficiencies in some health-care milieus, but these are normal parts of embodied human experience for all people of a certain age. Whether a medical development, technique, or procedure provides function or enhancement depends on the life stage of the individual. One illustration is hormone replacement therapy for menopausal women.

Hormone replacement therapy (HRT) is a treatment given to pre-, peri-, or postmenopausal women to "restore" the loss of hormones like estrogen and progesterone. HRT is carcinogenic and linked to an increase in the risk of stroke and venous thromboembolic events.[12] Hormone replacement therapy "has little if any benefit" according to the *Cochrane Heart Group* journal,[13] yet in the developed world women are often prescribed synthetic hormones to alleviate some of the effects of menopause—like sweating, decreased libido, and bone density loss. HRT does not eliminate menopause; it only masks the symptoms of a normal part of aging.

At the same time, hormone replacement therapy highlights health disparities worldwide. Women who die prematurely are not offered HRT for menopause because they do not live long enough to feel the effects of natural hormonal fluctuations. It is largely an offering for women who have secured an extended lifespan and desire medical intervention for a basic inconvenience. Overall, hormone replacement therapy does not meet a health-care need; it is a medical enhancement, at a particular stage of life, in developed countries. While there are cultural, personal, and social components attached to some age-related degenerations, possible alternatives can also form the ethical assessment of function or enhancement.[14]

Elective hip and joint replacement are now considered a "routine" procedure for people—usually older, white, middle-upper-class Americans with health insurance—who begin to have joint pain.[15] Elective hip and joint replacement do attend to the human need for mobility. Yet, joint pain is oftentimes related to lifestyle and can be prevented or reversed. Joint pain is more prevalent in the overweight and obese who place undue pressure on their joints through their excess weight.[16] Weight loss can alleviate the underlying issue. Non-invasive physical therapies are also an option. The elective nature of some hip and joint replacements, in addition to the presence of alternatives, indicates enhancement. It should also be remembered that not all elective procedures are successful, and many have negative medical externalities.

Incommensurate medical risk to clinical benefit can indicate enhancement. The *British Medical Journal* reports, "Major elective surgery contributes to intensive care occupancy, with a significant mortality rate."[17] Iatrogenic and nosological infections, side effects, and damage to the person—both physical and psychological—can accompany surgery, drugs, and manipulations of the body. While additional medical problems may be present in procedures that address function, the risks vis-à-vis exposure to other diseases and mortality for enhancement are disproportionate to the medical benefit. There is no clinical benefit for enhancement, since by definition it is not a *medical* concern.[18]

Biomedical ethics uses the paradigm of function and enhancement to identify health-care need or health-care want. Medical developments, techniques, and procedures that provide function are typically health-care needs. In contrast, medical developments, techniques, and procedures that enhance beyond what is necessary for human function, as stated above, are generally wants. In order to conserve resources, medical developments, techniques, and procedures that are health-care needs aimed at function should be prioritized before health-care wants that are enhancement.

[...]

Notes

1. Naomi Oreskes and Erik Conway, *Merchants of Doubt: How a Handful of Scientists Obscured the Truth on Issues from Tobacco Smoke to Global Warming* (London: Bloomsbury Publishing, 2010).
2. Andrea Vicini, "Is Transhumanism a Helpful Answer to Contemporary Bioethical Challenges?," lecture, Ethics Grand Rounds, University of Texas Southwestern Medical Center, Dallas, Texas, March 11, 2014, https://utswmed-ir.tdl.org/utswmed-ir/.

3. Erik Parens, "Is Better Always Good? The Enhancement Project," in *Enhancing Human Traits: Ethical and Social Implications*, ed. Erik Parens (Washington, DC: Georgetown University Press, 1998), 1–28.

4. Gerald P. McKenny, "Enhancements and the Quest for Perfection," *Christian Bioethics* 5, no. 2 (1999): 102.

5. Michael Hauskeller, "A Cure for Humanity: The Transhumanisation of Culture," *Trans-Humanities Journal* 8, no. 3 (2015): 131–47.

6. Nick Bostrom, "Human Genetic Enhancements: A Transhumanist Perspective," *Journal of Value Inquiry* 37, no. 4 (2003): 493–506.

7. Thomas Szasz, *The Medicalization of Everyday Life: Selected Essays* (Syracuse, NY: Syracuse University Press, 2007); Didier Fassin and Richard Rechtman, *The Empire of Trauma: An Inquiry into the Condition of Victimhood*, trans. Rachel Gomme (Princeton, NJ: Princeton University Press, 2009).

8. Howell and Sale, "Specifying the Goals of Medicine," 68–69.

9. Alexandre Baril and Kathryn Trevenen, "Exploring Ableism and Cisnormativity in the Conceptualization of Identity and Sexuality 'Disorders,'" *Annual Review of Critical Psychology* 11 (2014): 389–416; Eric Parens and Adrienne Asch, "The Disability Rights Critique of Prenatal Genetic Testing: Reflections and Recommendations," *Special Supplement Hastings Center Report* 29 (1999): S1–S22.

10. Daniel Callahan, "Sustainable Medicine," *Project Syndicate*, January 20, 2004.

11. Jean-Jacques Rousseau, *Discourse on the Origin of Inequality*, trans. Donald A. Cress (Indianapolis, IN: Hackett, 1992).

12. Collaborative Group on Epidemiological Studies of Ovarian Cancer, "Menopausal Hormone Use and Ovarian Cancer Risk: Individual Participant Meta-Analysis of 52 Epidemiological Studies," *Lancet* 385, no. 9980 (2015): 1835–42.

13. Henry Boardman et al., *Hormone Therapy for Preventing Cardiovascular Disease in Post-Menopausal Women* (Review) (New York: Wiley, 2015).

14. Pradeep K. Sacitharan, Sarah J. B. Snelling, and James R. Edwards, "Aging Mechanisms in Arthritic Disease," *Discovery Medicine* 14, no. 78 (2012): 345–52.

15. Sarah Derrett, Charlotte Paul, and Jenny M. Morris, "Waiting for Elective Surgery: Effects on Health-Related Quality of Life," *International Journal for Quality in Health Care* 11, no. 1 (1999): 47–57.

16. National Institute for Health and Care Excellence, "Offer Weight Loss Surgery to Obese People with Diabetes," *NICE*, November 27, 2014.

17. Jonathan Wilson et al., "Reducing the Risk of Major Elective Surgery: Randomised Controlled Trial of Preoperative Optimization of Oxygen Delivery," *BMJ* 318 (1999): 1099.

18. In 2015, a penis transplant raised ethical questions around offering elective, non-lifesaving surgeries that are medically risky. James Gallagher, "South Africans Perform First 'Successful' Penis Transplant," *BBC News*, March 13, 2015.

Review Questions

Directions: Refer to your readings to help respond to the questions and prompts below.

1. Visit your state's website. Under the Department of Health and Human Services division, search for ethical guidance documents for crisis standards of care and ethical allocation of medical resources/services during emergencies/disasters. If you cannot find your state, look at Michigan.gov. How does a state allocate health care resources in times of crisis? What are the moral theories or principles that they adhere to?

2. Using moral theories and principles, what criteria would you rely on if there was a shortage of pain medications? The article *"Social Ethics of Medicine: Allocation Resources, Health Insurance, Transplantation, and Human Subjects Research"* discusses the inevitability of rationing. Are there, or should there be, different criteria for pain medication (beneficence, mercy) or other medications? What about cost containment, as the article discusses?

3. No legal right to health care exists in the United States. This is controversial because many other nations offer universal health care. The concern is what counts as paying one's fair share. The first assigned article discusses social utility. It provides three reasons for this: society's interest, social good, and a matter of justice. Which could be the United States' most potent argument for universal health care?

4. Scotland utilizes the "opt-out" system for organ donation. What does this mean? Do you believe this could work in the United States? What are the legal and ethical rationales for your answer?

5. Considering the argument of health care want or health care need, how does bioethics distinguish between enhancement and function? Should it matter if the function is more aesthetic, such as removing excess skin after dramatic weight loss? Remember, excess skin can also impair function, increase the risk of infection, and affect mobility.

6. Why is relying on research evidence the gold standard for clinical decision-making and a legal standard for malpractice?

References

Jacobson v. Massachusetts, 197 U.S. 11 (1905)

Chapter 11

Health Care Professionals

Introduction to the Chapter

Health care professionals are unparalleled in their dedication to their work. The challenges and concerns embedded in health care are unlike those of other callings. Burnout, understaffing, mental and physical health pressures, civil and criminal lawsuits, physical violence, verbal assaults, and ever-present medical errors culminate in the nerves of highly trained individuals. Stress causes physical and behavioral changes.

These burdens can be eased by constructing healthy environments that foster well-being, accessibility to mental health care, lessening administrative toil, and strengthening public health. Health care professionals have spoken about their struggles and asked for change and help. Coping and communication are key.

The COVID-19 pandemic exposed many problems endemic to our health system. Physician and nurse burnout reached an all-time high. Clinical and nonclinical roles, crucial in maintaining delivery and safety in treatment, faltered. Society's views on health care, including an unwillingness to adhere to science, further strained providers.

Health care ethics manages mental health and increases skillful communication to work through personal and professional dilemmas.

It is imperative to strive to create healthy communication and respect.

Learning Outcomes

After reading this chapter, students will:

1. Define and integrate key terms into discussion, writing, assignments, and prompts.
2. Analyze relevant case law and statutes to predict future trends.
3. Integrate moral theories and principles into corresponding points to consider that extend from health care professionals, including ethics of public health, human rights approach to public health policy, workplace law, discrimination, privacy, cultural considerations, religious considerations, legal and illegal interview questions, federal regulations affecting professionals, employment discrimination, health and safety/

Occupational Safety and Health Administration (OSHA), consumer protection and collection, the Emergency Medical Treatment and Active Labor Act (EMTALA), medical records, professional liability/medical malpractice, and unique pressures in health care.

Key Terms

The following key terms will be introduced and used in this chapter.

- **Abuse:** physical, mental, or sexual harm done to a person through actions.
- **Conscience Clause:** a legal document that provides health care professionals with the right to refuse to assist in specific medical procedures they deem religiously or morally wrong.
- **Infectious Diseases:** bacteria, viruses, or other pathogens that can be spread from person to person or from animal to person.
- **Legal Record:** documentation of the legal happenings of a case, chart, or other evidence.
- **Neglect:** physical, psychological, or sexual harm done to a person through inaction.
- **Public Duties:** the responsibility to educate people about health, disease, prevention, detection, response, organization, and assistance to people and entire populations to promote general welfare.
- **Vital Statistics:** data about a specific region's mortality, morbidity, and birth rates.

Introduction to the Readings

The following readings focus on health care professional issues.

"Making Medical Decisions," by Saul Weiner, discusses essential information that physicians should use when treating patients, such as the clinical state, research evidence, patient preferences, and patient context. The author suggests that patient context, anything in patients' lives relevant to planning their care, is most overlooked.

"Pulling the Plug on the Conscience Clause," by Wesley J. Smith, outlines general principles that should protect medical professionals who must choose "conscientious refusal" of care based on provider moral beliefs.

"The Cost of Appearances," by Arthur W. Frank, points out research that shows that patients strive to make everyone else around them comfortable instead of relying on providers to support them. This is often done out of fear of being labeled hostile or disagreeable.

"The Racist Patient," by Sachin H. Jain, tells the story of an angry patient making racist comments. The physician reflects on the duty of treatment versus limitations, especially when denial of services is appropriate because of an unfit relationship.

Selection from "Making Medical Decisions"

Saul Weiner

Saul J. Weiner, Selection from "Making Medical Decisions," *On Becoming a Healer: The Journey from Patient Care to Caring about Your Patients*, pp. 129–134. Copyright © 2020 by Johns Hopkins University Press. Reprinted with permission.

> Medical decision making can be described as answering one question: "What is the best next thing for *this* patient at *this* time?"
>
> Simon Auster

All physicians who care for patients make medical decisions, sometimes dozens a day. And yet, as far as I am aware, hardly any of us have training in the process itself. I wish I'd learned in medical school that there are four types of information one should always consider: First, there's what you need to know to characterize a patient's *clinical state*, including their medical diagnoses, what treatments they're receiving, and how sick they are. This is the information you acquire by taking a medical history, doing a physical exam, looking at the medical record, ordering lab tests and other studies, and interpreting the results. The second is the *research evidence* for managing that clinical state, accessible in clinical decision support resources like UpToDate or federal websites with guidelines, and by looking directly at peer-reviewed journal articles.

The third, *patient preferences*, applies any time there are choices for evaluating or treating a medical condition that have differing implications for an individual's quality of life. Whereas physicians are best at knowing that treatment A is more effective than treatment B in a clinical trial, only patients can say which they'd prefer, depending on their particular circumstances and priorities. This is especially important when the stakes are high, such as whether to have surgery. However, the situation that comes up most frequently is how far to work up symptoms or findings that are probably not serious ... but just might be. Physicians vary greatly in whether they "chase" things, just watch them, or do something in between. Patients are often not consulted about what they would like. When I staff the urgent care clinic, I see countless people coming in with little puzzles. They range from odd lumps, bumps, and rashes, to quirky pains, to unexpected findings on X-rays and CT scans and slightly abnormal lab values. My colleagues who work up everything reduce the risk of missing a serious condition but put the patient through discomfort, inconvenience, anxiety, and potential complications of the evaluation itself. My more laissez-faire approach spares patients those stressors but may increase the chance that something significant is missed or caught too late. Hence the decision about how aggressively to evaluate a condition should include input from patients. Typically, I tell patients why I'm inclined to watch something rather than refer them for further testing right away, and ask if they have any questions or concerns.

Reflecting on this approach, a first-year resident asked, "So, what if your patient wants you to order what you regard as unnecessary tests anyway? What if they have garden variety lower back pain and tell you they want an MRI to see if they have a tumor, and won't sleep because of anxiety until they find out?" My initial response to such a patient is to ask more questions to be sure I've not missed something that could indicate their concerns are warranted. If it becomes evident that I haven't, I'll share with them my clinical reasoning so that they can appreciate why I'm not worried. I'll also tell them about the risk of false positives: an MRI of any part of the body can expose "incidentalomas" that get everyone worried but are generally better off left undiscovered. Often they just need this bit of medical education to change their mind. If that doesn't help, I'll explore with them the source of their anxiety and try to address what I can: Might they have an undiagnosed mood disorder that needs treating, or know someone who seemed to have a similar presentation and did have a tumor? Finally, if none of that works, there are two remaining options: Order a "therapeutic MRI" on the grounds that while it's not diagnostically indicated and could even confuse the picture, it may provide peace of mind. I'll advise them that their insurance company may not approve the test, in which case they'll have to pay for it out of pocket. Alternatively, I could decline on the grounds that I am not personally comfortable ordering a study that isn't clinically indicated and might escalate their anxiety. I'll remind them that they can seek a second opinion. Which of the two paths I take is a judgment call. Fortunately, it is rare in my experience for a discussion about preferences to get stuck at a point where we can't reach agreement.

The fourth type of information is *patient context*, which [...] refers to anything in patients' lives that is relevant to planning their care. In my experience, this is the one physicians forget about the most. And patients often don't speak up because they may not be aware that some aspect of their various life circumstances is important for the doctor to know about. For instance, someone who is taking a medication erratically because it costs too much may not know there are less expensive alternatives. Hence, physicians have to be on the lookout for signs—such as patients not refilling medications, missing appointments, or saying something like "Boy, it's been tough since I lost my job"—that might indicate the presence of a contextual issue affecting their care.

While these four types of information are all essential to clinical decision making, there are strong incentives for paying attention to the first two but not the third and fourth. You can spend your entire medical career mostly ignoring preferences and context while looking like a perfectly good doctor to anyone who audits your charts. Meanwhile, many of your patients are left miserable and unaware that their problems could be traced back to you. They'll rarely understand that there were reasonable alternatives to the painful surgery they agreed to, or that a less costly medication regimen for their diabetes than the one you selected could have kept them out of debt.

Take prostate cancer screening. My neighbor once asked me whether he should go along with his urologist's recommendation that he have a prostatectomy. His PSA had gone up, and a biopsy showed cancer, a word that frightened him. But not all prostate cancers are the same, and surgery can lead to incontinence and problems having sex. After I printed out a few papers and went over the data with him on patients with similar pathology findings—which indicated a low likelihood of spread—he decided to forgo treatment. Seventeen years later I still smile to myself with satisfaction when I see him out walking his dog, looking as healthy as ever.

It's easy to overlook patient preferences and context because health care quality measures focus almost exclusively on adherence to research evidence, which is also what counts in a court of law. But if the goal of medicine is to help people lead the lives they want to lead, they matter greatly. [...] Consider Ms. Dawson, described in the introduction, who was referred to the preoperative testing clinic prior to bariatric surgery for obesity. Her *clinical state* was that she had a body mass index of 43.6, with complications of diabetes and hypertension. Conservative attempts to lose weight hadn't worked. The *research evidence* indicated that bariatric surgery could lead to long-term remission of diabetes, improved cardiovascular health, relief from depression, and less joint pain. Based on this information, she'd signed a consent form that also described the medical risks of the procedure.

However, eliciting *patient context* (by asking her about her son when she mentioned she was looking forward to the surgery so she could better take care of him) revealed that she was the sole caregiver for a young man with advanced muscular dystrophy who relied on her to bathe and feed him. Because she'd need an open rather than a laparoscopic procedure owing to a prior history of abdominal adhesions from gallbladder surgery, she wouldn't be able to safely lift him for over a month. Her surgeons probably weren't aware of the bind she'd be in, likely because they hadn't asked about her life situation.

When Ms. Dawson was asked if someone else could care for her son while she recovered, she said absolutely not. Personally tending to him was her highest priority—her *patient preference*. With all four types of information considered, going to the operating room looked like a terrible plan and, at Ms. Dawson's request, her surgery was indefinitely postponed. Had she had the surgery, she might have lifted her son anyway, risking opening up a surgical wound. One day she would likely benefit from bariatric surgery, but not then.

Figure 11.1.1 illustrates, using a Venn diagram, how making clinical decisions entails integrating these four sources of information. I first came across it in 2004, a couple of years after it was published, but at the time it only had three rings. I wrote an editorial in the same journal illustrating the importance of including patient context and, years later, added a fourth ring to the diagram in *Listening for What Matters*.

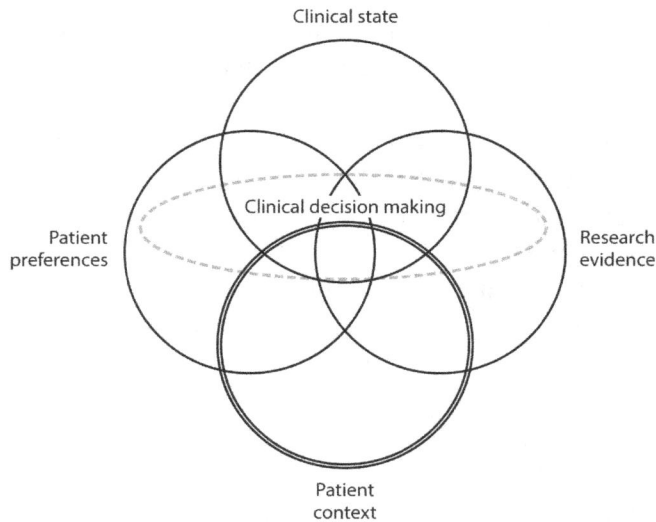

Figure 11.1.1   Clinical decision making should take into account and integrate the four types of information shown here.

My impression is that the major themes discussed [...]—problems with engaging, judgmentalism, and a lack of boundary clarity—all contribute to overlooking patient context and preferences. They result in a striking lack of caring. For instance, a patient requiring long-term anticoagulation was admitted to our hospital with an international normalized ratio (INR) of 9.0, an indication that he had somehow inadvertently ingested way too much warfarin (a blood thinner). He'd come in with a bleed in his shoulder joint, in a lot of pain. In the past, his INR was always between 2.0 and 3.0, where it should be. His doctors did all the right things technically, including giving vitamin K to reverse the effect of the medication and draining his shoulder. Remarkably, however, no one looked into why he had overdosed. Could he have early dementia that had progressed to a point where he could no longer take his medications safely? If so, is there someone to help him at home? Is his family even aware of what's happening? Does he have a pillbox? Is it time to switch to a different blood thinner that may not be as dangerous if you take too much, such as apixaban? No one asked these questions. The thought that comes to mind is: "Would you have overlooked them if this had been your grandpa?"

[...]

Pulling the Plug on the Conscience Clause

Wesley J. Smith

Over the past fifty years, the purposes and practices of medicine have changed radically. Where medical ethics was once life-affirming, today's treatments and medical procedures increasingly involve the legal taking of human life. The litany is familiar: More than one million pregnancies are extinguished each year in the United States, thousands late-term. Physician-assisted suicide is legal in Oregon, Washington, and, as this is written, Montana via a court ruling (currently on appeal to the state supreme court). One day, doctors may be authorized to kill patients with active euthanasia, as they do already in the Netherlands, Belgium, and Luxembourg.

The trend toward accepting the termination of some human lives as a normal part of medicine is accelerating. For example, ten or twenty years from now, the physician's tools may include embryonic stem cells or products obtained from cloned embryos and fetuses gestated for that purpose, making physicians who provide such treatments complicit in the life destruction required to obtain the modalities. Medical and bioethics journals energetically advocate a redefinition of death to include a diagnosis of persistent vegetative state so that these living patients—redefined as dead—may be used for organ harvesting and medical experimentation. More radical bioethicists and mental-health professionals even suggest that patients suffering from BIID (body-integrity identity disorder), a terrible compulsion to become an amputee, should be treated by having healthy limbs removed, just as transsexuals today receive surgical sexual reassignment.

The ongoing transformation in the methods and ethics of medicine raises profound moral questions for doctors, nurses, pharmacists, and others who believe in the traditional virtues of Hippocratic medicine that proscribe abortion and assisted suicide and compel physicians to "do no harm." To date, this hasn't been much of a problem, as society generally accommodates medical conscientious objection. The assisted-suicide laws of Oregon and Washington, for example, permit doctors to refuse to participate in hastening patient deaths. Similarly, no doctor in the United States is forced to perform abortions. Indeed, when New York mayor Michael Bloomberg sought to increase accessibility to abortion by requiring that all residents in obstetrics and gynecology in New York's public hospitals receive training in pregnancy termination, the law specifically allowed doctors with religious or moral objections to opt out through a conscience clause.

This comity permits all who possess the requisite talent and intelligence to pursue medical careers without compromising their fundamental moral beliefs. But that may be about to change. Tolerance toward dissenters of what might be called the "new medicine" is quickly eroding. Courts, policymakers, media leaders—even the elites of organized medicine—increasingly assert that patient rights and respect for patiencts' choices should trump the consciences of medical professionals. Indeed, the time may soon arrive when doctors, nurses, and pharmacists will be compelled to take, or be complicit in the taking of, human life, regardless of their strong religious or moral objections thereto.

A recent article published by bioethicist Jacob Appel provides a glimpse of the emerging rationale behind the coming coercion. As the Montana Supreme Court pondered whether to affirm a trial judge's ruling creating a state constitutional right to assisted suicide, Appel opined that justices should not only validate the "right to die" but also, in effect, establish a physician's duty to kill, predicated on the medical monopoly possessed by licensed practitioners. "Much as the government has been willing to impose duties on radio stations (e.g., indecency codes, equal-time rules) that would be impermissible if applied to newspapers," Appel wrote, "Montana might reasonably consider requiring physicians, in return for the privilege of a medical license, to prescribe medication to the dying without regard to the patient's intent." Should the court not thus guarantee access to assisted suicide, it would be merely creating "a theoretical right to die that cannot be meaningfully exercised."

Indeed, forcing medical professionals to participate in the taking of human life is already advancing into the justifiable stage. In Washington, a pharmacy chain refused to carry an abortifacient contraceptive that violated the religious views of its owners. A trial judge ruled that the owners were protected in making this decision by the First Amendment. But in *Stormans Inc. v. Salecky*, the Ninth Circuit Court of Appeals reversed the decision, ruling that a state regulation that all legal prescriptions be filled was enforceable against the company because it was a law of general applicability and did not target religion.

In a decision that should chill the blood of everyone who believes in religious freedom, the court stated: "That the new rules prohibit all improper reasons for refusal to dispense medication ... suggests that the purpose of the new rules was not to eliminate religious objections to delivery of lawful medicines but to eliminate all objections that do not ensure patient health, safety, and access to medication. Thus, the rules do not target practices because of their religious motivation." And since pharmacists are not among the medical professionals allowed by Washington's law to refuse participation in assisted suicide, *Stormans* would also seem to compel dispensing lethal prescriptions for legally qualified patients even though the drugs are expressly intended to kill.

It isn't just the courts. Many of the most notable professional medical organizations are also hostile to protecting medical conscience rights. In 2007, for example, the American College of Obstetricians and Gynecologists (ACOG) published an ethics-committee opinion denying its members the right of conscience against abortion:

> Although respect for conscience is important, conscientious refusals should be limited if they constitute an imposition of religious and moral beliefs on patients. ... Physicians and other healthcare providers have the duty to refer patients in a timely manner to other providers if they do not fed they can in conscience provide the standard reproductive services that patients request ... Providers with moral or religious objections should either practice in proximity to individuals who share their views or ensure that referral processes are in place. In an emergency in which referral is not possible or might negatively impact a patient's physical or mental health, providers have an obligation to provide medically indicated requested care.

If this view is ever mandated legally, every obstetrician and gynecologist in America will be required either to perform abortions or to be complicit in them by finding a willing doctor for the patient. And don't think that can't happen. A law enacted last year in Victoria, Australia (the Abortion Law Reform Act of 2008) imposes that very legal duty on every doctor. The law states:

> If a woman requests a registered health practitioner to advise on a proposed abortion, or to perform, direct, authorize, or supervise an abortion for that woman, and the practitioner has a conscientious objection to abortion, the practitioner must—(a) inform the woman that the practitioner has a conscientious objection to abortion; and (b) refer the woman to another registered health practitioner in the same regulated health profession who the practitioner knows does not have a conscientious objection to abortion.

Recent California legislation for what could be called euthanasia by the back door attempted to incorporate the same approach. As originally written, AB 2747 would have granted terminally ill patients—defined in the bill as persons having one year or less to live—the right to demand "palliative sedation" from their doctors. The bill was subversive on two fronts. First, it redefined a proper and ethical palliative technique, in which a patient who is near death, and whose suffering cannot otherwise be alleviated, is put into an artificial coma until natural death from the disease occurs. But as originally written, the bill redefined, as a method of killing, "the use of sedative medications to relieve extreme suffering by making the patient unaware and unconscious, while artificial food and hydration are withheld, during the progression of the disease, leading to the death of the patient." In other words, the bill sought to legalize active euthanasia via sedation and dehydration.

Second, it would have granted patients with a year or less to live the right to be sedated and dehydrated *on demand*. And it wouldn't matter whether the physician didn't believe that the patient's symptoms warranted sedation or whether he or she objected morally to killing the patient: Physicians asked by qualified patients to be terminally sedated would have had the duty to comply or refer. (The bill ultimately passed without these objectionable provisions and without the improper definition of palliative sedation.)

Here's another example of intolerance of medical conscience: In the waning days of the Bush Administration, the Department of Health and Human Services issued a rule preventing employment discrimination against medical professionals who refuse to perform a medical service because it violates their religious or moral beliefs. Based on the decibel level of the opposition, one would have thought that *Roe v. Wade* had been overturned. "That meddlesome regulation encouraging healthcare workers to obstruct needed treatment considered offensive," Barbara Coombs Lee, the head of Compassion and Choices, railed on her blog, "allows ideologues in health care to place their own dogmatic beliefs above all." Protecting the consciences of dissenting medical professions is "dangerous," she wrote, because "it's like a big doggy treat for healthcare bulldogs who would love to sink their teeth into other people's healthcare decisions."

It wasn't just overt true believers like Lee. Even before the final rule was published in the *Federal Register*, Hillary Clinton and Patty Murray introduced a bill to prevent the rule from going into effect. Immediately following its promulgation, Connecticut—joined by California, Illinois, Massachusetts, New Jersey, Oregon, and Rhode Island, and supported by the ACLU—filed suit to enjoin the regulation from being enforced. One of the Obama administration's first public acts was to file in the *Federal Register* a notice of its intent to rescind the Bush conscience regulation.

Newspaper editorial pages throughout the nation exploded, opening another front against the rule. The *New York Times* called it an "awful regulation" and a "parting gift to the far right" The *St. Louis Post-Dispatch* went so far as to state: "Doctors, nurses, and pharmacists choose professions that put patients' rights first. If they foresee that priority becoming problematic for them, they should choose another profession." In other words, physicians and other medical professionals who want to adhere to the traditional Hippocratic ethic should be persona non grata in medicine—an astonishing assertion.

Society is approaching a crucial crossroads. It seems clear that the drive to include death-inducing techniques as legal and legitimate methods of medical care will only accelerate in the coming years. If doctors and other medical professionals are forced to participate in these new approaches or get out of health care, it will mark the end of the principles contained in the Hippocratic Oath as viable ethical protections for both patients and medical professionals.

True, healthcare workers enjoy some state and federal legal conscience protections. But a cold wind is blowing, threatening to end the current comity. If Hippocratic medicine is to be salvaged, the rights of medical conscience need to be expanded and made explicit. With the understanding that there may be nuances in specific circumstances not discussed here, I suggest that the following general principles apply in crafting such protections:

- Conscience clauses should be legally binding.
- The rights of conscience should apply to medical facilities such as hospitals and nursing homes as well as to individuals.
- Except in rare and compelling circumstances in which a patient's life is at stake, no medical professional should be compelled to perform or participate in procedures or treatments that take human life.
- The rights of conscience should apply most strongly in *elective procedures*, that is, medical

treatments not required to extend the life of, or prevent serious harm to, the patient

- It should be the *procedure* that is objectionable, not the patient. In this way, for example, physicians could not refuse to treat a lung-cancer patient because the patient smoked or to maintain the life of a patient in a vegetative state because the physician believed that people with profound impairments do not have a life worth living.
- No medical professional should ever be forced to participate in a medical procedure intended primarily to facilitate the patient's lifestyle preferences or desires (in contrast to maintaining life or treating a disease or injury).
- To avoid conflicts and respect patient autonomy, patients should be advised, whenever feasible, in advance of a professional's or facility's conscientious objection to performing or participating in legal medical procedures or treatments.
- The rights of conscience should be limited to bona fide medical facilities such as hospitals, skilled nursing centers, and hospices and to licensed medical professionals such as physicians, nurses, and pharmacists.

It is a sad day when medical professionals and facilities have to be protected legally from coerced participation in life-terminating medical procedures. But there is no denying the direction in which the scientific and moral currents are flowing. With ethical views in society and medicine growing increasingly polyglot, with the sanctity of human life increasingly under a cloud in the medical context, and given the establishment's marked hostility toward medical professionals who adhere to the traditional Hippocratic maxims, conscience clauses may be the only shelter protecting traditional morality in medicine.

[...]

The Cost of Appearances

Arthur W. Frank

S ociety praises ill persons with words such as "courageous," "optimistic," and "cheerful." Family and friends speak approvingly of the patient who jokes or just smiles, making them, the visitors, feel good. Everyone around the ill person becomes committed to the idea that recovery is the only outcome worth thinking about. No matter what the actual odds, an attitude of " You're going to be fine" dominates the sickroom. Everyone works to sustain it. But how much work does the ill person have to do to make others feel good?

Two kinds of emotional work are involved in being ill. One kind I have written about takes place when the ill person, alone or with true caregivers, works with the emotions of fear, frustration, and loss and tries to find some coherence about what it means to be ill. The other kind is the work the ill person does to keep up an appearance. This appearance is the expectation that a society of healthy friends, coworkers, medical staff, and others places on an ill person.

The appearance most praised is "I'd hardly have known she was sick." At home the ill person must appear to be engaged in normal family routines; in the hospital she should appear to be just resting. When the ill person can no longer conceal the effects of illness, she is expected to convince others that being ill isn't that bad. The minimal acceptable behavior is praised, faintly, as "stoical." But the ill person may not feel like acting good-humored and positive; much of the time it takes hard work to hold this appearance in place.

I have never heard an ill person praised for how well she expressed fear or grief or was openly sad. On the contrary, ill persons feel a need to apologize if they show any emotions other than laughter. Occasional tears may be passed off as the ill person's need to "let go"; the tears are categorized as temporary outbursts instead of understood as part of an ongoing emotion. Sustained "negative" emotions are out of place. If a patient shows too much sadness, he must be depressed, and "depression" is a treatable medical disease.

Too few people, whether medical staff, family, or friends, seem willing to accept the possibility that depression may be the ill person's most appropriate response to the situation. I am not recommending depression but I do want to suggest that at some moments even fairly deep depression must be accepted as part of the experience of illness.

A couple of days before my mother-in-law died, she shared a room with a woman who was also being treated for cancer. My mother-in-law was this woman's second dying roommate, and the woman was seriously ill herself. I have no doubt that her diagnosis of clinical depression was accurate. The issue is how the medical staff responded to her depression. Instead of trying to understand it as a reasonable response to her situation, her doctors treated her with antidepressant drugs. When a hospital psychologist came to visit her, his questions were designed only to evaluate her "mental status." What day is it? Where are you and what floor are you on? Who is prime minister? and so forth. His sole interest was whether the dosage of antidepressant drug was too high, upsetting her "cognitive orientation." The hospital needed her to be mentally competent so she would remain a "good patient" requiring little extra care; it did not need her emotions. No one attempted to explore her fears with her. No one asked what it was like to have two roommates die within a couple of days of each other, and how this affected her own fear of death. No one was willing to witness her experience.

What makes me saddest is seeing the work ill persons do to sustain this "cheerful patient" image. A close friend of ours, dying of cancer, seriously wondered how her condition could be getting worse, since she had brought homemade cookies to the treatment center whenever she had chemotherapy. She believed there had to be a causal connection between attitude and physical improvement. From early childhood on we are taught that attitude and effort count. "Good citizenship" is supposed to bring us extra points. The nurses all said what a wonderful woman our friend was. She was the perfectly brave, positive, cheerful cancer patient. To me she was most wonderful at the end, when she grieved her illness openly, dropped her act, and clearly demonstrated her anger. She lived her illness as she chose, and by the time she was acting on her anger and sadness, she was too sick for me to ask her if she wished she had expressed more of those emotions earlier. I can only wonder what it had cost her to sustain her happy image for so long.

When I tried to sustain a cheerful and tidy image, it cost me energy, which was scarce. It also cost me opportunities to express what *was* happening in my life with cancer and to understand that life. Finally, my attempts at a positive image diminished my relationships with others by preventing them from sharing my experience. But this image is all that many of those around an ill person are willing to see.

The other side of sustaining a "positive" image is denying that illness can end in death. Medical staff argue that patients who need to deny dying should be allowed to do so. The sad end of this process comes when the person is dying but has become too sick to express what he might now want to say to his loved ones, about his life and theirs. Then that person and his family are denied a final experience together; not all will choose this moment, but all have a right to it.

The medical staff do not have to be part of the tragedy of living with what was left unsaid. For them a patient who denies is one who is cheerful, makes few demands, and asks fewer questions. Some ill persons may need to deny, for reasons we cannot know. But it is too convenient for treatment providers to assume that the denial comes entirely from the patient, because this allows them not to recognize that they are cueing the patient. Labeling the ill person's behavior as denial describes it as a need of the patient, instead of understanding it as the patient's *response* to his situation. That situation, made up of the cues given by treatment providers and caregivers, is what shapes the ill person's behavior.

To be ill is to be dependent on medical staff, family, and friends. Since all these people value cheerfulness, the ill must summon up their energies to be cheerful. Denial may not be what they want or need, but it is what they perceive those around them wanting and needing. This is not the ill person's own denial, but rather his accommodation to the denial of others. When others around you are denying what is happening to you, denying it yourself can seem like your best deal.

To live among others is to make deals. We have to decide what support we need and what we must give others to get that support. Then we make our "best deal" of behavior to get what we need. This process is rarely a conscious one. It develops over a long time in so many experiences that it becomes the way we are, or what we call our personality. But behind much of what we call personality, deals are being made. In a crisis such as illness the terms of the deal rise to the surface and can be seen more clearly.

One incident can stand for all the deals I made during treatment. During my chemotherapy I had to spend three-day periods as an inpatient, receiving continuous drugs. In the three weeks or so between treatments I was examined weekly in the day-care part of the cancer center. Day care is a large room filled with easy chairs where patients sit while they are given briefer intravenous chemotherapy than mine. There are also beds, closely spaced with curtains between. Everyone can see everyone else and hear most of what is being said. Hospitals, however, depend on a myth of privacy. As soon as a curtain is pulled, that space is defined as private, and the patient is expected to answer all questions, no matter how intimate. The first time we went to day care, a young nurse interviewed Cathie and me to assess our "psychosocial" needs. In the middle of this medical bus station she began asking some reasonable questions. Were we experiencing difficulties at work because of my illness? Were we having any problems with our families? Were we getting support from them? These questions were precisely what a caregiver should ask. The problem was where they were being asked.

Our response to most of these questions was to lie. Without even looking at each other, we both understood that whatever problems we were having, we were not going to talk about them there. Why? To figure out our best deal, we had to assess the kind of support we thought we could get in that setting from that nurse. Nothing she did convinced us that what she could offer was equal to what we would risk by telling her the truth.

Admitting that you have problems makes you vulnerable, but it is also the only way to get help. Throughout my illness Cathie and I constantly weighed our need for help against the risk involved in making ourselves vulnerable. If we did not feel that support was forthcoming, we suppressed our need for expression. If we had expressed our problems and emotions in that very public setting, we would have been extremely vulnerable. If we had then received anything less than total support, it would have been devastating. The nurse showed no awareness or appreciation of how much her questions required us to risk, so we gave only a cheerful "no problems" response. That was all the setting seemed able to support.

Maybe we were wrong. Maybe the staff would have supported us if we had opened up about our problems with others' responses to my illness, our stress trying to keep our jobs going, and our fears and doubts about treatment. We certainly were aware that our responses cut off that support. It was double or nothing;

we chose safety. Ill persons face such choices constantly. We still believe we were right to keep quiet. If the staff had had real support to offer, they would have offered it in a setting that encouraged our response. When we were alone with nurses in an inpatient room, the questions they asked were those on medical history forms. In the privacy of that room the nurses were vulnerable to the emotions we might have expressed, so they asked no "psychosocial" questions.

It was a lot of work for us to answer the day-care nurse's questions with a smile. Giving her the impression that we felt all right was draining, and illness and its care had drained us both already. But expending our energies this way seemed our best deal.

Anybody who wants to be a caregiver, particularly a professional, must not only have real support to offer but must also learn to convince the ill person that this support is there. My defenses have never been stronger than they were when I was ill. I have never watched others more closely or been more guarded around them. I needed others more than I ever have, and I was also most vulnerable to them. The behavior I worked to let others see was my most conservative estimate of what I thought they would support.

Again I can give no formula, only questions. To the ill person: How much is this best deal costing you in terms of emotional work? What are you compromising of your own expression of illness in order to present those around you with the cheerful appearance they want? What do you fear will happen if you act otherwise? And to those around the ill person: What cues are you giving the ill person that tell her how you want her to act? In what way is her behavior a response to your own? Whose denial, whose needs?

Fear and depression are a part of life. In illness there are no "negative emotions," only experiences that have to be lived through. What is needed in these moments is not denial but recognition. The ill person's suffering should be affirmed, whether or not it can be treated. What I wanted when I was most ill was the response, "Yes, we see your pain; we accept your fear." I needed others to recognize not only that I was suffering, but also that we had this suffering in common. I can accept that doctors and nurses sometimes fail to provide the correct treatment. But I cannot accept it when medical staff, family, and friends fail to recognize that they are equal participants in the process of illness. Their actions shape the behavior of the ill person, and their bodies share the potential of illness.

Those who make cheerfulness and bravery the price they require for support deny their own humanity. They deny that to be human is to be mortal, to become ill, and die. Ill persons need others to share in recognizing with them the frailty of the human body. When others join the ill person in this recognition, courage and cheer may be the result, not as an appearance to be worked at, but as a spontaneous expression of a common emotion.

Review Questions

Directions: Refer to your readings to help respond to the questions and prompts below.

1. Perform a search of recent news reports. What legal cases, issues, laws, or concerns have occurred that directly concern health care professionals?

2. Research the medication error case of RaDonda Vaught. First, is it ethical that she was sued civilly and prosecuted criminally for medication error? Second, how responsible should the hospital system be for such mistakes, especially in times of understaffing or computer-related issues? Lastly, the incident only came to light because of an anonymous tip. What does that say about the culture of the hospital and the medical profession as a whole?

3. Scientific discoveries prompt concern about how providers can manage their personal religious and moral belief systems in the workplace. Conscience clauses are legal documents that allow providers to refrain from providing certain services because of religious or moral beliefs. Yet the providers' responsibility to patients includes minimizing disruptions to care. When would you feel the need to sign a conscience clause? How would you go about inquiring about your job?

4. Employment law, particularly contracts and noncompete agreements, makes accepting dream jobs seem less than ideal. It is a necessity to have a competent attorney review documents to prevent civil or even criminal lawsuits. Consider who you could consult for these matters. You will want an attorney licensed in your state with experience, especially with health care entities. Can you find a few resources, perhaps using the state Bar websites that categorize attorneys by specialty area?

Chapter 12

Future Trends in Health Care

Introduction to the Chapter

Predicting future trends in health care bioethics involves considering advancements in medical technology, changes in societal values, and emerging ethical dilemmas. Here are some potential trends:

- Genomic Medicine: As genomic sequencing becomes more affordable and accessible, ethical questions surrounding privacy, consent, and possible discrimination based on genetic information will arise. Additionally, issues related to genetic editing and enhancement will become more prominent.
- Artificial Intelligence (AI) and Machine Learning: AI and machine learning algorithms continue to be included in health care for diagnostics, treatment planning, and personalized medicine. Ethical considerations include transparency of algorithms, accountability for errors, and ensuring that AI does not exacerbate existing health care disparities.
- Telemedicine and Digital Health: Expanding telemedicine and digital health platforms raises questions about patient-provider relationships, informed consent for remote care, and equitable access to health care services. Privacy and security concerns about collecting and storing patient data must also be addressed.
- End-of-Life Care and Medical Aid in Dying: Debates surrounding end-of-life care, euthanasia, and medical aid in dying will continue as society grapples with questions of autonomy, suffering, and the sanctity of life.
- Health care Equity and Access: Addressing health care disparities based on race, ethnicity, socioeconomic status, and geography will remain a central concern in bioethics. It is a priority to ensure equitable access to health care resources and to mitigate biases in medical decision-making.
- Neuroethics: Advancements in neuroscience, including brain-computer interfaces and cognitive enhancement technologies, will raise ethical questions about identity, privacy, and the potential to manipulate mental processes.
- Global Health Ethics: With increasing globalization and interconnectedness, bioethics

will need to address issues such as access to essential medicines, medical tourism, and the responsibilities of high-income countries toward global health equity.

- Environmental Health and Climate Change: Bioethics will intersect with environmental ethics as the health impacts of climate change become more severe. Questions about resource allocation, environmental justice, and the responsibilities of health care institutions to address climate-related health risks will arise.
- Biosecurity and Dual-Use Research: Concerns about bioterrorism, pandemic preparedness, and the ethical implications of dual-use research (research with both civilian and military applications) will remain essential areas of focus in bioethics.
- Emerging Biotechnologies: Advances in biotechnology, such as synthetic biology and tissue engineering, will raise novel ethical questions about manipulating living organisms and the boundaries of what it means to be human.

These trends suggest that bioethics will continue evolving in response to technological innovation, social change, and the pursuit of ethical principles in health care delivery and biomedical research. Ethicists, policymakers, health care providers, and the public must engage in thoughtful dialogue and moral deliberation to navigate these complex issues responsibly.

Accordingly, practitioners should reflect on history to better forecast ways to adjust to inevitable change. While our forefathers could not imagine how the world would change, they offer their experience in adaptation. Embracing history, social sciences, and other disciplines helps society avoid making the same mistakes twice. It provides future guidance. It teaches ways to think, consider, and evaluate.

The future of health care demands innovative agility, and it is imperative to learn from other disciplines: to think in different ways. It is often considered a "soft skill," but it is challenging to hardwire into brains.

This book, especially this chapter, is designed to be a living document. It should be kept out. It should be used. It should remain open to change. Careers in health care must remain available to change. Discoveries, technology, and humanity necessitate continual learning and evolution.

Consider the following technological advances in the readings. When you read this chapter, numerous breakthroughs will undoubtedly have been accomplished. Look up current bioethical issues. What is new? What is outdated? What should be included in this book or your studies?

When applying moral theories and principles to future trends in health, select the topic for consideration and consider the main goals of the following theories. How would utilitarianism (act and rule), Kantian ethics, natural law theory, Contract Theory, and virtue ethics view a possible future scenario?

Landmark cases, laws, and decisions that can be studied to help consider future trends in healthcare are:

Americans with Disabilities Act of 1990 and the Individuals with Disabilities Education Act (1990)

Civil Rights Act of 1964

Drug Amendments of 1962

Emergency Medical Treatment and Labor Act (EMTALA; 1986)

Federal Food, Drug, and Cosmetic Act (1938)

Food and Drug Act (1906)

Hill-Burton Hospital Survey and Construction Act (1946)

Occupational Safety and Health Act (1970)

Personal Responsibility and Work Opportunity Reconciliation Act (1966)

Social Security Act (1935), which later included Medicare, Medicaid, and professional standards review organizations (1972)

State police power: *Jacobson v. Massachusetts* (1905)

Title VI of the 1964 Civil Rights Act

Title VII, as amended by the Equal Employment Opportunity Act of 1972

Learning Outcomes

After reading this chapter, students will:

1. Define and integrate key terms into discussion, writing, assignments, and prompts.
2. Analyze relevant case law and statutes to predict future trends.
3. Integrate moral theories and principles into corresponding points to consider that extend from future trends in health care, including artificial intelligence, voice patterns in disease diagnosis, public health measures, socialized medicine, robots, telehealth, and sins of medicine.

Key Terms

Please address any new terms, ideas, and concepts discovered in your reading and research.

- **Living Document:** a piece of writing that needs to be completed. It is continually used, updated, revised, and edited. It is not static and reflects current and future changes.

Introduction to the Readings

The following readings focus on a few facets of future trends in health care. It can be difficult to have certainty about future health care trends; therefore, many provocative topics are shared. The breadth of potentiality demonstrates the vastness of ethical issues on the horizon.

"The Robot Will See You Now: Can Medical Technology Be Professional?" by William P. Cheshire Jr., MD, analyzes professionalism, automation, and ethical aspects of technology. It pays special attention to religious elements, such as the Christian belief that there is "a deeper meaning of health and illness ... and human life."

"Global Health Issues and Programs: Conceptual Tools," by Peter J. Brown and Svea Closser, highlights five conceptual tools related to public health in a large sphere, paying attention to medical anthropology.

"Seven Sins of Humanitarian Medicine," by David R. Welling, James M. Ryan, David G. Burris, and Norman M. Rich, pointedly calls out the messes left behind by predecessors because of the complex issues that often need to be considered. It claims that how the world practices humanitarian medicine can define us as a society.

"Bioexpectations: Life Technologies as Humanitarian Goods," by Peter Redfield, cites three examples of corporations' help with humanitarian concerns. It focuses on how companies attempt to fight famine only subsequently fail.

"Global Challenges and the Future of Healthcare," by David Lemberg, is a frightening piece about pathogens' spread, treatment, and adaptability. Conflicting information creates distrust, and people see prevention as an inconvenience, as they don't feel they will be affected.

"The Triumph—and Limits—of Socialized Medicine," by Peter Huber, is another look at the intelligence of microbes compared to the world's ability to fight them. Science has moved on, but policies to help people have fallen behind.

"Healthcare Issues in Contemporary Society, Part 1: The Possibility of Precision Medicine," by David Lemberg, discusses tailoring medical treatment to the characteristics of each patient. Using examples of cystic fibrosis and postmortem sperm retrieval, the article delves into numerous challenges.

"Healthcare Issues in Contemporary Society, Part 2: Health Disparities/Health Inequities and LGBT Populations," by David Lemberg, focuses on the need for more extraordinary data collection to understand better the population's needs, biases, and rights to health care.

The Robot Will See You Now: Can Medical Technology Be Professional?

William P. Cheshire, Jr., MD

William P. Cheshire, Jr., "The Robot Will See You Now: Can Medical Technology Be Professional?," *Ethics & Medicine*, vol. 32, no. 3, pp. 135–141. Copyright © 2016 by Bioethics Press. Reprinted with permission. Provided by ProQuest LLC. All rights reserved.

Doctors are not healthcare vending machines, but professionals who understand the difference between negative rights, such as the right to refuse treatment or be left alone, and positive rights, including entitlement to treatment.

–David Stevens[1]

Abstract

As innovative technology replaces more and more of what physicians do, the question arises whether there is any limit to the potential medical capabilities of technology at the bedside. Drug-dispensing kiosks, robotic surgery, computerized sedation devices, and other novel medical technologies bring practical advantages while also raising philosophical questions about the nature of the relationship between the patient and technology that serves as a proxy for the healthcare professional. Moreover, the shift in language from "professional" to "provider" accommodates a detrimental attitude that regards technical performance and human care to be interchangeable. This paper unpacks the

1. Stevens D. Medical martyrdom? How to defend your right of conscience. *Today's Christian Doctor* 2007; 38(3): 18–21.

meaning of professionalism from the perspective articulated by the Christian Medical & Dental Associations and examines its technical, ethical, and spiritual aspects vis-à-vis surrogate technology. A close examination of the meaning of professionalism finds that there are aspects of medical practice that are irreducibly human.

Introduction

"The hard part is giving up control," said I to the anesthesiologist. Astonished, he looked up from the chart and saw that I was still awake. Moments before, he had injected carefully measured doses of midazolam and propofol into my intravenous line. That is the last thing I remember.

Trust

The moment I went unconscious, my life was in the hands of my anesthesiologist, who throughout the surgical procedure diligently watched my vital signs, monitored my oxygenation, and ensured that air reached my lungs and that my blood pressure and heart rate remained stable. Anesthetic agents are no candy; they can cause breathing to stop and blood pressure to drop. If anything were to go wrong, he possessed the knowledge and skill to respond, reassess a complex situation moment by moment, and implement any of numerous medications or procedures as the condition required. Ingrained in that response would be care and concern. Later, when I awoke from surgery, I knew that I had been kept safe by my physician colleague who has dedicated his career to preserving life. The year was 1998.

Enter Automation

If I had had the procedure done 15 years later, my anesthetic might have been delivered and monitored, not by a physician, but by a computerized sedation system. In 2013 Johnson & Johnson introduced an innovative device called Sedasys®, a computer-assisted, personalized sedation system that administers intravenous propofol during select procedures, such as colonoscopies and upper endoscopies. The device monitors the patient's physical signs that indicate the level of sedation and adjusts the rate of drug delivery automatically. Designed to shorten the time of recovery from anesthesia, reduce cost, and increase efficiency, its workings feature alarms and safety locks to prevent dosing errors.[2],[3]

In 2016 Johnson & Johnson pulled Sedasys from the market.[4] One reason the device did not gain acceptance may have been the published findings that same year of a study that found a 13% increase in the risk of complications in patients who underwent colonoscopy with anesthesia services—typically with propofol—as compared to standard sedation with a benzodiazepine and narcotic.[5] As the determining factor in the study

2. Frankel TC. New machine could one day replace anesthesiologists. *The Washington Post*, May 11, 2015.
3. Rockoff JD. Robots vs. anesthesiologists. *The Wall Street Journal*, October 9, 2013.
4. Reader T. Anesthesia use for colonoscopy attracts new scrutiny. *HealthLeaders Media*, April 13, 2016.
5. Wernli KJ, Brenner AT, Rutter CM, Inadomi JM. Risks associated with anesthesia services during colonoscopy. *Gastroenterology* 2016; 150(4): 888–894.

was the choice of drug, not the delivery system, in principle the prospect of replacing the anesthesiologist with a machine remains.

Additional surrogate technologies knock at the hospital door. Increasingly, healthcare consumers are accessing healthcare resources via self-service interactive kiosks that assist with health data entry and provide health screening, including tests of vision, weight, blood pressure, and symptom checkers.[6,7,8] The FDA has even considered authorizing the use of prescription drug vending machines where consumers could enter a few answers to an online questionnaire, self-diagnose, and receive pharmaceuticals that currently require a medical examination and a prescription from a physician.[9,10]

Future generations of these and other technologies that substitute for tasks previously performed by physicians are likely to offer even more sophisticated capabilities. Like many past technological innovations, if used wisely, they can enhance efficiency and make possible new and better ways of delivering healthcare. Unlike previous technologies, they may have the potential to substitute for physicians personally. Can physicians be replaced by technology, or is there an irreducibly human aspect of medicine that should be defined, guarded, and preserved?

Professionalism

Physicians and other healthcare workers are professionals. They avow that they are competent and willing to care for the sick, and they commit to healing as their way of life. Professionals are not the same as service providers.

Physician ethicist Robert D. Orr has pointed out the confusing recent usage of the word "professional" to denote anyone who does something for money.[11] Widespread misapplication of this word has reduced the perceived meaning of professionalism in medicine. At the same time, the term "provider" has slipped into the culture of healthcare. Although the shift to calling physicians "providers" is well-intentioned as language inclusive of midlevel caregivers such as physician assistants and nurse practitioners, linguistic demotion to "provider" is, in fact, dismissive of the professionalism of all these groups.

Word choice matters. A provider, Orr observes, develops a contractual relationship with a consumer, whereas a healthcare professional develops a covenantal relationship with a patient. A provider learns a trade, gets a job, and pursues a business to gain a market share. A healthcare professional, by contrast, under-

6. Wrenn G, Kasiah F, Syed I. Using a self-service kiosk to identify behavioural health needs in a primary care clinic serving an urban, underserved population. *J Innov Health Inform* 2015; 22: 323–328.

7. Lowe C, Cummin D. The use of kiosk technology in general practice. *J Telemed Telecare* 2010; 16: 201–203.

8. Couret J. FDA approves SoloHealth station. BizJournals.com, June 5, 2012. Accessed at: http://www.bizjournals.com/atlanta/news/2012/06/05/fda-approves-solohealth-station.html

9. Mercola J. FDA wants prescription drug vending machines. Mercola.com, May 21, 2012. Accessed at: http://articles.mercola.com/sites/articles/archive/2012/05/21/fda-patient-kiosks.aspx#!

10. Zieger A. Consumer health IT tools could allow self-prescribing. HealthcareScene.com, March 23, 2012. Accessed at: http://www.hospitalemrandehr.com/tag/self-service-prescriptions/

11. Orr RD. Will you be a provider or a professional? *Ethics & Medicine* 2013; 29(3):147–150.

goes many years of difficult training and sacrifice, develops a practice, and pursues a vocation for the purpose of serving others.[11]

With that distinction in mind, one can more easily imagine technology stepping in to fulfill the role of a provider than a professional. Many of the functions of a provider can be approximated, if not replicated, by technology that stores and retrieves information, executes well-defined tasks with minimal error, and performs utilitarian services for monetary profit.

Considering the trajectory of innovation, it may be tempting to imagine that future improvements in technology will eventually bridge the gap between provider and professional. If the difference between a machine as provider and a human as professional is merely one of a difference in the degree of functional capacity, then there would seem to be no reason why a sufficiently advanced computer wired to mechanical attachments could not, in principle, satisfy the definition of a medical professional.

Furthermore, the belief that that gap had been bridged would likely erode the integrity of medicine. Attitudes toward human professionalism would be influenced even by the erroneous perception that an artificially intelligent robot with a stethoscope had nullified the practical distinction between a provider and a professional.

To explore this question explicitly, this essay will examine the meaning of professionalism as articulated by the Christian Medical & Dental Associations (CMDA).[12] A corresponding document for understanding the meaning of a provider might be the owner's manual that comes with the purchase of any automobile, computer, internet service device, vending machine, or coffee brewer, and will not be considered in detail here.

The Technical Aspect

Professionalism has, first of all, a technical aspect.[12] This begins with the acquisition of a large volume of knowledge that draws from multiple complementary disciplines. The technical aspect comprises a system for organizing and integrating this information, a method for analyzing evidence and assessing its reliability, and a way of evaluating its relevance to specific clinical problems. The professional continues to add to this knowledge, learns from experience, is prepared to reevaluate and, when appropriate, reject previously held theories when confronted by conflicting yet convincing new evidence.

In addition to knowledge, professionalism consists of technical skill. Examples include the exquisite dexterity required to thread a fine catheter safely through a patient's arterial arborizations and the precision of the surgeon's scalpel when slicing through living tissue to excise a tumor. Technical skill also involves communication, for example, the delicate choice of wording required to probe into sensitive topics of personal health or convey bad news.

Years of rigorous study are required to gain and perfect this technical competence. Scholarly learning continues throughout the lifetime of the professional, who seeks new knowledge and improvement in the

---

12. Christian Medical & Dental Associations, Professionalism Ethics Statement, April 24, 2014. Used with permission. The primary author was the author of this paper. Archived at: https://cmda.org/resources/publication/professionalism-ethics-statement

skills of application with ever-advancing proficiency. Aiming always toward excellence, professionals establish and enforce standards of practice.[13]

Each component of the technical aspect of professionalism could, in principle, be performed by sufficiently advanced technology. Already robotic surgery is gaining widespread acceptance based on a variety of outcome measures.[14][15] Advances in artificial intelligence might one day push the boundaries of some types of technical performance beyond human capability. As measured by technical competence, a robot might become at some future time an adequate medical provider, but technical competence alone does not make a medical professional.

The Ethical Aspect

Secondly, professionalism has an ethical aspect.[12] Professionalism involves the judicious application of technical knowledge and skill in order to heal and not to harm, in keeping with the principles of beneficence, non-maleficence, respect for persons and their autonomy, and justice. In other words, professionalism requires wisdom. Aristotle called this type of wisdom "phronesis," meaning practical virtue, which involves an ability to discern how and why to act morally as well as excellence of character. Neither sheer information, no matter how voluminous, nor mechanically-guided instrument movements, no matter how precise, are sufficient for phronesis, because clinical judgment and moral probity are also required. Phronesis entails vigilance in avoiding harm, whether that be preventable adverse outcomes or the use of immoral means to a desired end. Phronesis entails acting "with caution and forethought, protecting the patient's health, safety, and confidentiality."[12] Phronesis extends to "a stewardship responsibility to foster affordability and availability of care by applying medical or dental resources prudently."[12]

Phronesis is also concerned with the professional's personal character. Technology may be morally neutral, but the professional must not be. In relation to the patient, the healthcare professional possesses special expertise, and this asymmetrical power over the patient "must always be exercised for the patient's good."[12] The relationship of the healthcare professional to the patient is also one of moral equality. As a fellow human being, the healthcare professional is sensitive to the patient's vulnerability and responds with empathy. Professionalism also entails the discipline of communicating "respectfully with colleagues and team members, acknowledging the contributions of all."[12]

The CMDA position on professionalism states: "The doctor has the moral responsibility to respect the worth and dignity of all patients, who at all times are his or her equals as persons. Moral equality mandates mutual respect; there must be trust and integrity of communication combined with cooperation in giving and receiving care."[12] Accordingly, the healthcare professional "should treat patients without favoritism or

13. Cheshire WP, Hutchins JC. Professionalism in court: The neurologist as expert witness. *Neurol Clin Pract* 2014; 4: 335–341.

14. Jeong W, Kumar R, Menon M. Past, present and future of urological robotic surgery. *Investig Clin Urol* 2016; 57: 75–83.

15. Foote JR, Valea FA. Robotic surgical training: Where are we? *Gynecol Oncol* 2016 Jun 2, epub ahead of print.

discrimination"[12] and choose treatments that "accommodate the patient's perspective, as health is integrally related to the patient's life goals, needs, and personal values."[12]

This ethical aspect of professionalism departs from and surpasses what is possible through technology alone. Technology by its nature lacks the competence to weigh questions of value and purpose; this competence is held and exercised by technology's human designers and users.[16] Ethics, unlike a computer program, assigns to each possible action varying levels of priority according to moral judgments. The physician will drop whatever he or she is doing to respond immediately and assist someone who has suddenly stopped breathing. The computerized sedation system responds only in the way it has been programmed. To the computer, all electron pathways along its circuits are accorded equal weight. All available actions are morally equivalent. All programmed actions, whether injecting an ampoule of epinephrine or dispensing a cup of espresso, are accomplished with equal readiness.

The new field of affective computing challenges some of the distinctions between human communication and automatic computer programming. By decoding patterns of facial muscle activation and voice inflection, computer programmers can write code that adds to computer-generated speech a layer of intonation imitating human emotion.[17] Such software impersonates but does not reflect genuine compassion. Computers can be programmed to provoke emotional responses in humans but ultimately cannot comfort. Algorithms cannot care. This is why the CMDA statement exhorts the healthcare professional in attitude not to be "limited to the reductionistic tendencies of science or economics" but to "strive for ever-increasing moral discernment and knowledge of life's higher meanings and obligations."[12]

The Christian Aspect

In addition to the two previous aspects, which apply to all healthcare professionals—but not necessarily to robots—the Christian healthcare professional recognizes a third and transcendent aspect to medicine.[12] The CMDA statement on professionalism states that the Christian healthcare professional "appreciates and encourages a deeper meaning of health and illness in the context of the special value and eternal destiny of human life."[12] From this worldview perspective, "The Christian doctor appreciates that the patient's dignity derives from having been created in the image of God."[12] The significance of this truth for medicine, both historically and personally, is profound, for it means that every patient is a person of inestimable worth.

Through the Judeo-Christian tradition comes the principle that, in their actions toward all others, people of faith are responsible to a righteous, merciful, and loving God who is deeply concerned for the sick and suffering.[18] The Christian healthcare professional, therefore, is motivated by the expectation of divine judgment to do what is right and to do it well. But unlike the dictates of healthcare policy or law that enforce

16. Cheshire WP. When moral arguments do not compute: prospects for an ethics checker. *Ethics & Medicine* 2012; 28(2): 71–76.
17. Luneski A, Konstantinidis E, Bamidis PD. Affective medicine. A review of affective computing efforts in medical informatics. *Methods Inf Med* 2010; 49: 207–218.
18. Cheshire WP. Twigs of terebinth: The ethical origins of the hospital in the Judeo-Christian tradition. *Ethics & Medicine* 2003; 19(3): 143–153.

compliance through rules and out of fear, and unlike the cold, calculating code of computer programs, God's commands are backed by love, which infuses the Christian healthcare professional with an ethic of care that reaches farther than would be possible through one's own strength.

Furthermore, CMDA acknowledges that the Christian healthcare professional is imperfect. Knowing that he or she is accountable to God for the care provided fellow human beings, and despite diligent effort and the best of intentions, "medical care is sometimes imperfect or inadequate. Faith in Christ provides the doctor with humility, encouragement, and the inspiration to improve and persevere."[12]

Finally, the CMDA statement affirms that the Christian healthcare professional "knows that true wholeness consists not only of physical health and emotional well-being but ultimately in being in a right relationship with God through faith in Jesus Christ."[12] The Christian who is called to a healthcare profession "is given a ministry: humble service of others in a spirit of self-sacrificial love for all, including the neediest and the lowliest."[12]

Alongside the inspired and compassionate healthcare professional, technology made to function as a medical provider falls flat on its face. The swiftest and sleekest robots are spiritually inert. Machines cannot aspire. Erroneous automatons feel no remorse. Whereas technology might be crafted to imitate, and perhaps eventually substitute, for a *provider*, technology that mimics the *professional* can never be more than a caricature. As one physician news commentator put it simply, "Medicine needs human contact."[19]

Conclusion

Several months later I happened to pass my anesthesiologist colleague in the hallway. Embarrassed at my impoliteness for having fallen asleep during our conversation, I apologized. Graciously, he smiled. In that moment of shared humor, we acknowledged a uniquely human experience. We knew that undergoing anesthesia was something more than a temporary cessation of cerebral information input and output. We understood that delivering anesthesia to a human patient meant something more than flipping a switch and counting numbers.

19. Alvarez M. Will doctors be replaced by robots under ObamaCare? FoxNews.com, September 30, 2013.

Global Health Issues and Programs: Conceptual Tools

Peter J. Brown and Svea Closser

Peter J. Brown and Svea Closser, "Global Health Issues and Programs: Conceptual Tools," *Understanding and Applying Medical Anthropology: Biosocial and Cultural Approaches*, pp. 408, 450. Copyright © 2016 by Taylor & Francis Group. Reprinted with permission.

- Many medical anthropologists work in the field of global health, most often as consultants to specific programs. Since the World Health Organization's 1978 proclamation for primary health care (PHC), there have been efforts to institute basic health services and prevention programs on a worldwide basis. PHC represented a change from previous international health programs aimed at single disease eradication. The idea of PHC was to bring health *to the people,* to empower communities through health initiatives, and to decrease mortality through "horizontal" efforts (poverty alleviation and broad health programs)—as opposed to fighting disease through "vertical" programs (those focused only on one disease). PHC work requires sensitivity to local cultural beliefs and values, as well as cooperation with and empowerment of local people. Medical anthropology has made significant contributions to this field (Lane and Rubinstein 1996).
- Primary health care programs often center on mother and infant health. The child survival initiatives have used relatively simple technologies—oral rehydration therapy (ORT), childhood immunizations, promotion of breast-feeding, and the use of growth charts to identify malnourished children for supplementary feeding. These programs clearly work in lowering infant and child mortality (Basch 1990; Coreil and Mull 1990).

- Medical anthropologists study the culture and organization of global health programs themselves. There is a culture to global health programs and policies, just as there is a culture to clinical biomedicine. Health policies develop out of political processes, and local sociocultural contexts shape the implementation of programs. Medical anthropologists have shown that cultural factors *within the health program* are sometimes important obstacles to the success of a project (Foster 1987). An excellent example of an ethnography of a health policy and its implementation is Judith Justice's *Policies, Plans, and People* (1986).
- Some medical anthropologists strive to promote cooperation of traditional ethnomedical practitioners within international health programs. Traditional healers and lay midwives are health workers who often cooperate with biomedical practitioners. For example, Edward Green (1985) has helped organize and train local traditional healers in Swaziland to use oral rehydration therapy. Another area of substantial work is the supplementary training of traditional birth attendants (TBAs) in efforts to reduce maternal mortality (Cosminsky 1986).
- Anthropologists working with global health issues and programs must look beyond cultural differences that may influence the acceptance of health-innovations and analyze the political–economic circumstances that create health problems. Sometimes medical anthropologists working in global health projects are expected to be the experts in "culture" and to work toward the cultural acceptability of an innovation. Although this is important work, it is also important to explain the bigger picture. Political and economic constraints, a history of colonial exploitation, or unjust local governments can play significant causal roles in perpetuating health problems in the developing world—problems that Paul Farmer calls "structural violence" ([...]). The hallmark of anthropology is a holistic approach to understanding human societies and their problems—especially their health problems.

References

Basch, P. F. 1990. *Textbook of International Health.* Oxford: Oxford University Press.

Coreil, J., and Mull, J. D. (Eds.). 1990. *Anthropology and Primary Health Care.* Boulder, CO: Westview Press.

Cosminsky, S. 1986. Traditional Birth Practices and Pregnancy Avoidance in the Americas, in A. Mangay-Maglacas and J. Simons (Eds.), *The Potential of the Traditional Birth Attendant.* WHO Offset Publication No. 95. Geneva: World Health Organization.

Foster, G. 1987. Bureaucratic Aspects of International Health Agencies. *Social Science and Medicine* 25: 1039–48.

Green, E. C. 1985. Traditional Healers, Mothers, and Childhood Diarrheal Disease in Swaziland: The Interface of Anthropology and Health Education. *Social Science and Medicine* 20(3): 277–85.

Justice, J. 1986. *Policies, Plans, and People: Foreign Aid and Health Development.* Berkeley and Los Angeles: University of California Press.

Lane, S. D., and Rubinstein, R. A. 1996. International Health: Problems and Programs in International Health, in C. Sargent and T. Johnson (Eds.), *Medical Anthropology: Contemporary Theory and Method.* Westport, CT: Praeger.

Seven Sins of Humanitarian Medicine

David R. Welling, James M. Ryan, David G. Burris, and Norman M. Rich

David R. Welling et al., "Seven Sins of Humanitarian Medicine," *World Journal of Surgery*, vol. 34, no. 3, pp. 466–470. Copyright © 2010 by John Wiley & Sons, Inc. Reprinted with permission.

The Catholic Church during the Middle Ages had a list of seven cardinal sins.[1] Commission of any of these sins was considered to be a severe act. The list addressed many of our human foibles and included extravagance, gluttony, greed, sloth, wrath, envy, and pride. These "deadly" sins were more serious than the "venial" sins that we all commit more regularly. Forgiveness from the seven sins required confession, penitence, and extraordinary efforts. When considering the topic of humanitarian medicine, it has occurred to us that we could craft a list of seven areas of concern, seven mistakes that are common and continue to challenge those who go forth on humanitarian missions (box 1). With each area mentioned, we provide examples. Finally, we propose the ideal humanitarian mission, with its features.

The Seven Sins of Humanitarian Medicine

Sin #1: Leaving a mess behind

Sin #2: Failing to match technology to local needs and abilities

1. Seven deadly sins. *Wikipedia*. http://en.wikipedia.org/wiki/Seven_deadly_sins. Accessed March 26, 2009.

Sin #3: Failing of NGOs to cooperate and help each other, and to cooperate and accept help from military organizations

Sin #4: Failing to have a follow-up plan

Sin #5: Allowing politics, training, or other distracting goals to trump service, while representing the mission as "service"

Sin #6: Going where we are not wanted or needed and/or being poor guests

Sin #7: Doing the right thing for the wrong reason

Almost invariably, applicants for medical school when asked why they have decided to become a physician, give as an answer: "the desire to help others." Humanitarian medicine provides the almost perfect opportunity to do just that. To go to an area where good care is not available, to provide services that can make a huge difference in the health and welfare of a fellow human being, to provide this service freely and without personal gain—surely these sorts of activities can be life-altering for both provider and recipient of care. And yet we do not always successfully accomplish our goals of providing safe, modern, successful, appropriate care.

This article is in no way meant to denigrate the good works of those who participate in humanitarian missions. We salute all those in these sorts of activities, realizing that there often is real sacrifice made, including the sacrifice of time, money, and equipment. Occasionally, humanitarian missions can even expose us to serious disease, accidents, or assaults. We have great respect for all who go forth to serve. Surely those who aspire to help others almost always do so with honorable intent, and almost never set out to satisfy selfish desires. However, despite our good intentions, mistakes continue to be made, which we attempt to demonstrate in this paper. In our view, there are (at least) seven major opportunities for improvement in the art and science of humanitarian medicine.

The following are major reasons for failures in humanitarian medicine:

sin #1 · Leaving a mess behind. Complications can ruin everything. The death of a child can quickly erase the memories of a thousand successful operations. A good example of this principle is found in reviewing the story of Operation Smile. Operation Smile had been described as a "model charity." It was founded in 1982 to increase vastly the ability to treat cleft palate and cleft lip cases throughout the developing world. This humanitarian effort quickly gained popularity and traction. Supporters of this organization have even included Mother Theresa, Goldie Hawn, and Bill Gates. It became a well-funded charity. The problems with Operation Smile began in 1998 with the death of a child in China. It was alleged that "It was the direct result of a poorly run mission with far too much attention being paid to publicity and not enough to patient safety and standard operating techniques." Medical professionals at the Beijing hospital where Operation Smile conducted the mission also were severely critical, saying, " There was a high number of serious complications where children suffered from excessive bleeding or had to have emergency surgery because their palates had collapsed." Besides the criticism of the Chinese mission, there was a child who died because the oxygen supply had run out in Kenya, and another child died in Viet Nam of unrecognized asthma. This sort of adverse publicity has had a predictable, negative effect upon the organization, which continues to operate missions throughout the world. Major contributors withdrew offers of support, and the organization has under gone some serious restructuring and introspection as a result of these accusations. " After Operation Smile came to Bolivia, several children needed extensive follow-up care at San Gabriel Hospital," according to Dr. Roberto Rosa, a pediatric surgeon there who was sharply critical of Operation Smile and other charities. "This is a form of neo-colonialism," argued Dr. Rosa, saying that Operation Smile had committed "surgical safaris against our children," who are from poor families who are unlikely to complain.[2]

Perhaps some of the difficulty encountered by Operation Smile revolved around the complexity of the cases they attempted. As a rule, the more difficult cases should not be routinely done by humanitarian medicine transient teams, in our view. Sometimes "No" is the best answer when pressed. Surely it is wise to always review the capabilities of the team and never allow providers to do more than they should be doing, given limitations of equipment, time, etc. Numbers of cases performed should not be allowed to trump patient safety and proper monitoring. Large and complex cases should be reviewed and only performed when the team is convinced that the case can be done safely, and that the patient will receive good care when the humanitarian team is no longer on the scene. This implies a great degree of trust and cooperation with local health care providers, which Operation Smile apparently did not always have. We also believe that, ideally, visiting surgeons should be teaching local surgeons how to do the operations and have them fully onboard in the decision-making and care, especially if the visitors plan to leave patients with unresolved issues. If local surgeons feel that they lack expertise in a particular operation and ask for training by the visiting surgeons, then certainly that sort of training is sensible and more likely will have a positive outcome.

One good rule is to offer the types of procedures that are minimally invasive, to relieve immediate discomfort, and that require little follow-up care, especially for missions that are short-term. Thus, removal of abscessed teeth, removal of ingrown toenails, fitting of eyeglasses—simple acts of this sort will create good will and a positive memory of the care given, with little risk of leaving a mess behind.[3]

sin #2 · Failing to match technology to local needs and abilities. Despite what we may think, a vast part of our world does not have high-speed Internet access, or even electricity, or potable water. As we prepare to go off on a mission to a disadvantaged country, we ought to be asking ourselves how we might best go about helping. Generally, bringing the latest and the greatest new technology into a society that is impoverished can be more a cruel joke than a boon for the people. Yet, as we prepare to go, we generally like to surround ourselves with equipment that we normally use, and so this error is very easily understood. Here is a telling quote from a Belgian plastic surgeon, Dr. Christian Dupuis, who has volunteered to go to Southeast Asia for several months each year since the 1970s: "I have seen professors from fancy American universities teaching endoscopy skills in Laos to internists who don't have access to an endoscope. ..."[4] Perhaps this foible is somewhat tied into the desire to do a "first," as in doing the first laparoscopic adrenalectomy in the Amazon basin. It is more about bragging rights than about solid, needed care that will be sustainable after we leave.

2. R. Abelson, E. Rosenthal. Charges of shoddy practices taint gifts of plastic surgery. November 24, 1999. http://www.nytimes.com/1999/11/24/world/charges-of-shoddy-practices-taint-gifts-of-plastic-surgery.html?=health&spon=&pagewanted=l. Accessed March 26, 2009.

3. Minken SL, Colgan R, Barish RA, Doyle J, Brown PR, Welling DR. Waging peace: a medical military mission to Bosnia-Herzegovina. *Surg Rounds*. 2008;31:128–135.

4. Wolfberg AJ. Volunteering overseas: lessons from surgical brigades. *N Engl J Med*. 2006;354:443–445.

sin #3 · Failing of ngos to cooperate and help each other and to cooperate and accept help from military organizations. Nongovernmental organizations (ngos) are in a constant battle with each other as they compete for funding for their particular cause. If they can somehow show that their particular organization is doing more operations, or pulling more teeth, or treating more patients, this degree of activity can translate into getting more funds from the donors. It is well known that these organizations get into contests with each other and spend a good deal of energy and resources trying to look better than the competition. To quote Dr. Anthony Redmond, a British Professor of Accident and Emergency Medicine: "Teams must cooperate with each other. Competitive humanitarianism is destructive and very wasteful of resources, both human and material. There can be pressure, either real or imagined, to be seen to be doing something in the eyes of those who have sponsored the team. This must be resisted. Much useful work can be done away from the glare of publicity in support of the work of others."[5] One area that certainly could be improved is the attitude of ngos toward the military. Both U.S. and non-U.S. military capabilities for transportation of supplies and personnel, for setting up tent hospitals, for bringing in operating room capabilities and blood banks—this sort of amazing capability is available and has been proven effective throughout the world. And yet at times the ngos would appear to rather go without than to be seen working with someone in a military uniform. Ultimately, that attitude hurts the mission. We believe that both sides, military and nonmilitary, could do more to foster cooperation in this regard. Perhaps some progress is being made. Very recently, Navy Captain Miguel Cubano, who is presently serving as the U.S. Southern Command Surgeon, reported that ngos have been offered operating room time on board the usns *Comfort*, and a number of ngos were onboard as the ship was to sail into the Caribbean on its next mission, which began in April 2009 (Dr. Miguel Cubano, personal communication). This sort of planning, which is innovative and unusual, should be congratulated and encouraged in the future.

sin #4 · Failing to have a follow-up plan. A good example of this foible has been the activity of the U.S. military in Africa during the past several decades. We have had a yearly mission to a given area, a humanitarian effort, which is a wonderful and unforgettable opportunity for those lucky enough to be chosen to go along. The problem with these missions is that they have generally never gone back to the same place twice; thus, perversely, instead of helping people, perhaps these efforts actually cause the good people of Africa to resent our well-intentioned efforts. One of us (David Welling) was involved in a humanitarian mission, called Operation Red Flag, to northern Cameroon in March 2000. This mission lasted almost a month. It involved several hundred medical and support military personnel, mainly stationed in Germany, who were transported via C-17 and B-747 aircraft to Garoua, Cameroon. Tons of supplies were brought in, as well as vehicles and other ancillary equipment. We presented the hospital with a vast array of new equipment, including autoclaves and operating room tables. Our teams built an X-ray suite at the military hospital. Teams went to villages, where wells were drilled, vaccinations were given, teeth pulled, and eyeglasses distributed. We were very kindly hosted by the local populace, and when we finally left, dinners were held in our honor, toasts were made, and we said goodbye to our new friends. But what must the good people of Garoua think of those Americans now? Surely the supplies are long gone, and the equipment needs maintenance or replacement. Those who had our care no doubt need follow-up. It was almost a cruel joke, tantamount to taking a little child to Disneyland for 15 minutes, and then getting back into the car and leaving forever. We had given the

5. Lumley JSP, Ryan JM, Baxter PJ, Kirby N. *Handbook of the Medical Care of Catastrophes*. London: Royal Society of Medicine Press Limited; 1996:37.

citizens of Garoua just a taste of modern medicine, just a brief look at what might be. And then we left. Surely we should never have one-time-only missions. We should have an ongoing, regular visit schedule. We should see our patients again and again. We should know and have ongoing dialogue with our medical colleagues in these countries. None of this was done after the Cameroon mission. It is much better to pick one country and continue to serve it well, than to hopscotch all over Africa, going everywhere and truly getting nowhere.

sin #5 · Allowing politics, training, or other distracting goals to trump service, while representing the mission as "service." The U.S. Navy has two large hospital ships, the usns *Comfort* and the usns *Mercy*. The *Comfort* is berthed in Baltimore, Mary land, and the *Mercy* in California. Our Navy has fairly frequently used these ships to go on "humanitarian" cruises, as well as for response to natural and manmade disasters. For humanitarian missions, the *Comfort* usually goes to the Caribbean, while the *Mercy* goes to the South Pacific. Typically, at the end of a cruise, the Navy will announce the results of these missions, with invariably positive publicity. For example, a 2007 Caribbean tour by the *Comfort* involved more than 500 personnel and lasted several months; 98,000 patients were seen, 1,170 surgeries were performed, 32,322 shots were given, 122,245 prescriptions were filled, 24,242 eyeglasses were fitted, 3,968 teeth were pulled, and 17,772 animals were treated. Schools were built, and even the U.S. Navy Show Band participated.[6] On another mission, the *Mercy* left in May 2008, on a Southeast Pacific voyage, and after several months, reported that their providers had examined more than 90,000 patients and had performed almost 1,400 operations.[7] Obviously, for those aboard for these missions, this was a remarkable experience. But truly it was more about photo opportunities, training, diplomacy, and "showing the flag" than about service. These huge ships (894 feet long) are not well-suited to these missions. At times in the Caribbean, the *Comfort* was required to anchor a dozen miles offshore, relying on helicopters and smaller boats to ferry patients back and forth. Each port in the Caribbean was visited for about a week, and the visits were not always well-coordinated with local organizations, which at times were not even consulted. Thus, resources were not maximized. Even Fidel Castro weighed in on this mission and was quoted as saying this about our efforts, and he has a good point: "You can't carry out medical programs in episodes."[8] Interestingly, President Barack Obama, while attending a summit of the hemisphere's leaders in Trinidad and Tobago in April 2009, seemed to validate what Castro had previously inferred. President Obama felt that the United States could learn a lesson from Cuba, which for decades has sent doctors to other countries throughout Latin America to care for the poor. The policy has won Cuban leaders Fidel and Raul Castro deep goodwill in the region.[9] Apparently, the Cuban doctors have correctly realized that by staying in one place for a prolonged period of time, they can have maximum impact with the local populace. For a small and poor country, Cuba has made remarkable contributions to reducing infant mortality and helping disaster victims throughout the world. During the past four decades, some 52,000 doctors and nurses have been sent to 95 needy countries. Recently large numbers of doctors and nurses have been sent to Venezuela, with some subsequent discontent voiced by Cuban citizens, who now are noticing increased waiting times, and

6. http://www.southcom.mil/AppsSC/factfiles.php?id=6. Accessed April 20, 2009.

7. Davis KD, Douglas T, Kuncir E. Pacific Partnership 2008: U.S. Navy Fellows provide humanitarian assistance in Southeast Asia. *Bull Am Coll Surg.* 2009;94:14–23.

8. http://www.flacso.org/hemisferio/al-eeuu/boletines/02/86/rel_07.pdf. Accessed April 20, 2009.

9. Wilson S. Obama closes summit, vows broader engagement with Latin America. *Washington Post.* April 20, 2009; A6.

difficulty gaining access to routine care.[10] Cuba also has helped to establish medical schools in a number of third-world countries.[11]

These U.S. Navy missions must be great for training and for projecting power and showing the flag, but prob ably could be modified by using smaller ships and more frequent missions to the same places. The *Comfort* and the *Mercy* have never been proven able to reach a disaster site in a timely manner, and their attempts at humanitarian medicine have not always been convincing in the aggregate. The last usns *Comfort* mission to the Caribbean began on April 1, 2009.[12]

sin #6 · Going where we are not wanted or needed and/or being poor guests. Dr. Anthony Redmond teaches us that we need an official request to go into an area in need, asking for our specific help. He states this: "The pressure to do something immediately can be considerable. Emotive television and press reports galvanize public opinion into demands for immediate action. However, without recognized terms of reference and a clear mandate to enter and work in another country, foreign teams will at best be stranded at airports and at worst add considerably to the problems of an already beleaguered nation. Time spent in securing a safe passage through and identifying a task to be completed will result in a shorter journey to the scene."[5] Dr. Redmond also talks about the necessity of doing what the local officials want, instead of what we think they may need. "If assistance is to be most effective it has to be organized. Local officials are in charge and must be allowed to develop and execute their plans with foreign teams there as a resource and not a threat. When a team has gained local confidence and developed good local relationships they will have a better knowledge of local requirements. This process of 'bedding in' to the local network can be completed within 24 hours."[5] Mr. Jim Ryan, a surgeon from the United Kingdom and someone well-experienced in humanitarian medicine, relates seeing a whole team from Scandinavia, which had, with the very best of intentions, responded to the tsunami disaster in Sri Lanka without first getting permission from the government. Despite their great expertise and extensive equipment, they were sequestered and were not allowed to leave their compound, let alone go out and help the victims. As to how one should conduct oneself when on a humanitarian mission, a dose of humility might get us off on the right foot as we begin. Anything that looks like boorish behavior, or condescension, or a patronizing attitude—any such behavior is detrimental to our efforts and will leave an unpleasant memory of us for those who would be our patients and our colleagues. We need to be very careful with local customs and mores. How we dress, how we act, what we drink—all of these activities will define us to our hosts. We can learn much from third-world providers, as they maximize what they have in supplies, and innovate to give their patients the very best care possible. We should go with the desire to see a different way to render care, instead of insisting that our way is the only correct way possible.

sin #7 · Doing the right thing for the wrong reason. In *Murder in the Cathedral*, T.S. Eliot wrote about the various temptations that Thomas the Archbishop suffered through, and the very last was the most difficult. As Thomas proclaimed: "The last temptation is the greatest treason: To do the right deed for the wrong rea-

10. Lakshmanan, I. A. R. As Cuba loans doctors abroad, some patients object at home. *Boston Globe*. August 25, 2005. http://archive.boston.com/news/world/latinamerica/articles/2005/08/25/as_cuba_loans_doctors_abroad_some_patients_object_at_home/.
11. http://www.medicc.org/ns/index.php?s=46&p=12. Accessed May 20, 2009.
12. http://www.southcom.mil/appssc/factfiles.php?id=103. Accessed April 20, 2009.

son."[13] The list of wrong reasons to go off on a humanitarian mission is potentially a long list, and no doubt would vary somewhat from person to person. To name a few reasons not to go, one might include the desire to go on an unusual vacation, bragging rights for having done a "first," the desire to perform a large number of complex cases quickly (without the niceties of informed consent, proper monitoring, planned follow-up, and without training the local surgeons to do the procedures themselves), to gain fame, to have a free trip to an exotic land, or to somehow get an advantage in academia. The corollary to this last observation would be that we should go forth with pure motives, with a well-thought-out plan of action, including host nation physicians, avoiding the types of operations that lend themselves to long-term complications, and with a teachable, humble attitude.

Summary

We have listed some of the common mistakes and pitfalls that can beset those who would go on humanitarian missions, with thoughts about how we might improve in this regard. The importance of doing humanitarian medicine properly cannot be overemphasized. To maximize our effectiveness as humanitarian providers, more time should be spent thinking about the details of a given mission. Motives should be questioned. We ought to aggressively plan activities that will do the most good for our patients, and we ought to shun those activities that are more designed for our own personal aggrandizement. There is an inexhaustible demand for modern medicine throughout the world, and we face that demand with finite resources and human foibles. How we go about doing humanitarian medicine can define us, for better or for worse.

13. Eliot TS. Murder in the cathedral. In: Brooks C, Purser JT, Warren RF, eds., *An Approach to Literature*. 4th ed. New York: Appleton-Century-Crofts; 1964:816.

Selection from "Bioexpectations: Life Technologies as Humanitarian Goods"

Peter Redfield

Peter Redfield, Selection from "Bioexpectations: Life Technologies as Humanitarian Goods," *Public Culture*, vol. 24, no. 1, pp. 157–184, 337–340. Copyright © 2012 by Duke University Press. Reprinted with permission.

[...]

Case 2: Plumpy'nut and Therapeutic Food

In contrast to DNDi, my next three examples all feature corporations. As such they disrupt the nonprofit conventions of the aid world that figure humanitarian concern through charity and the gift. At the same time, these corporations participate in the greater flow of funding among multilateral and state agencies, philanthropic foundations, ngos, and concerned individuals. This "aid market" of donors and beneficiaries has its own calculus of exchange. Within it, sustainability is buoyed or limited by media exposure, finds a measure in grant cycles, and ultimately depends on noneconomic values such as humanitarian sentiment.

I begin with recent developments in "ready-to-use therapeutic food" (rutf), designed for small children facing malnutrition. The most prominent among these is a packaged mixture of peanuts, sugar, vegetable fat, and milk powder, patented by the French company Nutriset in the name of "nutritional autonomy" and licensed under the unforgettable name of Plumpy'nut. Plumpy'nut not only satisfies the nutritional needs of children in a palatable way but also remains simple to manufacture, easy to store, and hygienic to administer. The Nutriset website cheerfully explains the general logic of rutf:

As a ready-to-use food, Plumpy'nut® requires no preparation, no dilution in water prior to use, no cooking, and it can be consumed direct from the sachet. Because it can be used at home without any preparation, under the supervision of the mother or another member of the family, Plumpy'nut® makes it possible to treat the majority of children suffering from severe acute malnutrition without them needing to be hospitalized. This has made it possible to considerably increase the number of malnourished children treated, while improving adherence to the regularity of the treatment, and the recovery rate.[1]

A prepackaged super food can compensate for a lack of sanitation and expertise. Administered in the absence of nutritionists or hospitals—even a cooking fire or clean water—its hermetically sealed contents survive any manner of social disruption to arrive unspoiled. Plumpy'nut floats free from a functioning health system. In this sense it compensates for state inadequacies and extends the reach of international aid. Packaged in individual servings of 92 grams each, a carton of the substance can bring a child to targeted weight in six to ten weeks.

The subject of debate and discussion among humanitarian and development experts, such foodstuffs constitute a nutritional standing reserve, one circulating through an explicitly humanitarian market. Founded in 1986, Nutriset seeks to follow a commitment to "invent, produce and make accessible solutions for the treatment and prevention of malnutrition." It does so as a private company claiming an ethical purpose under the slogan "Nutritional autonomy for all." Based in Normandy, it remains of modest size, employing some 120 people and with 52 million euros in turnover in 2009. The company estimates that its star product has "treated" a million children, with another half million benefiting from supplemental alternatives. Nonetheless, Nutriset's owner ship of manufacturing license agreements has been the matter of some controversy (Motavalli 2009; Rice 2010). Who should control the rights to such a recipe? In its own small, sticky way, Plumpy'nut provokes similar ethical debates to those of commercial pharmaceutical production and poor populations, pitting intellectual property rights against humanitarian needs.

The large-scale deployment of rutfs under famine has likewise provoked disputes. In 2005 msf undertook a massive program in response to malnutrition in Niger, adopting a strategy of outpatient home-based care. Using rutfs rather than a standard inpatient therapeutic feeding center (tfc), the organization managed to treat some 63,000 children while achieving similar success rates (Tectonidis 2006). Nonetheless, the response generated criticism from those invested in a developmental approach and, consequently, invested in markets and their regulation by the state. Following a meeting with regional states and donors in Dakar, the un Office for the Coordination of Humanitarian Affairs (ocha) issued a press release calling such humanitarian aid "a temporary, inappropriate and expensive palliative."[2] msf fired back:

> Behind the generic term "humanitarian aid," it is free food distribution that is being stigmatized. Our United Nations colleague's concern is unjustified however; the figures even show that it is invalid: whereas international food aid in Niger represented 20% of national production in 1984, it is now down to no more than 2% twenty years later. ... Social welfare policies have negative effects that must also be taken into account. So why do the richest recommend to the poorest solutions that they are unable to apply at home? The poor of Maradi have to acquire food self-sufficiency, but not the poor of Paris? (Bradol 2006: 4)

Defining malnutrition as a medical problem, the group drew parallels with resistance to using antiretroviral drugs to combat hiv/aids in poor countries. In subsequent years, msf continued to advocate aggressively for an rutf approach and, by allocating more than $40 million annually, had moved into third place worldwide for such nutritional programs, after the European Commission and World Bank but ahead of Canada and the United States (msf 2009b: 10).

The debate over prepackaged foods mobilizes several threads of contemporary moral discourse. First and foremost, it asserts the value of ordinary human life, as directly measured in the body weight of malnourished children. However, in terms of a logic of state-based economic development its administration appears unsustainable, an ever-temporary substitute for economic exchange. The matter remains morally convoluted with regard to manufacture; although the material composition of the mixture lends itself to high mobility and local production, the patent protection of its formula and restrictive licensing mirror the intellectual property debates surrounding commercial drug manufacture. And yet when conceived as medicine, Plumpy'nut makes eminent sense. It offers a viable therapeutic alternative to clinical care in a tfc, one far more efficient in terms of scale. Although it might not reach all malnourished children within a population, and holds out little hope for "curing" chronic hunger, it undoubtedly saves many lives. As a humanitarian palliative, it appears to work quite well.

The emergence of rutfs reconfigures a classic biopolitical problem: that of scarcity and the threat of famine. Foucault (2007: 30–49) describes the problem of scarcity as a critical juncture of political economy, a site where a mercantilist system of prevention involving price controls and prescriptions against hoarding gave way to the expectation of a self-regulating market. From the perspective of liberal economics, security was best found in open circulation, not a restrictive effort to prevent a possible negative event. By allowing free trade, including hoarding, an optimal supply could be ensured, all through the counterintuitive action of permitting prices to rise as well as fall and attending to the natural fluctuations of flow. Thus care for the population could appear linked to a liberalized economy rather than a tightly controlled one. In liberal settings, political economy emerged as a crucial element in the biopolitical repertoire.

By contrast, the rutf approach accepts that market logic may shape reality of food supply through the self-regulation of price, but it refuses any threat to life that may result. Indeed, it distrusts the security that market correction promises, suspecting that it will leave behind a residue of victims. Thus when scarcity tips into famine, humanitarian concern triggers another circulation of sustenance for the starving, regulated by medical rationales rather than general economics. In this sense, Plumpy'nut anticipates real events and provides a ready-made response to them. It embodies a normative expectation that children should live and also an assumption that neither impoverished nation-states nor their attendant national markets can adequately secure a stable food supply. Medicine, not economics, will respond to exceptional malnutrition. At the same time, the emergence of rutf also extends humanitarian action beyond classic forms of famine response (de Waal 1997). Dispensing with the cumbersome infrastructure of clinical care, it concentrates health expertise into a packaged formula, the contents of which invite decentralized production and distribution. The humanitarian conscience now exceeds both state and market at the level of nutritional design. Significantly, its reach is simultaneously global and minimal: in place of the national somatocracy of postwar Europe, we have a mobile safeguard for elementary survival. [...]

Notes

1. For this and related quotations, see the Nutriset website: http://www.nutriset.fr/en/ (accessed May 16, 2011).
2. See also Jeffrey Sachs, Jessica Fanzo, and Sonia Sachs's post (2010) in response to a *New York Times* story. They emphasize both the need to distinguish among forms of hunger and the fact that Plumpy'nut addresses only acute food deprivation, not chronic or long-term malnutrition.

References

Bradol, Jean-Hervé. 2006. A new approach towards malnutrition. *Messages* 141 (July): 1–5.

De Waal, Alex. 1997. *Famine Crimes: Politics and the Disaster Relief Industry in Africa*. Oxford: James Currey.

Foucault, Michel. 2007. *Security, Territory, Population: Lectures at the Collège de France, 1977–1978*. Edited by Michel Senellart, translated by Graham Burchell. New York: Picador.

Motavalli, Jim. 2009. Let them eat Plumpy'Nut. *Foreign Policy*, October 8. http://www.foreignpolicy.com/articles/2009/10/08/let_them_eat_plumpynut.

msf (Médecins Sans Frontières). 2009b. "*Malnutrition: How Much Is Being Spent.*" msf Campaign for Access to Essential Medicines. http://www.msfaccess.org/our-work/malnutrition/article/898.

Rice, Andrew. 2010. The peanut solution. *New York Times Magazine*, September 2, MM36.

Tectonidis, Milton. 2006. Acute malnutrition: A highly prevalent, frequently fatal, imminently treatable, neglected disease. In *msf Activity Report 2005–2006*. http://www.doctorswithoutborders.org/publications/ar/report.cfm?id=3228.

Selections from "Global Challenges and the Future of Healthcare"

David Lemberg

[...]

Emerging Infectious Diseases

Ebola virus disease is the prototypical emerging infectious disease. Infectious diseases such as EVD, cholera, Rift Valley fever, and schistosomiasis are endemic worldwide and many of these disorders maintain a broad reservoir of agents with the potential for rapid dissemination.[1] In 2015, lower respiratory diseases remained the third most frequent cause of death around the world. Diarrheal diseases were the eighth and tuberculosis was the ninth most frequent cause of death globally.[2] However, in 2015, in low-income countries, lower respiratory diseases were the number one cause of death and diarrheal diseases were the second most frequent cause of death. In 2015, in low-income countries, HIV/AIDS was the fifth, tuberculosis the sixth, and malaria the seventh most frequent cause of death.[3] Despite more than a century of progress in combatting these disorders, infectious diseases continue to cause extensive human suffering, interfere with and inhibit social and economic development, and contribute to global instability.[4]

Emerging infectious diseases may be categorized as *newly emerging* and *reemerging* disorders. Newly emerging infectious diseases are those recognized in the human host for the first time and are newly appearing in the population. Reemerging infectious diseases have historically infected humans, but are rapidly increasing in incidence or geographic range.[5] Reemerging infectious diseases may appear in new locations, reappear after apparent control or elimination, or appear in drug-resistant forms.[6] Infectious diseases emerge via a two-step process: (1) introduction of the infectious agent into a new host population and (2) establishment and dissemination within the new host population.[7] Many emerging infectious diseases are *zoonoses*, that is, they emerged from animal populations to infect and spread among humans.[8] Zoonoses include some of the most challenging illnesses healthcare systems are confronting at present, such as human immunodeficiency virus (HIV), Ebola virus, H5N1 and H1N1 influenza viruses, and the SARS coronavirus.[9] Emerging infectious diseases transmitted by vectors such as mosquitos include malaria, West Nile virus infection, dengue fever, and Japanese encephalitis.

Human factors contributing to emergence of infectious diseases include migration, urbanization, increased air travel, increased vehicular traffic across regions, and dam building. For example, population movement from rural areas to cities may spread a previously localized infection.[10] Cities that serve as transportation hubs provide numerous additional routes for widespread dissemination of an emerging infectious disease. The spread of HIV, cholera, and dengue infections has been facilitated by these urban gateways.[11] Infections transmitted by mosquitos and other arthropods such as snails are often accelerated by expansion of standing water. Examples include Japanese encephalitis, a mosquito-borne disease whose incidence is closely associated with rice production and flooding irrigation. Outbreaks of Rift Valley fever, a mosquito-borne viral disease, in sub-Saharan Africa have been associated with dam-building projects that cause flooding. The altered ecological conditions and interactions between animals and humans facilitate transmission of Rift Valley fever.[12] The spread of schistosomiasis, caused by a parasitic worm whose intermediate hosts are certain freshwater snails, is similarly facilitated by flooding and overflow of freshwater in great lakes and rivers.[13] As well, the emergence of antibiotic-resistant bacteria such as MRSA (methicillin-resistant *Staphylococcus aureus*) is associated with "overuse of antibiotics in animals and inappropriate use in humans."[14] Overall, the circumstances of modern life "ensure that the factors responsible for disease emergence are more prevalent than ever before."[15] Yet, when planning and undertaking projects that are not specifically medical, the impacts of those projects on the environment and on population health are often not considered until after the fact.

Infectious pathogens demonstrate extraordinary adaptability in their capacity to replicate and undergo mutational change. These capabilities consistently provide temporary evolutionary advantages as against environmental factors, the human immune response, and antimicrobial drugs. Thus, as "infectious pathogens are evolutionarily dynamic," they possess the potential for "unpredictable and explosive global impact."[16] Animals, the environment, and insect vectors provide reservoirs for infectious pathogens and enable these microbes to become pervasive with the potential for future outbreaks.[17]

Therefore, countering the ever-changing threat of emerging infectious diseases necessarily entails effective public health measures. In the best case, countermeasures observe what has been termed the fundamental maxim of public health: "The health of the individual is best ensured by maintaining or improving the health of the entire community."[18] Essential public health services include the following:

- Assessment—monitoring health status, and investigating and diagnosing health hazards in the community
- Policy development—informing and educating people regarding health issues, and developing policies and plans that support individual and community health efforts
- Assurance of quality health services—enforcing laws and regulations, and evaluating accessibility, quality, and effectiveness of personal and population-based health services[19]

Strong public health fundamentals include ongoing surveillance of infectious diseases, laboratory detection, and epidemiologic investigation, including descriptive and analytical studies of the distribution and determinants of specific infectious diseases.[20] In order for surveillance to be effective, it must be specific, that is, associated with known agents of disease transmission and precise laboratory testing. Prevention and control programs are supported by applied research and public health infrastructure.[21] For example, as the accuracy of sequencing viral genomes improves and sequencing instruments become more portable, "real-time viral surveillance and molecular epidemiology will be routinely deployed on the front lines of infectious disease outbreaks."[22] As an example of a collaborative, transdisciplinary approach, the One Health global initiative links human health, animal health, and environmental health experts in efforts to develop and implement new approaches to prevention and control of zoonotic and vector-borne diseases.[23] One Health aims to foster collaborative relationships, improve communication between sectors, and coordinate disease surveillance activities. As well, One Health aims to develop uniform communications to the public regarding the interconnections between people, plants, animals, and our shared environment, and prevention and control of emerging infectious diseases. Overall, given their endemic characteristics, eradication of any of these disorders is unlikely. Preparation, readiness, international cooperation, and rapid response are the keys to effectively combatting the ongoing threat of emerging infectious diseases.

[...]

Notes

1. D. Satcher, "Emerging Infections: Getting Ahead of the Curve," *Emerging Infectious Diseases* 1, no. 1 (1995): 1–6, https://dx.doi.org/10.3201/eid0101.950101.
2. World Health Organization, *The Top 10 Causes of Death*, Updated January 2017, http://www.who.int/mediacentre/factsheets/fs310/en/.
3. World Health Organization, *The Top 10 Causes of Death: Leading Causes of Death by Economy Income Group*, http://www.who.int/mediacentre/factsheets/fs310/en/index1.html.
4. D. M. Morens and A. S. Fauci, "Emerging Infectious Diseases: Threats to Human Health and Global Stability," *PLoS Pathogens* 9, no. 7 (2013): e1003467, https://www.ncbi.nlm.nih.gov/pmc/articles/PMC3701702/.

5. S. S. Morse, "Factors in the Emergence of Infectious Diseases," *Emerging Infectious Diseases* 1, no. 1 (1995): 7–15, https://dx.doi.org/10.3201/eid0101.950102.

6. S. Fauci and D. M. Morens, "The Perpetual Challenge of Infectious Diseases," *New England Journal of Medicine* 366, no. 5 (2012): 454–461, http://www.nejm.org/doi/pdf/10.1056/NEJMra1108296.

7. S. S. Morse, "Emerging Viruses: Defining the Rules for Viral Traffic," *Perspectives in Biology and Medicine* 34, no. 3 (1991): 387–409.

8. Centers for Disease Control and Prevention (CDC), *A CDC Framework for Preventing Infectious Diseases: Sustaining the Essentials and Innovating for the Future* (Atlanta, GA: CDC, 2011), 7, https://www.cdc.gov/oid/docs/ID-Framework.pdf.

9. Ibid. 7.

10. Morse, "Factors in the Emergence of Infectious Diseases," 9.

11. Ibid.

12. Centers for Disease Control and Prevention, *Rift Valley Fever*, last updated October 19, 2016, https://www.cdc.gov/vhf/rvf/index.html.

13. X. H. Wu, S. Q. Zhang, X. J. Xu et al., "Effect of Floods on the Transmission of Schistosomiasis in the Yangtze River Valley, People's Republic of China," *Parasitology International* 57, no. 3 (2008): 271–276.

14. Fauci and Morens, "The Perpetual Challenge of Infectious Diseases." 459.

15. Morse, "Factors in the Emergence of Infectious Diseases," 13.

16. Fauci and Morens, "The Perpetual Challenge of Infectious Diseases," 455.

17. Ibid.

18. Satcher, "Emerging Infections," 3.

19. Institute of Medicine of the National Academies, *The Future of the Public's Health in the 21st Century* (Washington, DC: National Academies Press, 200), 99, https://www.nap.edu/catalog/10548/the-future-of-the-publics-health-in-the-21stcentury.

20. Centers for Disease Control and Prevention, *CDC Framework for Preventing Infectious Diseases*, 3.

21. Centers for Disease Control and Prevention, "Addressing Emerging Infectious Disease Threats: A Prevention Strategy for the United States," *Morbidity and Mortality Weekly Report* 43, no. RR-5, April 15, 1994, https://www.cdc.gov/mmwr/PDF/rr/rr4305.pdf.

22. Dudas et al., "Virus Genomes Reveal Factors," (referencing J. Quick, N. J. Loman, S. Duraffour et al., "Real-Time, Portable Genome Sequencing for Ebola Surveillance," Nature 530, no. 7589 (2016): 228–232.

23. Centers for Disease Control and Prevention, *One Health Basics*, last updated August 4, 2017, https://www.cdc.gov/onehealth/basics/index.html.

Selection from "The Triumph—and Limits—of Socialized Medicine"

Peter W. Huber

Peter Huber, "The Triumph—and Limits—of Socialized Medicine," *The Cure in the Code: How 20th Century Law is Undermining 21st Century Medicine*, pp. 3–5. Copyright © 2013 by Perseus Books Group. Reprinted with permission.

"There have been at work among us three great social agencies: the London City Mission; the novels of Mr. Dickens; the cholera." In *The Moral Imagination,* historian Gertrude Himmelfarb quotes this reductionist observation at the end of her chapter on Charles Dickens; her debt is to an English nonconformist minister, addressing his flock in 1853. It comes as no surprise to find the author of *Hard Times* and *Oliver Twist* honored in his own day alongside the City Mission, a movement founded to engage churches in aiding the poor. But what's *Vibrio cholerae* doing up there on the dais beside the Inimitable Boz?

It's being commended for the tens of millions of lives it's going to save. This vicious little bacterium has just launched the process of transforming ancient sanitary rituals and taboos into a new science of epidemiology. And that science will frame a massive—and ultimately successful—public effort to rid the city of a long list of infectious diseases.

Socialized medicine's finest hour arrived a century later, on October 16, 1975, by the marshes of Bhola Island, off the coast of Bangladesh. There, in the frame of three-year-old Rahima Banu, the World Health Organization finally cornered smallpox, the most efficient killer on the planet. Then as now, there was no known cure for the highly contagious disease, but vaccinating others on Bhola Island kept the virus from skipping to new human hosts, and little Rahima was the last one left.

In the 1960s, at the height of the Cold War, the Soviet Union and the United States had joined forces under the aegis of a United Nations affiliate to beat the disease. Over the course of the next two decades, they bought billions of doses of vaccine, deployed tens of thousands of workers, mobilized national armies to isolate infected regions, prohibited public meetings, quarantined hotels and apartment buildings, dispatched helicopters, airlifted refrigerators, sent in doctors and nurses, established rings of immunity around newly infected areas, and then tightened the rings until only one ring surrounding one little girl remained. And she, standing tiny but tall, finished off the most virulent strain of the virus on her own.

America underwrote much of the global war on smallpox and helped save hundreds of millions of lives worldwide, and because we no longer have to protect ourselves against smallpox, Americans today save as much every month in direct and indirect societal costs as their grandparents spent on the entire smallpox campaign. According to estimates made in 1994, every dollar spent on polio vaccine saved about five times as much in such costs. The measles immunization payoff was thirteen to one. In 2001, every dollar spent on immunization with five widely administered vaccines was saving an estimated $6 in direct medical costs and another $12 in costs of missed work, disability, and death. Socialized medicine's hundred-year war against germs did far more to improve human health and extend life expectancy than all the rest of medicine developed before or since.

But these triumphs of socialized medicine are behind us now. The medical future looks nothing like the medical past—the diseases are different, and so are the cures. While medical science moved on, Washington dug in. Our medical-regulatory complex—a briar patch of scientific and economic proscriptions, mandates, subsidies, and patents, plus one strange, little-known, but extremely important form of copyright—remains rooted in the scientific methods and public policies that coalesced between 1853 and the early 1980s. These policies, as outlined briefly in this [reading ...], were designed to regulate ignorance, not knowledge—the dearth of molecular medical science, not the science itself, nor its efficient, orderly development.

* * *

Pound for pound, bacteria, viruses, and other microbes contain far more intelligence than we do. They are the closest nature gets to pure code. They are also the most ancient, nimble, creative, and persistent developers of new code on the planet. They have survived planetary catastrophes ten thousand times longer than creatures like us have walked the earth. They probably outweigh all the rest of life combined. They thrive under the arctic permafrost, alongside thermal vents at the bottom of the ocean, under miles of rock, and most everywhere else on or anywhere near the earth's surface. Our own bodies host an estimated ten germs for every human cell.

A fistful of germs that specialize in dining on people evolved over the course of three thousand years of urban human history. These legacies of the distant medical past developed a molecular peg that fits neatly into some molecular hole that many of us share. Quite a number of them also found some ingenious way to provoke the sneeze, the violent diarrhea, or even the lustful itch that helps the germ spread. The cholera bacterium, for example, persuades cells in your gut that you've eaten a dangerous amount of salt, which must be flushed out with water sucked from your body.

Germs discovered the joys of socialism long before we did, and in health matters made communists of us all. An epidemic—from the Greek meaning "upon the people"—was the democracy of rich and poor incinerated indiscriminately by the same fever, or dying indistinguishably in puddles of their own waste. The crowded city served as septic womb, colony, and mortuary.

Smallpox was the Mao of microbes—it killed three hundred million people in the twentieth century alone. Sometimes called the first urban virus, it probably jumped from animals to humans in Egypt, Mesopotamia, or the Indus River Valley at about the same time that the rise of agriculture began drawing people together in towns and cities. Smallpox has also been called nature's cruelest antidote to human vanity. Princes broke out in the same pustules as paupers, reeked as foully of rotting flesh, and oozed the same blackish blood from all their orifices. Alongside millions of nameless dead lie kings of France and Spain, queens of England and Sweden, one Austrian and two Japanese emperors, and a czar of Russia.

When monarchs were dying alongside peasants, the language and politics of health and disease honestly tracked medical reality. The main threats to the "public health" threatened everyone. They also pointed to a compelling need for collective solutions. Disease was caused by invisible, external agents that individuals couldn't control on their own. We were all in the same us-against-it battle to the death. (Though the arrival of the invisible *it* was often blamed on foreigners—syphilis was the "French disease" for the English, "la maladie anglaise" for the French, the "Polish disease" for the Russians, and the "disease of the Christians" for the Arabs.)

For Dickens, the filth in the Thames River symbolized London's insidious taint, its ubiquitous, effluvial corruption. The urban pathologies he described in *Our Mutual Friend* in 1864 were as familiar to Londoners as the river. What social historians sometimes fail to note, however, is that here art imitated life. By the time Dickens was placing the Thames at the center of London's many ills, a new science—epidemiology—had already emerged to move the river far beyond metaphor.

* * *

[...]

Selection from "Healthcare Issues in Contemporary Society, Part I"

David Lemberg

[...]

The Possibility of Precision Medicine

In his state of the union address on January 20, 2015, President Barack Obama noted the possibility of "a new era of medicine—one that delivers the right treatment at the right time" and announced the launch of a new Precision Medicine Initiative. The Precision Medicine Initiative is intended to leverage advances in genomics as well as emerging methods for managing and analyzing large data sets to accelerate biomedical discoveries. The initial components of the Precision Medicine Initiative are (1) developing a voluntary national research cohort of a million or more Americans who will "contribute their health data to improve health outcomes, fuel the development of new treatments, and catalyze a new era of data-based and more precise medical treatment" (the *All of Us* Research Program) and (2) scaled-up efforts by the National Cancer Institute to "identify genomic drivers in cancer and apply that knowledge in the development of more effective approaches to cancer treatment." Data from large numbers of people are needed to identify genetic markers that may be predictive of a treatment response.

The goal of precision medicine has been described as the identification of a subset of patients with a common biological basis of disease, often defined by genomics, who are most likely to benefit from a specific drug. Precision medicine is not the creation of a drug or medical device that is unique to a specific patient. Rather, precision medicine represents tailoring medical treatment to the individual characteristics of each patient, based on "the ability to classify individuals into subpopulations that differ in their susceptibility to a particular disease ... or in their response to a specific treatment."

The pharmacological treatment of cystic fibrosis with ivacaftor is an example of precision medicine. Ivacaftor targets the protein encoded by a mutation in the cystic fibrosis transmembrane regulatory gene (CFTR). Ivacaftor increases the activity of the defective cell membrane channel regulatory protein and impacts the function of those transmembrane channels, with possible decreased pulmonary airway obstruction and improved lung function. Ivacaftor is effective in a subset of cystic fibrosis patients with a specific configuration of the affected transmembrane channel, and thus exemplifies a precision medicine framework that targets a drug to a precise subclass of patients.

A goal of precision medicine is to use information "about the genes, proteins, and other features of a person's cancer to diagnose or treat their particular disease." For example, the methodology of pharmacogenetics attempts to use a patient's genome to ascertain and prescribe the most effective, safest drug for that person. But randomized controlled trials are needed before primary care physicians are able to employ precision medicine at the level of the individual patient. Randomized comparisons "are the only way to reliably estimate the effects of tested therapies on clinical outcomes." Randomization assists in removing selection bias and provides an internal control for efficacy and safety. As well, randomization aids in the direct comparison between the experimental therapy and the existing standard of care. Overall, a primary as-yet-unanswered question regarding precision medicine relates to the demonstration of improvement in morbidity and mortality associated with specific diseases.

Assisted Reproductive Technologies: Postmortem Sperm Retrieval

Postmortem sperm retrieval (PMSR) is the medical practice of obtaining sperm for later use with assisted reproductive technologies. To ensure viability, sperm should be retrieved within twenty-four to thirty-six hours of death. After retrieval, sperm are typically frozen and stored at a sperm bank for future use. PMSR was first reported in 1980 in the case of a thirty-year-old man who had suffered a fatal brain injury in a motor vehicle accident. The first baby born as a result of posthumous conception was reported in 1999. Overall, requests for PMSR have been reported as increasing. For example, PMSR requests increased by 60 percent in the interval from 1997 to 2002.

Regarding legality of the procedure, in the United Kingdom, per the Human Fertilisation and Embryology Act of 1990, "a person's gametes must not be kept in storage unless there is an effective consent by that person to their storage and they are stored in accordance with the consent." In New Zealand, the National Ethics Committee on Assisted Human Reproduction has stated that "collection of sperm from a comatose or recently deceased person without that person's prior written consent is ethically unacceptable." Thus, in these countries, PMSR would not be permissible in the absence of prior consent of the decedent. In December 2016, in a case involving postmortem sperm retrieval, Israel's Supreme Court ruled that the right to procreate also applies to posthumous fertilization, but only the spouse of the deceased is entitled to decide on implementation of this right. Subsequently, in August 2017, Israel's Supreme Court approved the decision of a district court that the process of procreation utilizing a decedent's sperm could not be initiated by the parents of the deceased. In the United States, as of 2016, there was no federal law or state law that directly addressed PMSR.

In the absence of federal and state legislation in the United States, certain healthcare institutions and professional associations have created guidelines for PMSR. In New York, the Weill Cornell Medicine (WCM) Guidelines for PMSR states the institution only considers requests for sperm retrieval from the decedent's wife. The request should establish "convincing evidence that the man would have wanted to conceive children this way, and evaluation of the request should also be supported by unanimous agreement among available members of the immediate family." The WCM Guidelines specifies that the decedent's wife is "considered the only person for whom the sperm could be used for procreation." Regarding a decision to use retrieved sperm, the WCM Guidelines strongly recommends a one-year quarantine period after sperm retrieval, with psychological counseling and reassessment of decision making prior to attempting assisted reproduction. The Ethics Committee of the American Society for Reproductive Medicine has stated that healthcare institutions are not obligated to participate in PMSR and should develop written policies "regarding the specific circumstances in which they will or will not participate in such activities." The American Bar Association formally adopted the Model Act Governing Assisted Reproductive Technology (Model Act) on February 11, 2008. The Model Act specifies that gametes shall not be collected from deceased individuals or from preserved tissues unless written consent was obtained prior to death.

Thus, overall, PMSR entails numerous biomedical issues and poses numerous biomedical ethical challenges. These ethical concerns relate to the legality of PMSR, requirement for prior consent of the decedent, requests by persons such as a family member or same-sex partner for sperm retrieval or use of retrieved sperm in assisted reproductive technologies, rights and responsibilities of healthcare institutions and providers, and the rights of a child conceived via PMSR. As with other novel biomedical technologies, engagement of the public in policy discussions at the state and federal level will help ensure that social, cultural, and religious norms are considered and included as appropriate legislation is developed concerning new arenas of healthcare delivery.

[...]

Selection from "Healthcare Issues in Contemporary Society, Part II"

David Lemberg

[...]

Health Disparities/Health Inequities and LGBT Populations

Lesbian, gay, bisexual, and transgender (LBGT) persons experience unique health disparities and health inequities. In 2011, the IOM published *The Health of Lesbian, Gay, Bisexual, and Transgender People: Building a Foundation for Better Understanding*. The IOM report focused on the health of sexual-minority populations and assessed current levels of scientific knowledge regarding the health status of LGBT populations.[1] The IOM report emphasized the need to collect more national data to "fully understand the health needs of U.S. LGBT populations."[2]

The report noted that LGBT persons have been subject to discrimination within the healthcare system.[3] As well, LGBT individuals are disproportionately affected by stigmatization and victimization.[4] In 2012, HHS published the HHS LGBT Issues Coordinating Committee 2012 Report.[5] The HHS report noted that research suggests that LGBT individuals and families may face significant disparities in access to healthcare and health coverage. HHS objectives in 2012 included informing the National Institutes of Health and the broader research community "about important areas in which to advance biomedical research on LGBT health."[6]

However, despite these initiatives, healthcare practitioners, healthcare service providers, and medical researchers report a lack of knowledge regarding health disparities and health inequities that impact LBGT populations.[7] Healthy People 2020 identified numerous health disparities affecting LBGT persons,[8] including the following:

- A higher prevalence of HIV infection, mental health issues, and suicide among transgender people
- LGBT populations have high rates of tobacco, alcohol, and other drug use
- Lesbians are less likely to obtain preventive services for cancer
- Lesbians and bisexual females are more likely to be overweight or obese
- LGBT youth are more likely to be homeless
- LGBT youth are two to three times more likely to attempt suicide
- Elderly LGBT individuals encounter additional barriers to health owing to isolation and a lack of social services and culturally competent providers

Health inequities impacting LGBT persons include lack of health insurance, fear of discrimination from providers, insufficient availability of healthcare providers with appropriate training in the health needs of LGBT individuals,[9] and decreased access to quality preventive care.[10]

To begin to redress health disparities and health inequities experienced by LGBT individuals, the IOM report recommended that the National Institutes of Health implement "a research agenda designed to advance knowledge and understanding of LGBT health."[11] Priority research areas included demographic research, health inequities, and transgender-specific health needs.[12] The IOM recommended that data on sexual orientation and gender identity be collected in federally funded surveys administered by HHS. As well, data on sexual orientation and gender identity should be collected in EHRs.[13] In terms of healthcare practice, providers are encouraged to use gender neutral language when discussing a patient's personal relationships. Further, healthcare practitioners should provide statements regarding equal treatment for all patients and include partners (per the patient's instructions) in treatment planning.[14] Standardized intake forms should include additional identifiers for sexual orientation, gender identity, and alternative family units.[15] Additionally, professional education of physicians, nurses, and allied healthcare providers should include specific training regarding how to better serve LGBT patients and how to redress health disparities and health inequities that affect LGBT persons.[16]

Bias in Healthcare Delivery

Bias (or prejudice) may be defined as an unjustified negative attitude toward another based on that person's group membership.[17] Health disparities/health inequities among members of racial/ethnic minorities, those in lower socioeconomic groups, and LGBT persons may often be perpetuated by bias in healthcare delivery.[18]

As well, health disparities/health inequities exist in a "broader historical and contemporary context of social and economic inequality, prejudice, and systematic bias."[19]

Thus, healthcare providers, as all other persons, are likely influenced in their racial and ethnic attitudes by pervasive social trends.[20] Despite the explicit commitment to deliver care equally, some studies suggest that implicit stereotyping and bias on the part of healthcare providers can impact their judgment and behavior when they interact with stigmatized patients.[21] For example, evidence of implicit (unconscious) race bias among physicians was first formally documented in 2007.[22] Utilizing clinical vignettes of a "50-year-old male patient presenting to the emergency department with chest pain and an electrocardiogram suggestive of anterior myocardial infarction," physicians' implicit biases were strongly associated with treatment choices regarding thrombolysis (use of medication to dissolve clots formed in blood vessels). Specifically, as the degree of antiblack bias on a race preference *Implicit Association Test* (IAT)[23] increased, "recommendations for thrombolysis for black patients decreased."[24] As well, implicit bias against blacks (as measured by the race preference IAT) was "positively correlated with likelihood of recommending thrombolysis for white patients."[25] More recently, an assessment of the literature worldwide demonstrated that more than two-thirds of studies reviewed found evidence of racism among healthcare providers. For example, eleven vignette-based studies found that "race influences the medical decision making of healthcare practitioners, whereas eight studies found no association."[26] Recommendations for redress included a "systematic approach to monitoring racism among healthcare providers" and concurrent implementation of evidence-based antiracism approaches that counter stereotypes, build empathy and perspective taking, develop personal responsibility, and "promote intergroup contact and intercultural understanding within healthcare settings."[27]

Importantly, members of racial/ethnic minorities report greater dissatisfaction with their healthcare providers, particularly when the providers are not of the same ethnicity/race, and perceive significantly more bias in healthcare delivery compared with whites. Compared with whites, members of racial/ethnic minorities, including Hispanic Americans, African Americans, and Asian Americans, reported greater difficulty in communicating with their healthcare providers, were approximately fourteen times as likely to believe they would receive better healthcare if they were of a different race or ethnicity, and were more likely to feel treated with disrespect during a healthcare visit.[28]

As well, regarding LGBT persons, sexual minority status is "a marker of elevated risk for mental, physical, and sexual health problems."[29] The health of LGBT individuals may be compromised by chronic stress associated with minority status, legal barriers to health insurance, providers who receive minimal training in culturally competent care of LGBT persons, and experiences and expectations of discrimination within the healthcare system.[30] As an example of healthcare provider bias, research has demonstrated that "implicit preferences for heterosexual over lesbian and gay people are pervasive among a majority of health care providers."[31] Further, implicit stereotyping of LGBT older adults persists in the healthcare delivery system, and "these biases contribute to health disparities."[32] Such nonconscious stereotyping may manifest in acts of victimization and discrimination, as when "a transgender patient is denied care or when a hospital fails to allow a same-sex life partner to be at the patient's bedside in the intensive care unit."[33] Overall, for all individuals, such experiences of bias encountered in the delivery of healthcare services are likely to influence subsequent interactions with the healthcare community and may lead even to the avoidance of needed care.[34]

Recommendations for remedying bias include increasing the proportion of underrepresented U.S. racial and ethnic minorities among healthcare professionals and promoting consistency and equity of care through use of evidence-based guidelines.[35] Most professional educational interventions utilize a two-step approach that includes (1) making students aware of their implicit biases and (2) providing instruction in strategies "to either reduce the activation of implicit associations, or control how those associations influence judgment and behavior."[36] Strategies employed include bias awareness strategies, control strategies, and perspective-taking strategies. For example, control strategies are directed toward controlling automatic responses to members of minority groups and utilizing affirming egalitarian goals, seeking common-group identities, and relating to the patient as an individual via counterstereotyping.[37] As well, bias reduction should be promoted at the institutional level by utilizing positive intergroup contact across group boundaries, that is, across provider–patient and student-faculty boundaries.[38] The ultimate goal of training students and healthcare professionals to reduce implicit bias "is to reverse the disparities in care that many stigmatized patient groups receive."[39]

Universal Healthcare and a Right to Healthcare

Whether healthcare is a right or a commodity has remained an open question in the United States, the only industrialized nation that, as of 2017, did not have universal health insurance coverage.[40] A right to health, which is distinct from a right to healthcare, may be located in the World Health Organization (WHO) Constitution, signed on July 22, 1946, by representatives of sixty-one countries, including the United States.[41] The WHO Constitution declared the following:

> The enjoyment of the highest attainable standard of health is one of the fundamental rights of every human being without distinction of race, religion, political belief, economic or social condition. ... Governments have a responsibility for the health of their peoples which can be fulfilled only by the provision of adequate health and social measures.[42]

It may be reasonably stated that the WHO constitution does not propose a right to health as such. But [...] the WHO constitution's asserted obligation or duty of a government regarding the health of its peoples (a term more inclusive than "citizens") implies the existence of a corresponding right.[43] A right to health could be declared but would be aspirational rather than practical, as "health" is necessarily a complex phenomenon and based on a wide variety of independent variables. Further, an individual's health status is not fixed over time and an assertion of a "right" to all of those states becomes problematic. A right to health, as a *positive* right, would obligate the government (the *debtor*) to provide the circumstances, including the services, that would facilitate attainment of health. But as health is a quality and healthy states vary from person to person and within individuals over time, the duties inherent in a right to health would not be fixed or even specifiable on a continual basis. Thus, the "right" itself may not be a legitimate right as characterized by well-accepted rights frameworks.[44]

A *right to healthcare,* in contrast to a right to health, could be quantified and operationalized. A right to healthcare would necessitate equal access to appropriate services and would mandate the achievement of equity in health states.[45] Equal access to healthcare services would require establishing a minimum standard for everyone. Thus, nations with universal healthcare systems operationalize a right to healthcare by making an identical "basket of services" available to all people. Provision of a minimum standard of services represents an entitlement without financial or other considerations. The minimum standard is comprehensive and includes preventive and public health services as well as medical care. The scope is society-wide, including both individuals and populations, that is, communities, cities, and states.[46]

Examples of universal healthcare systems include Britain's National Health Service (NHS) and Canada Medicare. The NHS launched on July 5, 1948, and was grounded in three core principles: meeting the needs of everyone, being free at the point of delivery, and being based on clinical need rather than ability to pay.[47] By fulfilling these core principles, the NHS was intended to address inequities in healthcare and inequities in health states across society.[48] As of 2016, the NHS in England was dealing with more than 1 million patients every thirty-six hours, covered everything, and employed more than 1.5 million people.[49] In a 2017 international comparison of healthcare systems, the Commonwealth Fund rated the United Kingdom's NHS first overall among eleven high-income countries, including the United States, Australia, Canada, Sweden, France, and Germany.[50]

The NHS ranked first in care process, which rates performance in the areas of prevention, safety, coordination of care, and patient engagement. As well, the NHS ranked first in equity, denoting relatively small differences among lower- and higher-income adults regarding access, affordability, and timeliness of care. Of note, the NHS ranked tenth in healthcare outcomes. For example, five-year breast cancer relative survival rate was 81 percent, compared with the top rate of 89 percent obtained in Norway, Sweden, and the United States. Five-year colon cancer relative survival rate was 56 percent in the U.K., compared with the top rate of 69 percent obtained in Australia.[51] But "over the past decade the U.K. saw a larger decline in mortality amenable to healthcare (i.e., a greater improvement in the measure) than the other countries studied."[52] The U.K. had made a major investment in the NHS, increasing healthcare spending from 6.7 percent of gross domestic product (GDP) to 9.9 percent of GDP in 2015,[53] as part of efforts to place primary care at the center of NHS modernization and support a comprehensive program of quality improvement.[54]

In Canada, Medicare refers to the nation's publicly funded healthcare system, which is based on thirteen provincial and territorial health insurance plans rather than a single national plan.[56] The legislative origins of Canadian Medicare are located in the Hospital Insurance and Diagnostic Services Act of 1957 (HIDSA),[56] which established universal hospital coverage by means of implementing national standards and cost-share transfers from the federal government to the provinces, and the Medical Care Act of 1966 (MCA),[57] which established universal medical care insurance, again implementing national standards and cost-share transfers. Per the 1966 legislation, a medical care insurance plan of a province was required to furnish insured services "upon uniform terms and conditions to all insurable residents of the province." The number of insurable residents of the province who were entitled under the plan to insured services was to be "not less than 90% of the total number of insurable residents of the province." This minimum was to be expanded to 95 percent on July 1, 1970. Further, the plan must not impose any minimum period of residence or any waiting period greater than three months "before persons who are or become residents of the province are eligible for or entitled to insured services."[58] Overall, the phrase "uniform terms and conditions" established the universality of healthcare insurance in Canada.

Subsequently, in 1977, the shared-cost format was replaced by block funding from the Canadian federal government to the provinces. This change resulted in a proliferation of direct patient charges, including user charges and extra-billing.[59] In response to these infringements on universal coverage, Health and Welfare Canada issued a document in 1983 stating the following:

> The Government of Canada believes that a civilized and wealthy nation, such as ours, should not make the sick bear the financial burden of health care. Everyone benefits from the security and peace of mind that come with having prepaid insurance …. The costs of care should be borne by society as a whole. That is why the Government of Canada wishes to reaffirm in a new Canada Health Act our commitment to the essential principle of universal health insurance.[60]

The Canada Health Act (CHA) was passed on April 1, 1984, combining and updating the HIDSA and MCA. The CHA incorporated restrictions specifically added to deter direct patient charges and "provide citizens of all provinces with access to health care regardless of ability to pay."[61] By doing so, the CHA established the requirement of accessibility in addition to the "four existing criteria of public administration, comprehensiveness, portability, and universality."[62]

Thus, Britain's NHS and Medicare in Canada are two examples of universal healthcare implemented via single-payer systems. In Britain, the single payer is the national government, which establishes the budget for NHS England. Funding for the NHS comes directly from taxation. In Canada, the single payers are the thirteen healthcare insurance plans administered by the provinces and territories. The federal government provides healthcare funding to the provinces and territories via the Canada Health Transfer.[63] Other universal healthcare systems, such as those implemented in Germany and the Netherlands, utilize multipayer formats. In Germany, health insurance is required for all citizens and permanent residents. Coverage is provided by competing not-for-profit, nongovernmental health insurance funds in the statutory health insurance system (SHI) or by private health insurance. Funding for the SHI derives from compulsory contributions. As of 2015, the uniform contribution rate was 14.6 percent of gross wages.[64] In the Netherlands, the national government partly finances the health insurance basic benefit package via general taxation and payroll levies, as well as the compulsory health insurance system for long-term care, for which municipalities and health insurers are primarily responsible. In addition to statutory coverage, 84 percent of the population (as of 2015) purchases supplementary insurance covering benefits such as dental care, physiotherapy, and the full cost of copayments for pharmaceuticals.[65] Overall, a variety of universal healthcare systems have been implemented among the Organisation for Economic Co-operation and Development member countries.[67]

Other nations not typically considered affluent, including Ghana and Rwanda, are moving toward the goal of universal healthcare coverage. Ghana had passed mandatory national health insurance legislation (Act 650) in 2003 and launched nationwide implementation in 2004.[68] As of 2012, the general government expenditure on healthcare was 5.2 percent of the nation's GDP and encompassed 57 percent of all healthcare expenses. Private expenditures on healthcare were 43 percent of the total.[69] The Ghana National Health Insurance Scheme (NHIS) system is a "pro-poor policy and offers a generous benefit package," but many poor people have difficulty paying registration fees and premiums. As a result, as of 2012, the NHIS still was utilized more by higher-income groups.[70]

In Rwanda, in 1999, the government introduced a pilot community-based health insurance (CBHI) program in several districts and extended the program to all thirty districts in 2005.[71] In 2010, the government implemented a CBHI contribution policy[72] based on socioeconomic stratification, revising the prior regressive structure in which all households had paid equal premiums.[73] Rwanda's CBHI is structured on community ownership and management. Membership is voluntary and renewable annually. The expansion of CBHI, in association with malaria and HIV programs and community health and quality assurance programs, led to improvement in assisted delivery rates from 39 percent in 2000 to 52 percent in 2008 and a reduction in infant mortality rate from 139 per 1000 live births in 2005 to 62 in 2008.[74] (The 2016 estimate was 56.8.[75]) Under age five mortality rate declined from 152 per 1,000 population in 2005 to 103 in 2008.[77] (The rate in 2015 was approximately 42.[78]) As of 2017, Rwanda's near-universal healthcare system, financed by tax revenue, foreign aid, and voluntary premiums stratified by income, covered more than 90 percent of the population.[79]

Achieving universal healthcare in the United States will require broad public support. As of mid-2017, a Kaiser Health Tracking poll reported that 53 percent of Americans favored a single-payer system in which a single government plan would provide health insurance.[80] Additional public support would help to counter opposition from insurers, the medical care industry, and large segments of organized medicine.[81] Further, implementing a single-payer model, as in "Medicare for All," would require adopting large-scale tax increases.[82] As of 2017, adoption of a national single-payer healthcare system did not seem likely in the immediate future, and states were considering their own approaches. As against federal inaction, individual states such as New York and California were considering single-payer legislation. Examples of such legislation include A05062 ("New York Health Act"),[83] which passed the New York state assembly on June 1, 2016, and SB-562 ("The Healthy California Act"),[84] which passed the California senate on June 1, 2017. As of mid-2018, neither bill had made any further legislative progress.

However, worldwide, universal healthcare is recognized as a social good.[85] Importantly, as demonstrated by the social gradient of health,[86] short- and long-term improvement across a range of health indicators requires not only access, affordability, and delivery of healthcare services, but also public policies directed toward the social determinants of health. If the WHO constitution[87] could be utilized as a foundation for public policy, creating a moral context for action in the healthcare arena, then policies regarding healthcare would include "social measures" targeting inequities in income, housing, early childhood development, education, neighborhood construction and the built environment, and the work environment. Such a comprehensive approach would improve individual health, population health, and global economic health.[88]

[...]

BOX 12.8.1
Case Study: Health Disparities/Health Inequities

In scenario A, Daisy, a fifteen-year-old girl, has sustained a left ankle injury during a Saturday morning high school soccer match. Her parents, who were attending the match, drive her to the local hospital, a large suburban complex associated with the state university system. Daisy is seen in the emergency department, and x-rays show a bony abnormality. Follow-up computed tomography (CT) demonstrates a fracture of the tibia with mild displacement. Closed reduction of the displaced fracture is performed using general anesthesia. Daisy does well following the procedure and is placed in a cast. Later, she begins a course of physical therapy and learns how to perform cross-training exercises. Ultimately, premature closure of her tibial growth plate has been prevented and she achieves full function. Daisy is able to return to soccer team activities four months after her injury.

In scenario B, Daisy has sustained a left ankle injury during a Saturday morning high school soccer match. Her coach phones Daisy's mother, a cafeteria worker at a skilled nursing facility. Thirty minutes later Daisy's mother arrives. Two of Daisy's friends help her into her mother's car, and mother and daughter drive off in search of an urgent care center. They wait more than two hours to be seen by a harried physician's assistant, and then wait another thirty minutes for x-rays to be taken. CT is not performed. A pediatric orthopedist is not available and closed reduction is not done. Daisy does receive a cast and crutches. She is given a prescription for physical therapy, but Daisy knows this will not happen as her mother works and is not available to drive Daisy to appointments. Daisy makes a slow, painful recovery. Three months later she concludes that her ankle function is not the same as prior to her injury. She arranges with a friend to be driven to urgent care, where follow-up x-rays show premature closure of the tibial growth plate. Daisy never returns to sports. Five years later she is told during an employment physical examination that her left leg is one-quarter of an inch shorter than her right leg.

Ethical Analysis

1. Compare and contrast the outcomes in scenario A and scenario B in the context of health disparities and health inequities.
2. Discuss the possible long-term impacts of Daisy's outcomes in scenario B on Daisy herself, her community, and society as a whole.
3. From the perspective of the biomedical ethical principle of justice, discuss whether scenario B Daisy has a right to obtain a similar level of healthcare services as those obtained by scenario A Daisy. Discuss the social determinants of health that need to be addressed to achieve greater healthcare equity in scenario B.

[...]

References

1. Institute of Medicine, *The Health of Lesbian, Gay, Bisexual, and Transgender People: Building a*

Foundation for Better Understanding (Washington, DC: National Academies Press, 2011), http://www.nationalacademies.org/hmd/Reports/2011/The-Health-of-Lesbian-Gay-Bisexual-and-Transgender-People.aspx.

2. Ibid., 132.
3. Ibid., 75.
4. J. W. Buckey and C. N. Browning, "Factors Affecting the LGBT Population When Choosing a Surrogate Decision Maker," *Journal of Social Services Research* 39, no. 2 (2013): 233–252.
5. U.S. Department of Health and Human Services, *HHS LGBT Issues Coordinating Committee 2012 Report*, https://www.hhs.gov/programs/topic-sites/lgbt/enhanced-resources/reports/health-objectives-2012/index.html.
6. Ibid.
7. Buckey and Browning, "Factors Affecting the LGBT Population," 246.
8. Healthy People 2020, *Lesbian, Gay, Bisexual, and Transgender Health*, https://www.healthypeople.gov/2020/topics-objectives/topic/lesbian-gay-bisexual-and-transgender-health.
9. Institute of Medicine, *The Health of LGBT People*, 297.
10. L. Mollon, "The Forgotten Minorities: Health Disparities of the Lesbian, Gay, Bisexual, and Transgendered Communities," *Journal of Health Care for the Poor and Underserved* 23, no. 1 (2012): 1–6.
11. Institute of Medicine, *The Health of LGBT People*, 6.
12. Ibid.
13. Ibid., 9.
14. K. A. Bonvicini and M. J. Perlin, "The Same but Different: Clinician-Patient Communication with Gay and Lesbian Patients," *Patient Education and Counseling* 51, no. 2 (2001): 115–22.
15. Mollon, "The Forgotten Minorities," 4–5.
16. Ibid., 5.
17. B. D. Smedley, A. Y. Stith, and A. R. Nelson, eds., *Unequal Treatment: Confronting Racial and Ethnic Disparities in Health Care* (Washington, DC: National Academies Press, 2003), 10.
18. E. N. Chapman, A. Kaatz, and M. Carnes, "Physicians and Implicit Bias: How Doctors May Unwittingly Perpetuate Health Care Disparities," *Journal of General Internal Medicine* 28, no. 11 (2013): 1504–1510.
19. R. L. Johnson, S. Saha, J. J. Arbelaez et al., "Racial and Ethnic Differences in Patient Perceptions of Bias and Cultural Competence in Health Care," *Journal of General Internal Medicine* 19 (2004): 101–110.
20. Smedley, Stith, and Nelson, *Unequal Treatment,* 490.
21. C. A. Zestcott, I. V. Blair, and J. Stone, "Examining the Presence, Consequences, and Reduction of Implicit Bias in Health Care: A Narrative Review," *Group Process and Intergroup Relations* 19, no. 4 (2016): 528–542, 529.
22. R. Green, D. R. Carney, D. J. Pallin et al., "Implicit Bias among Physicians and Its Prediction of Thrombolysis Decisions for Black and White Patients," *Journal of General Internal Medicine* 22, no. 9 (2007): 1231–1238.

23. G. Greenwald, D. E. McGhee, and J. L. K. Schwartz, "Measuring Individual Differences in Implicit Social Cognition: The Implicit Association Test," *Journal of Personality and Social Psychology* 74, no. 6 (1998): 1464–1480.

24. Green et al., "Implicit Bias among Physicians," 1235.

25. Ibid., 1237.

26. Y. Paradies, M. Truong, and N. Priest, "A Systematic Review of the Extent and Measurement of healthcare provider racism," *Journal of General Internal Medicine* 29, no. 2 (2014): 364–387.

27. Ibid., 383.

28. Ibid.

29. Zestcott, Blair, and Stone, "Examining the Presence, Consequences, and Reduction of Implicit Bias in Health Care," 529.

30. K. S. Collins, D. L. Hughes, M. M. Doty et al., *Diverse Communities, Common Concerns: Assessing Health Care Quality for Minority Americans. Findings from the Commonwealth Fund 2001 Health Care Quality Survey* (Washington, DC: Commonwealth Fund, 2002), http://www.commonwealthfund.org/publications/fund-reports/2002/mar/diverse-communities–common-concerns–assessing-health-care-quality-for-minorityamericans.

31. J. A. Sabin, R. G. Riskind, and B. A. Nosek, "Health Care Providers' Implicit and Explicit Attitudes Toward Lesbian Women and Gay Men," *American Journal of Public Health* 105, no. 9 (2015): 1831–1841.

32. Ibid., 1831.

33. Ibid., 1840.

34. M. B. Foglia and K. I. Fredriksen-Goldsen, "Health Disparities among LGBT Older Adults and the Role of Nonconscious Bias," *Hastings Center Report* 44, no. 5 (2014): S40–S44.

35. Ibid., S42.

36. Ibid., S43.

37. Smedley, Stith, and Nelson, *Unequal Treatment,* 20.

38. Zestcott, Blair, and Stone, "Examining the Presence, Consequences, and Reduction of Implicit Bias in Health Care," 535.

39. Ibid.

40. Ibid., 536.

41. Ibid., 537.

42. E. C. Schneider, D. O. Sarnak, D. Squires et al., *Mirror, Mirror 2017: International Comparison Reflects Flaws and Opportunities for Better U.S. Health Care* (Washington, DC: The Commonwealth Fund, 2017), http://www.commonwealthfund.org/interactives/2017/july/mirror-mirror/.

43. World Health Organization (WHO), "Constitution of the World Health Organization," in *Summary Report on Proceedings, Minutes, and Final Acts of the International Health Conference Held in New York from 19 June to 2 July 1946* (New York: WHO, 1948), http://apps.who.int/iris/bitstream/10665/85573/1/Official_record2_eng.pdf.

44. Ibid., 100.

45. W. N. Hohfeld, *Fundamental Legal Conceptions as Applied in Judicial Reasoning, and Other Legal Essays* (New Haven, CT: Yale University Press, 1919), 38.

46. Ibid., 65–72.

47. M. Susser, "Health as a Human Right: An Epidemiologist's Perspective on the Public Health," *American Journal of Public Health* 83, no. 3 (1993): 418–426.

48. Ibid., 420.

49. National Health Service (NHS), Principles and values that guide the NHS, http://www.nhs.uk/NHSEngland/thenhs/about/Pages/nhscoreprinciples.aspx.

50. Susser, "Health as a Human Right," 420.

51. National Health Service (NHS), *About the National Health Service (NHS)*, http://www.nhs.uk/NHSEngland/thenhs/about/Pages/overview.aspx.

52. Schneider et al., *Mirror, Mirror 2017.*

53. Ibid., 24.

54. Ibid., 9.

55. Office of National Statistics, *UK Health Accounts: 2015*, https://www.ons.gov.uk/peoplepopulationandcommunity/healthandsocialcare/healthcaresystem/bulletins/ukhealthaccounts/2015.

56. T. Doran and M. Roland, "Lessons from Major Initiatives to Improve Primary Care in the United Kingdom," *Health Affairs* 29, no. 5 (2010): 1023–1029.

57. Government of Canada, Canada's Health Care System, https://www.canada.ca/en/health-canada/services/canada-health-care-system.html.

58. J. G. Turner. "The Hospital Insurance and Diagnostic Services Act: Its Impact on Hospital Administration," *Canadian Medical Association Journal* 78, no. 1 (1958): 768–770.

59. Department of Medical Economics, The Canadian Medical Association, "The Medical Care Act: Bill C-227," *Canadian Medical Association Journal* 95, no. 21 (1966): 1107–1108.

60. Ibid., 1108.

61. O. Madore, *The Canada Health Act: Overview and Options*, CIR 94-4E. Library of Parliament, Canada, Parliamentary Information and Research Service, revised May 16, 2005, https://lop.parl.ca/content/lop/researchpublications/944-e.pdf.

62. Ibid., 5.

63. Ibid.

64. G. P. Marchildon, "The Three Dimensions of Universal Medicare in Canada," *Canadian Public Administration* 57, no. 3 (2014): 362–382.

65. Department of Finance, Canada, *Canada Health Transfer*, https://www.fin.gc.ca/fedprov/cht-eng.asp.

66. E. Mossialos, M. Wenzl, R. Osborn et al., *2015 International Profiles of Health Care Systems* (Washington, DC: The Commonwealth Fund, 2016), 69, http://www.commonwealthfund.org/~/media/files/publications/fund-report/2016/jan/1857_mossialos_intl_profiles_2015_v7.pdf.

67. Ibid., 115.

68. Organisation for Economic Co-operation and Development, *Members and Partners*, http://www.oecd.org/about/membersandpartners/#d.en.194378.

69. Fusheini, "The Politico-Economic Challenges of Ghana's National Health Insurance Scheme Implementation," *International Journal of Health Policy Management* 5, no. 9 (2016): 543–552.

70. Garshong and J. Akazili, *Universal Health Coverage Assessment: Ghana*, Global Network for Health Equity, July 2015, http://gnhe.org/blog/wp-content/uploads/2015/05/GNHE-UHC-assessment_Ghana1.pdf.

71. Ibid., 11.

72. Ministry of Health, *Annual Report: Community Based Health Insurance* (Kigali: Government of Rwanda, 2012), 8, http://www.moh.gov.rw/fileadmin/templates/Docs/CBHI-Annual-Report2011–2012f-3__1_.pdf.

73. Ministry of Health, *Rwanda Community Based Health Insurance Policy* (Kigali: Government of Rwanda, 2010), https://images.indiegogo.com/medias/1274880/files/20140301080253-mutual_policy.pdf.

74. Ministry of Health, *Annual Report*, 9.

75. Ministry of Health, *Rwanda Community Based Health Insurance Policy*, 6.

76. Central Intelligence Agency, *The World Factbook, 2016*, https://www.cia.gov/library/publications/the-world-factbook/rankorder/2091rank.html.

77. Ministry of Health, *Rwanda Community Based Health Insurance Policy*, 6.

78. The World Bank, *Mortality Rate, Under-5 (per 1,000 Live Births)*, https://data.worldbank.org/indicator/SH.DYN.MORT?locations=RW.

79. E. Porter, "In Health Care, Republicans Could Learn from Rwanda," *New York Times*, July 7, 2017, https://www.nytimes.com/2017/07/18/business/economy/senate-obamacare-rwanda.html.

80. Kaiser Family Foundation, *Polling: Data Note: Modestly Strong but Malleable Support for Single-Payer Health Care*, July 5, 2017, http://www.kff.org/health-reform/poll-finding/data-note-modestly-strong-but-malleable-support-for-single-payer-health-care/.

81. J. Oberlander, "The Virtues and Vices of Single-Payer Health Care," *New England Journal of Medicine* 374, no. 15 (2016): 1401–1403.

82. Ibid.

83. New York State Assembly, A05062 Summary, http://assembly.state.ny.us/leg/?default_fld=&bn=A05062&term=2015&Summary=Y&Actions=Y&Votes=Y&Text=Y.

84. California Legislative Information, SB-562. The Healthy California Act, https://leginfo.legislature.ca.gov/faces/billNavClient.xhtml?bill_id=201720180SB562.

85. J. Rodin and D. de Ferranti, "Universal Health Coverage: The Third Global Health Transition?" *The Lancet* 380, no. 9845 (2012): 861–862.

86. M. G. Marmot, R. Fuhrer, S. L. Ettner et al., "Contribution of Psychosocial Factors to Socioeconomic Differences in Health," *Milbank Quarterly* 76, no. 3 (1998): 403–448.

87. WHO, "Constitution of the World Health Organization."

88. J. Frenk and D. de Ferranti, "Universal Health Coverage: Good Health, Good Economics," *The Lancet* 380, no. 9845 (2012): 863–864.

Review Questions

Directions: Refer to your readings to help respond to the questions and prompts below.

1. How can we use previous history, legal precedence, and failures to help forecast future trends?
2. What is the most critical area in the future of bioethics? How would the major moral theories apply to this argument?
3. Many of the significant laws are federal and, thus, applicable to the entire United States. What are some more specific state laws where you live? What local trends might these laws help us to anticipate? How will you stay current on medical and legal changes throughout your career?
4. Why does the law always seem to follow scientific advances? Will the United States ever be able to have a law before a new technology emerges?
5. Should the future of health care embolden or scare future providers more than the history of it? What, if anything, seems more daunting about the future? It is said that we can learn a lot from history. What are some of health care and medicine's most important historical lessons?
6. Check out the following links. What do you think about these future trends?

Bioethics Seminar – Semester B | TAU-bioethics-center Voice Patterns

https://www.americanhealthlaw.org/publications/health-law-hub-current-topics/artificial-intelligence-and-health-law Artificial Intelligence

https://www.cdc.gov/phlp/news/current.html Public Health Law News